The Broad Scope of Ego Function Assessment

WILEY SERIES IN GENERAL AND CLINICAL PSYCHIATRY

The Broad Scope of Ego Function Assessment
Edited by Leopold Bellak and Lisa A. Goldsmith

THE BROAD SCOPE OF EGO FUNCTION ASSESSMENT

Edited by
Leopold Bellak
Lisa A. Goldsmith

A Wiley-Interscience Publication
JOHN WILEY & SONS
New York • Chichester • Brisbane • Toronto • Singapore

Library of Congress Cataloging in Publication Data:

Main entry under title:

The Broad scope of ego function assessment.

(Wiley series in general and clinical psychiatry)
"A Wiley-Interscience publication."
Includes indexes.
1. Mental illness—Diagnosis. 2. Personality
assessment. 3. Ego (Psychology) I. Bellak, Leopold,
1916–   II. Goldsmith, Lisa A.   III. Series.

RC469.B76   1984   616.89′075   84-3726
ISBN 0-471-89198-3

Printed in the United States of America

10 9 8 7 6 5 4 3 2 1

Contributors

CLAUDIO AGUE, M.D.
University of Berne
Berne, Switzerland

JON G. ALLEN, PH.D.
Staff Psychologist
C. F. Menninger Memorial Hospital
Topeka, Kansas

J. ROBERT BARNES, M.D.
Clinical Assistant Professor of Psy-
  chiatry
Louisiana State University
New Orleans, Louisiana

WILLIAM BARRY, PH.D.
Professor
School of Psychology
Faculty of Social Sciences, and
Professor
Faculty of Health Sciences
University of Ottawa
Ottawa, Ontario, Canada

LEOPOLD BELLAK, M.D.
Clinical Professor of Psychiatry
Albert Einstein College of Medicine/
  Montefiore Medical Center
Bronx, New York, and
Clinical Professor of Psychology
Postdoctoral Program in Psycho-
  therapy and Psychoanalysis
New York University
New York, New York

MICHELINE BOIVIN, M.A.
Counseling Psychologist
Centre de Services Sociaux de
  l'Outaouis
Hull, Quebec, Canada

JAMES BUSKIRK, M.D.
Staff Psychologist
C. F. Menninger Memorial Hospital
Topeka, Kansas

v

MARY CERNEY, PH.D.
Staff Psychologist
C. F. Menninger Memorial Hospital
Topeka, Kansas

EDWARD CHARLES, M.A.
Assistant Professor of Clinical Psychology and Psychiatry
Columbia University College of Physicians and Surgeons
New York, New York

JACK CHASSAN, PH.D.
J. B. Chassan Consultations
Private Practice
Montclair, New Jersey

JEAN A. CIARDIELLO, ED.D.
Director, Program Planning and Evaluation
Adjunct Professor of Psychiatry
University of Medicine and Dentistry of New Jersey
Community Mental Health Center of Rutgers Medical School
Piscataway, New Jersey

LUC CIOMPI, M.D.
Director of Socio-Psychiatric University Clinic
University of Berne
Berne, Switzerland

LOLAFAYE COYNE, PH.D.
Assistant Director, Hospital Research
C. F. Menninger Memorial Hospital, and
Director, Statistical Laboratory
The Menninger Foundation
Topeka, Kansas

ALV A. DAHL, M.D.
Lecturer in Psychiatry
Oslo University School of Medicine
Oslo, Norway

JEAN-PIERRE DAUWALDER, M.D.
Private Dozent
Socio-Psychiatric University Clinic
University of Berne
Berne, Switzerland

JOHN P. DOCHERTY, M.D.
Chief
Psychosocial Treatments
Research Branch
National Institute of Mental Health
Rockville, Maryland

GERARD J. DONNELLAN, PH.D.
Clinical Psychologist
Private Practice
Lexington, Massachusetts

KENNETH FEINER, M.A.
Graduate Student
Yeshiva University
New York, New York

SUSAN FIESTER, M.D.
Visiting Scientist
Division of Extramural Research
National Institute of Mental Health
Rockville, Maryland

SIEBOLT FRIESWYK, PH.D.
Director of the Post-Graduate Psychotherapy Program
Faculty Member of the Topeka Institute for Psychoanalysis
Post-Doctoral Clinical Psychology Program, and
Staff Psychologist
The Menninger School of Psychiatry
C. F. Menninger Memorial Hospital
Topeka, Kansas

WILLIAM A. FROSCH, M.D.
Vice Chairman
Department of Psychiatry
Cornell University Medical College, and Medical Director
Payne-Whitney Clinic
New York Hospital
New York, New York

HELEN K. GEDIMAN, PH.D.
Adjunct Associate Professor
Postdoctoral Program in Psychotherapy and Psychoanalysis
New York University
New York, New York

LISA A. GOLDSMITH, PH.D.
Assistant Professor in Psychiatry (Psychology)
Albert Einstein College of Medicine/ Montefiore Medical Center
Bronx, New York

LOUIS N. GRUBER, M.D.
Associate Professor of Psychiatry
City of Faith Medical Research Center
Oral Roberts University
Tulsa, Oklahoma

MARVIN HURVICH, PH.D.
Chairman
Department of Psychology
Long Island University
Brooklyn, New York

N. WILLIAM KEARNS, M.D.
Section Chief
C. F. Menninger Memorial Hospital
Topeka, Kansas

MYRA E. KLEIN, M.ED.
Research Associate
Program Planning and Evaluation
University of Medicine and Dentistry of New Jersey
Community Mental Health Center of Rutgers Medical School
Piscataway, New Jersey

JAMES A. KNIGHT, M.D.
Professor of Psychiatry
Louisiana State University Medical Center
New Orleans, Louisiana

LEAH BLUMBERG LAPIDUS, PH.D.
Associate Professor
Clinical Psychology Program
Columbia University Teachers College
New York, New York

MICHAEL J. MADIGAN, M.D., PH.D.
Resident in Psychiatry
Timberlawn Hospital
Dallas, Texas

AUGUSTINE MEIER, PH.D.
Assistant Professor
University of St. Paul
Ottawa, Ontario, Canada

BARNETT MEYERS, M.D.
Assistant Professor
Department of Psychiatry
Cornell University Medical College
New York, New York

HARVEY MILKMAN, PH.D.
Professor
Department of Psychology
Metropolitan State College
Denver, Colorado

DORIS M. MODLY, R.N., M.S.N.
Assistant Professor
Psychiatric-Mental Health Nursing
Case Western Reserve University
School of Nursing
Cleveland, Ohio

THOMAS M. MURPHY, M.D.
Director
Inpatient Diagnostic Unit
Children's Hospital
The Menninger Foundation
Topeka, Kansas

GAVIN NEWSOM, M.S.W.
Admissions Director
Adult Services
The Menninger Foundation
Topeka, Kansas

PETER NOVOTNY, M.D.
Staff Psychiatrist
C. F. Menninger Memorial Hospital
Topeka, Kansas

E. OPGENOORTH, PH.D.
University of Vienna
Vienna, Austria

SAMUEL OSHERSON, M.D.
Instructor
Department of Psychiatry
Harvard Medical School, and
Curator of Longitudinal Studies
Harvard University Health Services
Cambridge, Massachusetts

RICHARD L. RUBENS, PH.D.
Psychoanalyst (private practice),
    and
Supervisor and Faculty Member
National Institute for the Psy-
    chotherapies, and
Adjunct Assistant Professor
Department of Clinical Psychology
Teachers College of Columbia Uni-
    versity
New York, New York

JONETTE MUSZYNSKI SAWYER,
    R.N., M.S.N.
Tallahassee, Florida

PATRICIA J. SCHRODER, R.N., M.A.
Associate Director of Nursing
C. F. Menninger Memorial Hospital
Topeka, Kansas

P. SCHUSTER, M.D.
University of Vienna
Vienna, Austria

LIESELOTTE SCHWINDL, PH.D.
University of Vienna
Vienna, Austria

VERNON SHARP, M.D.
Assistant Clinical Professor of Psy-
    chiatry
Vanderbilt University School of
    Medicine
Nashville, Tennessee

SHAWN SOBKOWSKI, M.ED.
Research Associate
Program Planning and Evaluation
University of Medicine and Den-
    tistry of New Jersey
Community Mental Health Center of
    Rutgers Medical School
Piscataway, New Jersey

GERALD TARNOFF, M.D.
Staff Psychologist
C. F. Menninger Memorial Hospital
Topeka, Kansas

CATHERINE TREECE, PH.D.
Instructor in Psychology
Department of Psychiatry
Harvard Medical School at the Cam-
    bridge Hospital
Cambridge, Massachusetts

MARGARET S. WOOL, M.S.W.,
    A.C.S.W.
Clinical Social Worker
Department of Psychiatry
Rhode Island Hospital
Providence, Rhode Island

Series Preface

This series of books is addressed to psychiatrists, mental health specialists, and other serious students of the behavioral sciences. It is inspired by the genius of Adolf Meyer, who introduced psychobiology to psychiatry and charted the course, recently reformulated by George L. Engel, of the biopsychosocial model. Each book may consider the importance of any level of human behavioral interaction—community, family, interpersonal, individual, psychological, psychoanalytic, physiological, biochemical, and genetic or constitutional. Each level is respected on its own terms; no book in this series will fall victim to the fallacy of reductionism.

All aspects of psychiatric disorders, including theoretical, empirical, and therapeutic, are considered. Specific research studies, with their practical applications, are also included. It is our intention that the books in this series be comprehensive, thorough, rigorous, systematic, and original.

MAURICE R. GREEN
ROBERT W. RIEBER

New York University Medical Center
New York, New York

College of Physicians and Surgeons
  of Columbia University
and John Jay College of the City University of
  New York
New York, New York

Preface

In 1973, Bellak, Hurvich, and Gediman published *Ego Functions in Schizo-phrenics, Neurotics, and Normals* (New York: Wiley), the culmination of five years of work done under a major research grant from the National Institute of Mental Health (Grants MH 14260-03 and MH 18395-01, 02, and 02SI, Leopold Bellak, Principal Investigator). This work presented the rationale for a descriptive yet quantifiable approach to the assessment of dynamic personality functions. Included were an account of research using that approach and a guide and scoring scheme for Ego Function Assessment (EFA).

It was gratifying to find that EFA met a receptive audience—in the United States and elsewhere—and generated a considerable body of research on the part of those who shared our interest in the systematic evaluation of dynamic personality functions. The current volume updates the previous work by reporting in one collection widely diverse studies using this approach. An attempt is also made to give some direction to the future use of EFA and its development as an instrument. The present authors have found further evidence of EFA's validity, reliability, and flexibility; we hope it will continue to prove useful to the work of clinicians and researchers alike.

This volume is divided into five parts. Part 1 constitutes a series of papers by Bellak and one by Goldsmith that discuss the theoretical and conceptual underpinnings of ego function assessment (EFA), providing the broad frame of reference for its use. Bellak establishes the usefulness of EFA as a diagnostic approach, as a guide in formulating a treatment strategy, and as a prognostic tool; he also indicates its potential for implementing research.

Goldsmith's article outlines the place of ego function assessment in psychoanalytic theory in light of the current critiques of the structural model.

The main body of the volume brings together diverse strands of research in which EFA was used as an assessment instrument. Part 2 includes a variety of studies that demonstrate EFA's value in assessing the outcome and efficacy of psychotherapy and drug treatment; Part 3 includes several studies that document EFA's function in diagnosis and clinical assessment; and Part 4 includes a wide range of research applications.

The studies reported in Part 2 contribute to EFA's foundation as a psychometric tool, establishing its reliability and validity as a rating scale. Additionally, there are three studies in this section that have begun the extension of EFA to European samples, thereby facilitating cross-cultural comparisons, fulfilling one of the aims of the first volume (Bellak et al., 1973).

Docherty and Fiester's study, the first chapter of the section addressing issues in psychotherapy research, used EFA as the central instrument for assessing the relationship between ego function constructs and specific aspects of treatment outcome in a schizophrenic sample. The authors were able both to compare their findings to those of Bellak et al. (1973) and to specify the implications of their findings for treatment planning. The papers submitted by investigators from the Menninger Foundation are part of a large research project designed to define and quantify those patient variables that predict the outcome of long-term psychiatric hospital treatment. In the Menninger investigations EFA was used to generate a profile of patient functioning that might prove to be of use to clinicians in forecasting important treatment developments. As part of the same project, the relationship of Bellak's scales to a symptom rating scale was investigated for the purpose of relating intrapsychic change to symptomatic change; additionally, EFA was one of the instruments used to assess the degree of change at the time of follow-up. Finally, the Menninger group adapted and broadened the scales so that they could be used with hospital records and thus need not be limited to interview data.

Both Dahl's and Schwindl et al.'s works have clear cross-cultural implications. Dahl investigated EFA's reliability in a sample of Norwegian subjects and explored its usefulness in differentiating diagnostic subgroups, while Schwindl, Opgenoorth, and Schuster used EFA to evaluate the effect of lithium treatment on personality structure in a Viennese population. In the same spirit, Ciompi, Ague, and Dauwalder devised a modified version of EFA to evaluate psychodynamic changes in psychotherapy. The modified form was applied to a French population and seemed to testify to EFA's usefulness and applicability, with specific attention given to issues of reliability and validity.

Three papers by Bellak and colleagues address EFA's use in research on psychoanalysis. In the context of psychotropic drug research, Bellak, Chassan, Gediman, and Hurvich utilized EFA as the major instrument with which to compare the effects of Valium and a placebo in a setting of psychoanalytic psychotherapy. With Meyers, Bellak considered the role of EFA in articulating those dimensions prognostic of analyzability, and, finally, Sharp and Bellak introduced EFA as a methodology to monitor the psychoanalytic process, with the specific focus on incorporating EFA as an objective tool in the supervisory situation.

Wool, in the interest of improving upon a standardized instrument specifying selection criteria for brief forms of psychotherapy, used both the selection questionnaire and Bellak et al.'s Ego Function Assessment of Object Relations. Interestingly, Bellak's measure of Object Relations—a variable of crucial importance in determining suitability for brief treatment—was shown to be superior to the instrument specifically designed for the purpose of patient selection.

Finally, Modly was able to integrate EFA with a phenomenological perspective in the context of a therapeutic and diagnostic encounter with a schizophrenic patient. This integration seemed particularly useful in articulating what could otherwise have been amorphous, nonverbal material.

Part 3 begins with two detailed and sophisticated investigations of the patterning of ego function variables as they relate to drug choice (Milkman and Frosch) and specific patternings of defect in drug abusers from the perspective of adaptation (Treece). Further, both papers integrate findings within the rich psychoanalytic literature on the addictions.

A number of studies have made clinical use of EFA in other than the traditional psychiatric setting. Gruber, Barnes, Madigan, and Knight not only incorporated EFA in screenings for civil service applicants but showed its usefulness with a nonpsychiatric population, and they further went on to amplify the Reality Testing scale for use in this population. Ciardiello, Klein, and Sobkowski used EFA to identify critical variables in the rehabilitative process of chronically schizophrenic patients. With careful and elaborate statistical analysis, they were able to isolate specific dimensions of ego impairments and strengths as these relate to vocational functioning and planning for rehabilitation.

Sawyer used an abbreviated form of EFA to identify ego function profiles of manic-depressive individuals in remission. While not incorporating a double-blind design, the study has heuristic value for delineating specific areas of dysfunction in this broad diagnostic group. (It is interesting that both Schwindl et al. and Sawyer, independently studying populations of affectively disordered patients, obtained comparable findings in regard to several dimensions of ego functioning.) Studies by both Bellak and Goldsmith, Charles, and Feiner applied EFA as an adjunct to diagnosis. Bellak used the EFA model to articulate the dimensions of MBD and to articulate the interface of such dimensions with psychopathological symptoms, while Goldsmith, Charles, and Feiner attempted to identify patterns of ego functioning in borderline patients.

The last study in this section, conducted by Goldsmith, investigated the relationship between humor and suicide lethality, regarding humor as a manifestation of the capacity for adaptive regression and suicide lethality as a manifestation of pathological regressive processes. ARISE, a clinical rating scale derived from EFA, was employed as one of a series of measures to assess the potential for adaptive regression and proved to be the most useful instrument in that battery.

We turn in Part 4 to the application of EFA as a research methodology in the study of particular personality variables. Donnellan's study, which leads off this section, is an initial application of EFA to children. He employed EFA in the study of fantasy and symbolization in a latency-age child. Specifically, using an N of 1 design, he applied the ARISE scale and his own symbolization scale to monitor the course of a child's psychotherapy.

Following this is a study conducted by Meier, Barry, and Boivin that was designed to examine ego function patterns in families with schizophrenic offspring. This study's most distinctive feature is its exhaustive consideration of reliability; it provides important support for EFA's psychometric properties.

Rubens and Lapidus's investigation of patterns of arousal in schizophrenic and control group subjects demonstrated a striking relationship between patterns of modulation of arousal as reflected in a psychophysiological measure—GSR patterns—and a psychological one—Bellak et al.'s stimulus barrier ratings. By identifying an association between the psychophysiological mechanism and the psychodynamic construct of stimulus barrier, this study gives added validation to the particular construct of stimulus barrier as defined by Bellak et al. (1973). Finally, through a lengthy exploration of the psychological implications of life transitions and career changes, Osherson ultimately considers EFA, in conjunction with coping response theory, to be the most useful means of organizing his theoretical and preliminary findings and for directing subsequent research.

Part 5 focuses on the potentialities for further development and application of EFA. The hope is to make it clear that EFA is an instrument that can presently be used in an open-ended and free-wheeling way. Another hope is that Ego Function Assessment will continue to stimulate research and further codification, and perhaps be used in the manner of the Wechsler Adult Intelligence Scale—where the clinical interview is supplemented by devices that permit the testing of specific processes via criterion measures.

The appendix following Part 5, reprinted from the original volume on ego function research, enables the reader to become acquainted with the interview guides for eliciting and assessing ego functions, a process we hope the current volume further encourages.

LEOPOLD BELLAK
LISA A. GOLDSMITH

Larchmont, New York
New York, New York
April 1984

Acknowledgments

The editors are greatly indebted to Helen Siegel, M.A., for her essential role as liaison between the editors, and between the editors and contributors. She was instrumental in the organization and editing of the volume and kept track of the innumerable aspects and complex correspondence involved. Similarly, the book could hardly have progressed without the help and coordination of Marlene Kolbert.

The editors also gratefully acknowledge the invaluable comments and suggestions of Drs. Joseph Richman, Jane Tucker, and Fred Pine. To Evelyn Post, Lillian Rothenberg, and Janet Stott, our sincere thanks for the typing of this manuscript; their patience, fortitude, and good will were unwaivering, and our debt to them is appreciable. We are also grateful to Sylvia Davidson, librarian of the psychiatry library at Albert Einstein College of Medicine, for her help in researching several items in the manuscript.

Finally, the editorial assistance of Kenneth Feiner was such that it is hard to imagine having completed the manuscript without him.

L.B.
L.A.G.

Contents

The Broad Scope
of Ego Function
Assessment

PART ONE

The Basic Concept of Ego Function Assessment (EFA)

CHAPTER ONE

An Overview

LEOPOLD BELLAK

Systematic assessment of personality in clinical psychiatry and psychology has typically been a two-edged sword. In clinical psychiatry, descriptive methods, usually without any concern for reliability and validity, have predominated. The classical mental status examination is a good example of this approach. Diagnostic efforts related to classifications, such as those incorporated in DSM-III, are of more use for administrative and epidemiological purposes, however, than for clinical ones. Of all these efforts, DSM-III is the most ambitious. Originally, the authors attempted operational definitions, but, by their own admission, had to fall back on simply descriptive ones. Their purpose serves primarily to allow for some ease and precision of communication between different clinicians, basically dealing with interrater reliability rather than validity. To attain something in the way of objective criteria, a great deal of meaningfulness was sacrificed and much clinical usefulness lost.

Psychologists attempted assessment primarily by means of two kinds of tests: first, projective devices, outstandingly the Rorschach and the T.A.T. and graphomotor tests, and second, a variety of questionnaires, of which the MMPI is the most widely used. The so-called objective tests, namely, the questionnaires and inventories, attained a good deal of reliability and sometimes some validity, but the meaningfulness of their computerized items often remains highly questionable. The Rorschach and the T.A.T., on the

3

other hand, although valuable tools in the hands of the very well trained, never attained satisfactory validity and reliability measures.

Adding to these difficulties is the fact that the validity or usefulness of the diagnostic categories themselves have been questioned. Problems in diagnosing schizophrenia by the typical psychiatric interview or by psychological tests and questionnaires may arise specifically from the fact that, as I have suggested for a long time, we are probably dealing not with an entity, but rather with the final common path of *a variety* of disturbances (Bellak, 1958; 1979).

My attempt to develop an instrument for the assessment of ego functioning began with a long-standing interest in schizophrenia. When an extensive review of the literature (Bellak, 1948) and an attempt to study schizophrenics via their somatotypes (Bellak & Holt, 1948) or psychological inventories (Bellak & Parcell, 1946) failed to establish any means of diagnosing schizophrenics, it was then that I formulated the ego-psychological-multifactorial psychosomatic theory of schizophrenia (Bellak, 1949). According to this conception, schizophrenia is viewed as a syndrome with various possible etiologic or pathogenic pictures that share, as a final common path, a serious impairment of the ego. It became apparent that different patients exhibited different patterns of impairment in their ego functioning and so it seemed most useful to assess each ego function independently. I first described this approach in a paper in 1949 and continued to address it in a series of subsequent publications (Bellak, 1952; 1958) and eventually in the volume *Ego Functions in Schizophrenics, Neurotics, and Normals* (Bellak, Hurvich, & Gediman, 1973).

Although ego function assessment (EFA) indeed had its origins in the attempt to deal rationally with the problems presented in the schizophrenias, the need for an assessment that can be descriptively, operationally, and dynamically meaningful is compelling. In the present volume some of these areas are given particular focus. EFA has been utilized in such different contexts as forensic psychiatry, selection and evaluation of major executives as well as political figures and civil servants, the assessment of drug effects, the assessment of analyzability, the evaluation of research in psychotherapy, as well as in the monitoring of the psychotherapeutic process itself (see chapters in Part 2).

Of all these, of course, the role of ego function assessment in psychiatric diagnosis is the one that stands in the foreground.

REFERENCES

Bellak, L. *Dementia praecox: the past decade's work and present status: A review and evaluation.* New York: Grune & Stratton, 1948.

Bellak, L. A multiple-factor psychosomatic theory of schizophrenia. *Psychiatric Quarterly,* 1949, *23,* 738–755.

Bellak, L. *Manic-depressive psychosis and allied disorders*. New York: Grune & Stratton, 1952.

Bellak, L. Toward a unified concept of schizophrenia. *Journal of Nervous and Mental Disease*, 1955, *121*, 60–66.

Bellak, L. (Ed.) *Schizophrenia: A review of the syndrome*. New York: Logos Press; distributed by Grune & Stratton, 1958.

Bellak, L. *The Thematic Apperception Test, Children's Apperception Test, and Senior Apperception Technique in clinical use*. (3d and rev. ed.) New York: Grune & Stratton, 1975.

Bellak, L. (Ed.) *The disorders of the schizophrenic syndrome*. New York: Basic Books, 1979.

Bellak, L., & Holt, R. R. Somatotypes in relation to dementia praecox. *American Journal of Psychiatry*, 1948, *104*, 713–724.

Bellak, L., Hurvich, M., & Gediman, H. *Ego functions in schizophrenics, neurotics, and normals*. New York: Wiley, 1973.

Bellak, L., & Parcell, B. The prepsychotic personality in dementia praecox; study of 100 cases in the Navy. *Psychiatric Quarterly*, 1946, *20*, 627–637.

Basic Aspects of Ego Function Assessment

LEOPOLD BELLAK

EGO FUNCTIONS AS CONSTRUCT

Psychoanalysis as a body of theory has followed several models. The still most widely accepted one is the tripartite model of structural theory. The structures, or as some would prefer it, the systems, are the ego, id, and superego. Ego psychology has in recent years become so prominent that it often tends to obscure the fact that a full metapsychological description—structural as well as dynamic, economic, genetic, and adaptive—is necessary for a full understanding of human behavior. In the ensuing description of ego functions, this fact has to be kept in mind.

If one keeps in mind that the ego is merely a useful construct of clinical working apparatuses, it becomes obvious that any discussion of ego functions involves some willingness to break this concept down into more or less arbitrary subdivisions. However, it should be noted that psychoanalysis and ego psychology, for that matter, do not differ in this respect from other sciences. In all of them, however precise, we employ more or less convenient fictions in an attempt to understand phenomena. The only object for discussion would be the nature and characteristics of the process and functions underlying this concept.

Many psychoanalysts have listed and discussed ego functions: Hartmann in 1939, Anna Freud in 1945, myself in 1949, Beres in 1956, and Arlow and Brenner in 1964, to mention some of the major ones. In addition, several investigators have developed scales for measuring or assessing ego functions. In 1952 I suggested that ego strength be appraised with a scale based on data from the life history and symptomatology. Green (1954) also offered a scoring guide for assessing 10 functions in 1954, and others have followed.

As early as 1952, my aim was to define ego functions in operational terms. The model was based on a subtest analysis, akin to the Wechsler-Bellevue Intelligence Test (WAIS). I envisioned ego function subtests that could be summed up in an ego function quotient, analogous to the intelligence quotient. I had already learned from Frederick L. Wells, one of my preceptors in 1941, and the then dean of American psychologists, that the pattern of subfunctions is more important than the numerical IQ. He and Gordon Allport, another of my teachers, agreed on the superiority of an idiographic or personally unique approach over an actuarial or general classificatory nomothetic one.

Predicated on my earlier work on the Global Ego Strength Scale (Bellak & Rosenberg, 1966; Bellak, Hurvich, and Gediman, 1973) together with a number of colleagues, selected 12 ego functions in the context of a study on ego functions in schizophrenic, neurotic, and well-functioning individuals. We attempted to employ a number of distinctions that would encompass those dimensions currently recognized as the most important. It is a matter of choice among workers as to how many and what concepts seem necessary and sufficient to encompass what are currently understood as the major manifestations of ego functioning.

The selection of 12 ego functions emerged from attempts to describe and rate behavior from taped 2-hour interviews. A group of raters would listen independently, formulate constructs, and rate them. By a prolonged process of trial and error, we finally arrived at 12 ego functions that we felt were both necessary and sufficient in understanding and describing people. Adopting the principle of parsimony, "necessary and sufficient" means that we did not feel we needed more and could not comfortably do with less. It does not mean that we might not be able to think of more or sometimes fewer.

Even so, there is a degree of circularity in defining the ego by its functions, as it involves a decision to classify functions in a particular way and then to call this class of functions ego. If we can define these functions in a manner that allows for measurement, and subsequently relate the ratings to other aspects of behavior, this process need not lead us in a circle.

The ego has been conceptualized in psychoanalytic theory as one of the three major structures of mental apparatus. Generally, structures relate to patterns of organization, schemata, agencies, and apparatuses. Functions typically refer, on the other hand, to activities and processes. While structures usually refer to relatively fixed substitives, functions are depicted as systematic variations within these.

The concept of structure is most usefully viewed as a specific process, which is characterized by a slow rate of change, and involves an organization of elements and a characteristic style of response (Rapaport, 1957), in contrast to a rigid, static entity or faculty. It is only by virtue of *relatively* stable structures that predictions of behavior are possible.

Ego function constructs may refer to mental contents, processes, or outcomes. A sound basis for understanding and perhaps classifying them is in terms of the processes involved. Outcomes are underscored when it is stated that an individual manifests serious adaptive failure in a given ego function area. The usefulness of such a statement is increased when there is a specification of relevant drives, superego factors, external circumstances, conflicts associated with the disturbance, and the extent of ego function disruption. Of course, ego functions are intimately related to biological substratum. Lack of maturation, intoxication, various neurotransmitters such as dopamine and catecholamine, and, of course, structural changes (Bellak, 1979) can vitally affect the nature of ego functions.

The vantage point one assumes in the study of ego functions can typically be bifurcated along the following lines: focusing on both the adaptation to the environment and inner processes. In other words, ego functions can be formulated operationally, where the emphasis is on adaptation and a natural science approach, and subjectively, where the focus is on personal meanings and psychic reality.

Ego functions differ in the extent to which they are subject to regression. As is true for many aspects of ego functioning, there is a substantial stability in the adaptive level of ego functioning characteristic for a given individual. It is also true that the adaptive adequacy of ego functioning varies more in some people than in others, and, indeed, the readiness with which fluctuations occur is an important aspect of personality functioning.

The adaptive level of ego functioning is generally more stable in well-functioning individuals than in those who show marked psychopathology. In fact, one criterion of ego strength proposed by Hartmann (1953) is the extent to which ego functions *resist* regressive changes under stress.

Serious and protracted ego function regressions have been observed in some patients during the course of psychoanalysis. These seem to occur in individuals who have a predisposition for severe ego function regression as a result of preexisting ego defects. These may result from congenital ego weaknesses due to structural damage, that is, as part and parcel of anatomical damage or, for example, from pathological object relations, resulting from the failure to establish normal identifications. Another important basis for ego defects is the overreliance on splitting mechanisms in early childhood; splitting interferes with the integration of affects, self, and object images and with the organization and integration of the ego, as Kernberg (1975) has pointed out.

More immediate triggers for serious ego regressions include defensive reactions to threatening situations, the implementation of secondary gains, as well as attempts at a belated mastery of earlier conflicts.

Let me make this matter of ego function fluctuation a bit more concrete again. In assessing ego functions in our research, we found it necessary to describe people in terms of current, characteristic, highest, as well as lowest level of functioning, if we were to describe their level of adaptation adequately. When we plotted the profiles of one person on these four levels, it became especially obvious that some people showed a large span between highest as well as between current and characteristic level, on one or more ego functions, whereas others displayed only small differences. This fact allows us to predict the relative stability or instability of one or more crucial personality characteristics. For the clinician this may have implications as to whether a person is likely to regress in some ways and not in others. For the specialist concerned with personnel assessment of one kind or another, instability or soundness of judgment under stress, for example, may be an important factor to note. From a clinical or theoretical viewpoint our observations of ego function fluctuations over time graphically illustrate that apparent qualitative differences between normal, neurotic, and psychotic functions may be a matter of quantitative fluctuations. Hence, what becomes critical is the systematic assessment of the processes underlying any particular ego function deficit.

Although it is generally recognized that ego functions are interdependent, clinical experience indicates that ego function deficits tend to be discrete rather than global. The question, then, is, "How much discreteness or possibility of independent variation is there among ego functions, and under what conditions?"

One important factor is the level of personality differentiation. *The less differentiated the personality, the greater the tendency for a number of ego functions to show maladaptive features at the same time.* Many kinds of difficulties and traumata, which result in developmental arrest, increase the intercorrelation among ego functions at a low level of adaptive adequacy. For example, when the mechanism of splitting is relied on excessively for defensive reasons early in life, the resulting split between various aspects of the person's self-representations and object representations will influence and retard the subsequent development of object constancy, the level of object relations, the scope of synthetic functioning, the development of sense of self, and the strength of repression and other high-level defenses. Defective sensory and neurological equipment can result in a lowering of the adaptive level of many ego functions, just as a range of early disturbances in the mother–infant relationship can impair differentiation and integration processes (Spitz, 1959; Provence and Lipton, 1962; and Mahler and Furer, 1968).

I have already mentioned that the major ego functions are multidimensional and complex, rather than unitary and simple. This introduces an additional level of complexity to the study of the interrelationships among ego functions, as we not only have to consider the interrelationships among, for example, reality testing and synthesis, but must also be concerned with the variations in the component factors of each major function.

Thus, depending on such factors as which drive derivatives are involved, what superego aspects become activated, what is the nature and degree of environmental press or stress, a person's adaptive level with regard to a given ego function can vary considerably. For example, a patient may demonstrate good, that is, highly adaptive judgment in a variety of situations, but, under certain rather specific circumstances, may tend to engage in sexual behavior that is markedly inconsistent with good judgment. The implications are that the term *good judgment* often needs to be qualified by additional information.

In our empirical study we found some ego functions to be more highly related than others for the group of schizophrenics. A principal components factor analysis showed four related groupings of ego functions. One factor, Reality of Relations, included Reality Testing, Judgment, and Sense of Reality. A second factor, Socialization, included Object Relations and Regulation and Control of Drive. A third factor, Adaptive Thinking, involved Thought Processes and Adaptive Regression. The last group factor, Integration, comprised Synthesis, Adequacy of Defenses, and Autonomous Functioning. Whether another sample of schizophrenic patients would show a similar grouping of factors can only be determined by assessing another possibly large group by the same methods used in the original study.

Having gone into some detail on ego functions, it should be noted that a discussion of such functions should not lead anyone to disregard other aspects of personality. In the research study we also appraised id and superego functioning on scales similar to the ego functions scales. It is clear that ego functions can be interfered with as a result of strong drive, superego factors, and the workings of other ego functions, especially the defensive operations. Reality testing, for instance, can be impaired by strong drive pressure, as when a hungry person perceives food-related aspects of a situation to a significantly greater degree than does a satiated person. Superego aspects can affect reality testing, as when a guilt-ridden individual sees every policeman as a threatening figure. Certainly the synthetic function can be influenced by these characteristics. Despite such complexities, ego functions emerge as important personality variables that can be rated by independent judges with a relatively high degree of reliability and construct validity for clinical and other purposes. As stable structures, ego functions can be understood and are amenable to experimentation and merit a great deal of research consideration.

In terms of the current psychoanalytic scene, psychoanalysis has gone through a series of theoretical reexaminations within the last decade (Bellak, 1982). Although the major event was the rise of object relations theory on the American scene, especially predicated on the work of Margaret Mahler and

Edith Jacobson, and elaborated by Kernberg, other aspects of psychoanalytic theory have also been subject to a good deal of criticism, particularly with regard to the metapsychological theory in general and the structural model in particular. Kubie was among the first to question the value of metapsychology and some of its "mechanistic" assumptions. Psychoanalytically trained psychologists, such as George Klein, Robert Holt, and, most recently, Roy Schafer, have been particularly critical of the economic model while also challenging the need for a tripartite model. Schafer has proposed an action language model that could serve as a substitute for metapsychological and tripartite conceptualizations.

If adoption of alternative conceptualizations is the criterion of their value, then it appears that the majority of psychoanalytic theorists have not found these substitutes for classical Freudian conceptions constructive. I personally believe that if one keeps in mind that id, ego, superego are merely constructs or working hypotheses, their value remains unparalleled.

In particular, in defining the ego by its functions, operational criteria are met. The concept of ego functions is of direct clinical use in bridging the descriptive and the dynamic. The concept permits one to understand, predict, and control—and that is as much as one can ask of a concept.

EGO FUNCTION ASSESSMENT: A BRIDGE BETWEEN DESCRIPTIVE AND DYNAMIC PSYCHIATRY

Ego psychologists, psychoanalysts, and general psychiatrists alike are well versed in and share common notions as to many of the specific functions of the ego. Hence, the relevance of ego function assessment (EFA), which, being predicated on an operational definition of the ego, is a method of evaluation based on principles with which every psychiatrist and psychologist is familiar.

As previously mentioned, symptom checklists are often used in descriptive psychiatry to assess mental status or overall psychological functioning. These itemized lists may well make sense to the computer, which grinds out factors or clusters on the basis of mathematical affinity, but for the practicing therapist such printouts have little relevance or coherence in that they fail to contribute to an understanding of psychodynamics or etiology, treatment, and prognosis. Assessment of ego functions, however (precisely because definitions of these functions serve as the conceptual framework of the psychoanalytic construct of the ego), is a method that permits one who is psychodynamically oriented to further relate ego functions to the nature of drive qualities and quantity, as well as to the entire matrix of interlocking psychoanalytic hypotheses.

For clinicians who are not psychoanalytically oriented, EFA may be conceptualized as a mental status examination with substantial practical usefulness. EFA, however, gives a broad-spectrum profile of the personality—

much broader than most mental status tests—with specific information as to the nature and degree of ego dysfunctions and how these deficits may affect other areas of ego functioning.

Not only does EFA act as a bridge between descriptive and dynamic psychiatry, it also bridges the gap between various schools of psychology and psychiatry. Various psychologists and psychiatrists have stressed the learned aspects of thinking and communication patterns—patterns that are, of course, influenced by the innate anatomical and physiological characteristics of the organism. The ego has often been defined as an aggregate of percepts or learned patterns of behavior. To the extent that these learned patterns of behavior can be affected by newly experienced perceptions, so can the structure of the ego be modified and changed, even if at a slow rate. Thus, EFA has broad clinical application and is compatible with various approaches to the understanding of the mind and the treatment of its dysfunctions.

BACKGROUND: HISTORICAL DEVELOPMENT OF EFA

In a research project sponsored by NIMH, a study was made of the ego functioning of 100 subjects—50 schizophrenic patients, 25 neurotic patients, and 25 normal subjects—for the purpose of defining the major, currently recognized manifestations of ego functioning (Bellak, Hurvich, & Gediman, 1973). The assessment procedure consisted of a 2-hour, semistructured clinical interview with each subject, designed to elicit information relevant to past and present ego functioning; it also included a survey of family history. The interview was videotaped and, subsequently, two or more clinicians listened to and independently evaluated it. The study took three years, and a large team of researchers, by a prolonged process of trial and error, finally arrived at a list of 12 ego functions they considered to be both necessary and sufficient to describe the personality of the individual. Each of these 12 ego functions was then defined in terms of its major component factors, and separate procedures were developed to measure the adequacy of each function.

MAJOR EGO FUNCTIONS

In selecting these 12 major ego functions, it was recognized that a degree of choice is always exercised when categories of functions are delineated for the purpose of ordering observable phenomena. Furthermore, just as it is generally recognized that ego function can be influenced by drives or by superego factors, so there also exists some degree of overlap between the ego functions themselves. For example, sound judgment requires both good reality testing and good impulse control. Nevertheless, distinctions among the major currently recognized manifestations of ego functioning can be made.

The 12 functions (with their various components) that were eventually selected are as follows:

1. *Reality Testing.* The components are (a) the distinction between inner and outer stimuli; (b) accuracy of perception (including orientation to time and place and interpretation of external events), and (c) accuracy of inner reality testing (psychological mindedness and awareness of inner states).

2. *Judgment.* The components are (a) awareness of appropriateness of, and likely consequences of, intended behavior (anticipation of probable dangers, legal culpabilities, and social censure or disapproval) and (b) extent of manifest behavior as a reflection of the awareness of these likely consequences.

3. *Sense of Reality of the World and of the Self.* The component factors are (a) the extent to which external events are experienced as real and as being embedded in a familiar context (degree of derealization, déjà vu, trancelike states); (b) the extent to which the body (or parts of it) and its functioning and one's behavior are experienced as familiar, unobtrusive, and belonging to (or emanating from) the individual: (c) the degree to which the person has developed individuality, uniqueness, and a sense of self and self-esteem; and (d) the degree to which the person's self-representations are separated from his or her object representations.

4. *Regulation and Control of Drives, Affects, and Impulses.* The components are (a) the directness of impulse expression (ranging from primitive acting out through neurotic acting out to relatively indirect forms of behavioral expression) and (b) the effectiveness of delay and control, the degree of frustration tolerance, and the extent to which drive derivatives are channeled through ideation, affective expression, and manifest behavior.

5. *Object (or Interpersonal) Relationships.* The components are (a) the degree and kind of relatedness to others and investment in them (taking account of withdrawal trends, narcissistic self-concern, narcissistic object choice or mutuality); (b) the extent to which present relationships are adaptively or maladaptively influenced by, or patterned on, older ones, and serve present, mature aims rather than past, immature ones; (c) the degree to which the person perceives others as separate entities rather than as extensions of himself or herself; and (d) the extent to which the person can maintain object constancy (i.e., sustain relationships over long periods of time and tolerate both the physical absence of the object and frustration, anxiety, and hostility related to the object).

6. *Thought Processes.* The components are (a) the adequacy of processes that adaptively guide and sustain thought (attention, concentration,

anticipation, concept formation, memory, and language) and (b) the extent of relative primary–secondary process influences on thought (degree to which thinking is unrealistic, illogical, and/or loose).

7.   *Adaptive Regression in the Service of the Ego.*   The components are (a) relaxation of perceptual and conceptual acuity and other ego controls with a concomitant increase in awareness of previously preconscious and unconscious contents (first phase of an oscillating process) and (b) the induction of new configurations that increase adaptive potentials as a result of creative integrations (second phase of the oscillating process).

8.   *Defensive Functioning.*   The components are (a) the degree to which defensive components adaptively or maladaptively affect ideation and behavior and (b) the extent to which these defenses have succeeded or failed (degree of emergence of anxiety, depression, and/or other dysphoric affects indicating weakness of defensive operations).

9.   *Stimulus Barrier.*   The component factors are (a) a threshold for, sensitivity to, or awareness of stimuli impinging on various sensory modalities (primarily external, but including pain) and (b) the nature of response to various levels of sensory stimulation in terms of the extent of disorganization, avoidance, withdrawal, or active coping mechanisms employed to deal with them.

10.   *Autonomous Functioning.*   The components are (a) degree of freedom from impairment of apparatuses of primary autonomy (functional disturbances of sight, hearing, intention, language, memory, learning, or motor function) and (b) degree of, or freedom from, impairment of secondary autonomy (disturbances in habit patterns, learned complex skills, work routines, hobbies, and interests).

11.   *Synthetic–Integrative Functioning.*   The components are (a) degree of reconciliation or integration of discrepant or potentially contradictory attitudes, values, affects, behavior, and self-representations and (b) degree of active relating together and integrating of psychic and behavioral events, whether contradictory or not.

12.   *Mastery–Competence.*   The components are (a) extent of competence, that is, the person's performance in relation to his or her existing capacity to interact with and master his or her environment and (b) the extent of sense of competence, that is, the person's expectation of success or the subjective side of actual performance (how well the person believes he or she can do).

RATING OF EGO FUNCTIONS

To describe impressions of an individual's ego functioning in a quantitative form, it was necessary in the creation of EFA to develop a rating scale for each of the 12 ego functions and their various components. Each function was rated on a scale of 1 to 7—1 representing the poorest or minimal level of functioning and 7 representing the optimal level of functioning. It should be noted that these extremes rarely exist in reality; 11 represents "average" functioning as defined by absence of any notable pathology but short of optimal functioning. (An alternate scoring method rates ego functions on a scale of 1 to 13.) A manual was designed that contains detailed and specific anchor definitions for alternate points on a scale between 1 and 7, each point describing a more primitive or more advanced level of ego functioning. The manual contains such rating scales for each of the various components that make up any ego function.

In assessing ego function of reality testing, for example, each of the components, (a) distinction between inner and outer stimuli, (b) accuracy of perception, and (c) reflective awareness and inner reality testing, would be individually rated. The scoring of reality testing component "a" (distinction between inner and outer stimuli) would be as follows:

Point 1 (Maximal Impairment).   Hallucinations and delusions pervade. Minimal ability to distinguish events occurring in dreams from those occurring in waking life, and inability to distinguish among idea, image, and hallucination. Perceptual experience is grossly disturbed (e.g., moving things look still and vice versa).

Point 2.   Hallucinations and delusions are severe but limited to one or more content areas. Patient may show considerable doubt about distinguishing whether an event really happened in his or her mind or in a dream.

Point 3.   Illusions are more likely to be found than hallucinations. Patient may be aware of seeing and hearing things that are not there but knows that others do not see or hear them.

Point 4.   Projections of inner states onto external reality are more likely than frank hallucinations or delusions. A "stimulus-bound" reality testing may occur at the cost of libidinal investments and gratification.

Point 5.   Confusion about inner and outer states occurs mainly on awakening, going to sleep, or under severe stress.

Point 6.   Inner and outer stimuli are well distinguished. Occasional denial of external reality in the service of adaptation.

Point 7.   Clear awareness of whether events occurred in dreams or waking life. Correct identification of the source of cognitive and/or perceptual content as being idea or image, and accurate identification of its source as internal or external. Distinction between outer and inner percepts holds up even under extreme stress. Checking perceptions against reality occurs with a very high degree of automaticity.

(See Appendix A for further elaboration of rating and scoring procedures.)

Once ego functions have been rated, they may be graphed; this permits easy visualization of the patient's psychological state. A graph with an indication of the ranges of normal, neurotic, borderline, and psychotic functions allows the clinician to appreciate at a glance the strengths and weaknesses of different ego functions and assists in diagnosis. (See Sharp & Bellak, Chapter 16, this volume.)

EGO FUNCTION ASSESSMENT AS A DIAGNOSTIC APPROACH

Diagnosis is, indeed, a many-splendored thing! In part, it belongs to the areas of general classification theory, nosology, and semantics—a subject that Martin Katz (1971) wrote a particularly good book on. In part, diagnosis is a social-psychological phenomenon, and Karl Menninger (1970) has written about the dangers of attaching labels, the social stigma that accompanies the labeling process, and the stereotyped thinking that it is likely to produce in the diagnostician, who often becomes the victim of his or her own prophesies. Despite the sympathy I have for the dangers of labeling, especially in view of the invasion of privacy that occurs in the context of third-party payments and similar threats that accompany the use of computer systems, I nevertheless feel that the advantages still outweigh the disadvantages in the labeling process. In this chapter I primarily address myself to the clinical and methodological aspects of diagnosis.

Above all, I think of a diagnosis as a heuristic hypothesis—a guiding framework that helps one to investigate a particular phenomenon. This implies that it must be flexible and subject to constant correction as new data emerge. A diagnostic hypothesis must help one *to understand, to predict,* and *to control.* In our field, understanding means finding causal connections, etiology, and pathogenesis. Clinically, prediction means prognostic statements and control means treatment, therapeutic control. When I speak of diagnosis, I am speaking of *nomothetic* labels and *idiographic* ones, that is, class statements, and some that hold true specifically just for a given patient.

Diagnosis must also permit one to make collateral inferences; that is, if one finds *A,* presumably one ought to also find *B, C,* and *D* covarying. Etymologically, "diagnosis" means one should be able to ascertain a difference, to differentiate (e.g., for Hippocrates, the difference between a stone in the bladder and an intestinal obstruction). For methodologists this means *discriminant validity,* that is, being able by means of certain criteria to discriminate between one condition and another.

A diagnosis should also enable one to make *postdictions,* which falls in the domain of predictive validity. That is, it should be possible, from the patient's current symptoms, to postdict what must have occurred in his or her past. Conversely, it should be possible from a history alone to predict what the patient's symptomatology *ought* to be. Incidentally, this process often highlights the limitations of our hypotheses, and frequently they are very marked. For instance, it is often very difficult to predict from history alone what drive manifestations the patient will exhibit, what his or her defenses against them will be, or what intricate mixture of the two we will find. Such an attempt involves quantitative propositions, which we are ill equipped to formulate at this time.

Psychoanalysis may do a little better than other fields with regard to understanding, prediction, and control, as it consists of an interrelated theory of personality, a theory of psychopathology, and a theory of psychotherapeutic technique, each of them predicated on interlocking propositions. For instance, if one has a patient suffering from premature ejaculation, it is possible to make the collateral inference that he probably also suffers from voyeurism, perhaps from erythrophobia, is probably impulsive, and also exhibits a number of oral characteristics (in light of the passivity involved in his chief complaint).

In general psychiatry we do not at present have adequate testable propositions, as witnessed, for instance, in the problems of diagnosing schizophrenia. It is possible to speak of two basic trends in the attempts to diagnose schizophrenia. One is primarily concerned with increasing the *reliability* of the diagnosis, and the other is concerned with establishing the *validity* of the diagnosis. Those familiar with the tenets of scientific methodology may argue that it is essential to strive for a combination of reliability and validity in one's findings. That is certainly true in theory, but very often not so in practice. There are a vast number of psychological and psychiatric questionnaires that have great reliability but very questionable validity. That is, if a test is administered to the same person by the same tester a second time, or administered to the same person by a different tester a second time, similar findings are very likely to be made. However, it is regrettable that often the degree to which the test measures what it purports to measure is in question, because construct validity as well as criterion-related validity is poor. Further, such tests do not correlate well with findings from other measurements or with clinical judgment. There are a whole host of factor analytic data for which the same may be said. They are found again and again with great reliability, but the statistical factors generated by the computer make no sense to the clinician.

In essence, the position underlying the search for reliability in the diagnosis of schizophrenia rests on the basic assumption that there is such an entity as "schizophrenia" and that all one needs to do is to agree on the necessary signs and symptoms defining it. If, however, this concept is not valid, then its reliability is meaningless. As long as we do not have experimental verification of the psychoanalytic hypotheses or generally accepted biological data for the construct validity of the diagnosis, be it schizophrenia, depression, or other psychiatric conditions, then psychiatric diagnosis remains either in the area of unsupported hunches or is purely descriptive and of limited usefulness.

It is on this basis that I suggested EFA as a bridge between descriptive and dynamic psychiatry and etiologic propositions. It is possible to assess the pattern of ego functions of "normal" subjects, and of a variety of neurotics and psychotics, in terms that can be and have been operationally defined. These ego function patterns permit an idiographic characterization of an individual patient as well as his or her classification within a group; that is, one can have both an individual profile and one that can be assigned by numerical rating to a class defined as neurotic or borderline or psychotic.

Diagnostic Patterns

EFA is helpful in enabling a clinician to qualify a nomothetic generic diagnosis with a series of hierarchical statements. For instance, the diagnosis of "schizophrenic syndrome" may be accompanied by statements such as "poor impulse control" and "poor judgment." This could target a need for close supervision of particular patients and/or the need for medication. By contrast, in another patient, inner reality testing might be judged to be very good, that is, the patient is aware of being ill and recognizes his or her poor outer reality testing. In this case it is useful to keep in mind Goldstein's (1970) findings, that patients with such awareness are often further impaired by phenothiazines. I would be especially hesitant to administer phenothiazines if awareness of being ill is accompanied by a poor "sense of self" and feelings of depersonalization, because phenothiazines may exacerbate a feeling of being "spaced out."

Any time that poor impulse control and relatively intact thinking are found in conjunction with a history of asocial behavior, the patient should be carefully examined for evidence of minimal brain dysfunction (Bellak, 1979). A careful personal and family history with regard to MBD should be taken in conjunction with a standard neuropsychological and neurological examination.

Assessing prognosis should be greatly aided by an analysis of ego function patterns. A patient with a universally and chronically low profile can be expected to profit minimally from what we have to offer, and is probably in need of rehabilitation efforts and a more highly structured environment. A patient in whom reality testing, judgment, and impulse control remain relatively intact, even in the acute episode, can probably be helped, with rehabilitation, to live constructively in the community, working on some simple job, even if his or her other functions are relatively poor.

The nature of a patient's object relations needs special scrutiny. Their assessment is important for a detailed and sophisticated diagnosis of the primary condition itself, for the kind of therapy suggested, and for the nature of the recovery one can expect.

REFERENCES

Arlow, J., & Brenner, C. *Psychoanalytic concepts and the structural theory*. New York: International Universities Press, 1964.

Bellak, L. A multiple-factor psychosomatic theory of schizophrenia. *Psychiatric Quarterly,* 1949, *23,* 738–755.

Bellak, L. *Manic-depressive psychosis and allied disorders.* New York: Grune & Stratton, 1952.

Bellak, L. Psychiatric aspects of minimal brain dysfunction in adults: Their ego function assessment. In L. Bellak (Ed.), *Psychiatric aspects of minimal brain dysfunction in adults.* New York: Grune & Stratton, 1979.

Bellak, L. *Current status of classical Freudian psychoanalysis.* Lessons 9, 10, and 11, Directions in Psychiatry. Hatherleigh Company, 1982.

Bellak, L., Hurvich, M., & Gediman, H. *Ego functions in schizophrenics, neurotics, and normals.* New York: Wiley, 1973.

Bellak, L., & Rosenberg, S. Effects of two antidepressant drugs on depression. *Psychosomatics,* 1966, *7,* 106–114.

Beres, D. Ego deviation and the concept of schizophrenia. In R. Eissler et al. (Eds.), *The psychoanalytic study of the child,* Vol. XI. New York: International Universities Press, 1956.

Eissler, K. Notes upon the emotionality of a schizophrenic patient and its relation to problems of technique. In R. Eissler et al. (Eds.) *The psychoanalytic study of the child,* Vol. VIII. New York: International Universities Press, 1953, pp. 199–251.

Freud, A. *The ego and the mechanisms of defense.* New York: International Universities Press, 1946.

Goldstein, M. J. Premorbid adjustment, paranoid status, and patterns of response to phenothiazines in acute schizophrenia. *Schizophrenia Bulletin,* 1970, *I* (Experimental Issue No. 3).

Green, S. The evaluation of ego adequacy. *Journal of Hillside Hospital,* 1954, *3,* 199–203.

Hartmann, H. *Ego psychology and the problem of adaptation.* New York: International Universities Press, 1939; 1958.

Hartmann, H. Contributions to the metapsychology of schizophrenia. In *Essays and ego psychology.* New York: International Universities Press, 1953; 1964.

Katz, M. *The role and methodology of classification in psychiatry and psychopathology.* (Proceedings of a conference, Washington, D.C., November, 1965.) Washington, D.C.: Government Printing Office, 1971.

Kernberg, O. *Borderline conditions and pathological narcissism.* New York: Jason Aronson, 1975.

Mahler, M., & Furer, M. *On human symbiosis and the vicissitudes of individuation.* New York: International Universities Press, 1968.

Menninger, K. Syndrome, yes; disease entity, no. In R. Cancro (Ed.), *The schizophrenic reactions.* New York: Brunner/Mazel, 1970.

Murray, H. A. *Explorations in personality.* New York: Oxford University Press, 1938.

Provence, S., & Lipton, R. *Infants in institutions.* New York: International Universities Press, 1962.

Rapaport, D. Cognitive structures. In M. Gill (Ed.), *The collected papers of David Rapaport.* New York: Basic Books, 1957; 1967.

Spitz, R. *A genetic field theory of ego formation.* New York: International Universities Press, 1959.

CHAPTER THREE

The Broad Scope of Ego Function Assessment

LEOPOLD BELLAK

CLINICAL APPLICATION OF EFA

As it is based solely on clinical data, the unobtrusive nature of ego function assessment renders it highly adaptable to many different clinical situations. For example, in the initial interview the dialogue between the doctor and patient can be permitted to flow without the patient feeling he or she is being "tested"—a sensation that may arouse considerable anxiety in some individuals. By the same token, EFA can be used in the course of ongoing therapy (psychotherapy or analysis) without the quality of treatment being affected. This is an especially important consideration for psychoanalysts who are particularly reluctant to invade the privacy of the patient–doctor relationship—an element that is fundamental and crucial to the treatment process.

EFA As a Valid Quantitative Technique

Bellak et al. (1973) demonstrated in their research study that on a 13-point scale, the interrater reliability between two judges formally evaluating 100 individuals—50 schizophrenic patients, 25 neurotic patients, and 25 normal subjects—ranged between .61 for the ego function of stimulus barrier and

.88 for autonomous functioning, with a mean correlation of .77. Although these figures are derived from the use of the specifically designed interview manual described earlier, ratings based on ordinary psychotherapeutic sessions allow for an interrater reliability of .72. Furthermore, these rated assessments of the patient's ego functions related meaningfully to what was known about the subject from other sources: For example, patients who had been diagnosed as schizophrenic by other criteria, when assessed blindly using the EFA method, were seen to have lower ego functions than subjects previously diagnosed as neurotics, and the neurotics, in turn, had lower ego functions than normals.

Use of EFA in Psychiatric Evaluation

Psychiatric evaluation of a patient in terms of mental status, dynamic diagnosis, potential treatability, and long-range prognosis is one of the most crucial functions carried out by clinicians in the field. Many important and far-reaching decisions are made on the basis of the initial interview. In the psychiatric emergency room, for example, the patient is interviewed by a psychiatrist who will formulate a diagnosis and arrive at a treatment plan. Decisions will be made regarding the following questions: Should the patient be hospitalized or treated in an outpatient setting? Is psychotherapy appropriate? If so, should this be supportive therapy, insight therapy, or psychoanalysis? Should the patient be put on a particular psychotropic drug? These decisions obviously have many ramifications that affect not only the patient but often the family as well.

EFA, by pinpointing the specific problem areas within the individual's psychic makeup, often leads to an understanding of the underlying dynamics and suggests the likely etiology as well, both of which carry direct implications in terms of treatment and, ultimately, prognosis. If, for example, a patient who presents with depression is demonstrated by EFA to have a particular difficulty in the area of object relations, and if this patient has suffered a recent object loss such as the death of a spouse or close friend, these factors point immediately to a dynamic understanding of the patient's current withdrawal and regression.

Since EFA permits the clinician to identify the nature of the present personality disturbance and gives some notion of the levels of functioning over time, it is also obviously a crucial aid in making accurate judgments regarding the treatment plan. The more precise the conceptualization and planning of the treatment, the more therapeutic success and the fewer impasse situations and prematurely terminated cases can be expected.

EFA in Crisis Intervention

As Bellak and Small (1978) have pointed out, the crux of the effectiveness of brief psychotherapy, emergency psychotherapy, and crisis intervention lies in explicit, careful conceptualization of the dynamics and structure of the patient and his or her complaints.

The more disturbed the patient, the more important it is that one have a clear picture of his or her assets and liabilities in order to gauge the prospective effectiveness of various psychotherapeutic methods. With severely disturbed individuals, it is important to utilize the intact aspects of the personality for the improvement of the poorly functioning ones.

EFA is especially useful for this process. A profile may show that autonomous functions are intact (despite poor reality testing and poor judgment) and can be utilized in a workshop setting to provide structure and improvement of the more impaired functions. Poor impulse control may immediately suggest pharmacotherapy, at the very least, in combination with psychotherapy. Poor synthetic–integrative functioning with a low rating in thought processes will militate against the use of insight therapy and speak in favor of a largely supportive, educational, and rehabilitative intervention.

EFA in Predicting Analyzability

In most cases it is possible to make an accurate assessment of a patient's analyzability by making an informal inquiry of the 12 ego functions, as opposed to a systematic and structured interview with the use of the rating manual. Various aspects of each ego function should be kept in mind with regard to a patient's ability to utilize the psychoanalytic treatment. Consider the ego function of reality testing as an example.

One aspect of reality testing involves the ability to distinguish internal from external stimuli. Absence of this capacity, as manifested in an extreme by hallucinations, is obviously a contraindication to putting a patient in analysis. A less blatant form of confusion between internal and external stimuli occurs when the perception of present reality is distorted in terms of the internalized past. The degree to which this confusion exists will determine a patient's ability to utilize the analytic mode. For example, if infantile fantasies or object representations determine his or her response to current situations to a large degree, this patient may well develop unmanageable transference reactions or engage in severe acting out.

Intra- and interpersonal validation of perceptions is another important component of reality testing that involves the comparison of one's own perceptions with those of others. A defect in this operation would lead to highly idiosyncratic beliefs or delusions that, if severe, might also render the psychoanalytic mode ineffective.

Inner reality testing involves the patient's ability to become aware of and understand his or her internal reality without losing an appreciation of external reality. This internal perceptiveness or "psychological-mindedness" would be compromised by impaired defensive functioning. For example, excessive use of denial or projective and introjective mechanisms would limit the patient's ability to explore his or her inner reality and therefore limit the analytic results.

Reality testing is also critical to other aspects of the process of psychoanalysis: free association, for example, is achieved by the process of adaptive regression, which permits the suspension of secondary processes and the retrieval of unconscious material. At the same time, observing reality testing is required for the recognition and understanding of external and internal reality based on the data of association. Reality testing is also obviously indispensable to the understanding and working through of the transference. When it is defective, severely distorted transference phenomena may develop. (A detailed discussion of the remaining 11 ego functions and their relevance in determining analyzability is given in Chapter 15 of this book.)

Use of EFA in the Choice of Psychopharmacologic Agents

EFA can be extremely valuable in determining analyzability, and it is equally valuable in assessing the appropriateness of other types of treatment. For example, EFA can be very helpful in making decisions concerning the use of psychotherapeutic drugs. Because it has been demonstrated that certain of the psychopharmacological agents have specific target symptoms, and these symptoms are often a manifestation of the disturbance of one or more ego functions, one would obviously be better equipped to prescribe a drug that will have the desired therapeutic effect by determining which of the specific ego functions are deficient in a particular patient. For example, it has been shown that certain phenothiazines affect thought processes and reality testing, as well as impulse control. Thus, if one had a schizophrenic patient with hallucinations, delusions, loose associations, and uncontrollably aggressive behavior, one might well think of prescribing such a drug to facilitate further treatment.

In other instances, where there is a disturbance in the sense of self—for example, in a borderline patient—phenothiazines may be contraindicated because of their tendency to aggravate this disturbance in nonpsychotic individuals. The choice of two combined drugs and their dose levels might be determined with the aid of EFA. For example, the depressed patient who historically presents evidence of psychotic thinking could be treated with tricyclic antidepressants with phenothiazines added, depending on changes in thought processes and sense of reality.

Use of EFA in the Evaluation of the Ongoing Treatment Process

Not only is EFA of crucial value in formulating a dynamic diagnosis and a specific treatment plan, it is also of substantial use in monitoring the ongoing treatment process.

Monitoring Drug Therapy

In monitoring drug therapy, the patient should obviously be evaluated first before beginning the drug. Once the drug is instituted, EFA should be administered at various intervals to see if there has been any change in the level of ego functioning, and, if so, which specific functions have been affected. This can be of help not only in determining the effects of the drug, but in making a retrospective diagnosis, because response to drugs can constitute a useful touchstone for diagnosis.

Monitoring the Psychotherapeutic Process

The use of EFA in ongoing psychoanalysis has proved highly beneficial. The administration of EFA at regular intervals not only can introduce the desirable element of precision to the ongoing analytic work, but also can provide a broad overview of specific trends in the treatment and a focus for predicting future trends. This also makes possible more methodical planning of future treatment goals.

OTHER APPLICATIONS OF EGO FUNCTION ASSESSMENT

The demand for an accurate method of evaluating personality and its dysfunctions is not limited to the clinical context alone. There are many situations that require psychiatric assessment. Within the field of psychiatry, for example, there has been a recent demand for a means of establishing a professional standards review, such as a peer review whereby clinicians would have the opportunity to evaluate each other's work as a means of ensuring high-quality medical care. Psychiatric research almost invariably requires a reliable method of before-and-after evaluation.

Outside the field—in the courtroom, for example—a psychiatrist's testimony or opinion is often crucial. It is also sought in cases of insurance claims and other matters involving third-party payments.

EFA in Peer Review

EFA constitutes the ideal "test instrument" for monitoring the psychotherapeutic process, and it is also a valuable tool—since it does not distort or disrupt the actual treatment—for the evaluation of psychoanalysis or psychotherapy by psychiatrists other than the primary physician. In practice, a patient in treatment with one analyst or therapist could be interviewed any time by another clinician and both therapists could make their independent EFA ratings. If there were two peers evaluating a third colleague's patient, they could "conference" their findings (conferencing of findings is an accepted method among researchers) and report the agreed ratings as a basis for comparison with those arrived at by the treating therapist. Utilizing this method of objective evaluation would further protect the treating therapist from arbitrary or poor ratings. In turn, it would be quite feasible, after independent ratings, for the treating analyst and the evaluating analyst to conference their separate assessments. This procedure would bring to the psychotherapeutic treatment process the often missed richness of shared observations, which play so constructive a role in other fields of medical practice and research.

EFA and Psychotherapy Research

The recent establishment of the research foundation of the American Psychoanalytic Association strongly reflects the thrust of new interest in clinical analytic research—an area in which EFA holds great promise. The

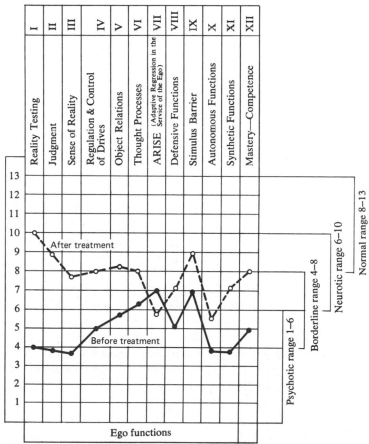

Figure 3.1.   Comparison of combined EFA scores of a patient rated by two evaluators before and after two years of psychoanalytic therapy. 1 = maximal impairment; 13 = optimal functioning. (Reprinted with permission from Bellak and Sheehy, 1976.)

Table 3.1. Comparison of Combined EFA Scores of a Patient Rated by Two Evaluators Before and After Two Years of Psychoanalytic Therapy

| | Combined EFA Scores, by Time of Evaluation | | |
| | Before Therapy | After Therapy | |
Ego Function			Significance[a]
Reality testing	4.0	10.0	$p < .01$
Judgment	4.0	9.0	$p < .01$
Sense of reality	4.0	8.0	$p < .01$
Regulation and control of drives, affects, and impulses	5.0	8.0	$p < .05$
Object relations	6.5	8.5	n.s.
Thought processes	8.0	8.5	n.s.
ARISE	7.5	6.0	n.s.
Defensive functioning	5.0	7.5	$p < .05$
Stimulus barrier	7.5	9.0	n.s.
Autonomous functioning	5.0	5.5	n.s.
Synthetic-integrative functioning	4.0	7.5	$p < .01$
Mastery-competence	4.0	8.0	$p < .01$

Source: Reprinted with permission from Bellak and Sheehy (1976).

[a] By chi-square test with correction for continuity.

usefulness of EFA as a tool in monitoring and evaluating the ongoing analytic or psychotherapeutic process has been mentioned. In terms of psychotherapy of any kind, the effect of interpretive and interpersonal efforts can be studied at close range while an objective record of general progress or deterioration is assembled to provide corrective feedback on the treatment process.

An accurate method for assessing the patient's psychological state at the commencement and termination of treatment is obviously crucial to the design of psychiatric research for the study of psychotherapy. A graph illustrating the application of EFA to before-and-after evaluation in psychotherapy research is shown in Figure 3.1. Figure 3.1 and Table 3.1 illustrate the ego functioning for one of 30 patients rated validly and reliably by independent observers before and after 2 years of psychoanalysis (Bellak & Sheehy, 1976).

EFA of Psychological Test Data

Test data reporting has been a notorious problem with no clear-cut relationship between primary data and inferences and, frequently, no consistent frame of reference.

EFA has been used by Bellak (1974) to examine individual test data, for example, data from the Thematic Apperception Test, the Children's Apperception Test, and the Senior Apperception Test. It has also been utilized for test reporting in his Diagnostic Test Report Form (1974).

A graph of ego functions permits the pictorial representation of the test findings as well as a profile for EFA as it emerges behaviorally during the testing.

EFA, in this case, may be able to promote more uniform and, in general, more easily comparable data than those provided by psychological tests.

EFA in General Medicine and Surgery

EFA might be useful for research in psychosomatic medicine by offering some definitions of personality characteristics of patients with asthma, ulcerative colitis and ileitis, and other disorders.

For liaison psychiatrists the evaluation of one specific ego function (the sense of self) might help prevent postoperative psychoses, especially in plastic surgery, but also in amputations, major abdominal surgery, and kidney dialysis.

EFA in the Extratherapeutic Context: Communication with Third Parties

Outside the field of psychiatry there is frequent demand for a method of accurate psychiatric evaluation. The use of EFA ratings to report behavioral and operational concepts to an interested, nonpsychiatric audience, such as county medical societies, insurance companies, and members of the courtroom, would make it possible to communicate important information while at the same time protecting the privacy of the individual patient or defendant.

EFA in Forensic Psychiatry

The history of forensic psychiatry has been mostly a regrettable one marked by an unfortunate pattern. One or more are psychiatrists hired by the defense and one or more by the prosecution; then the psychiatrists on each side promptly find the appropriate psychiatric diagnosis for their employers. In the process they project an embarrassing picture of psychiatry.

To improve this situation, psychiatric evidence should be removed from the adversary process. What is needed is a pool of psychiatrists trained and certified in forensic psychiatry. From this pool the court could draw by lot two or more psychiatrists who would make their findings available to the court, rather than to either the defense or the prosecution. Employing EFA in such a setting would provide a method that bridges the chasm between psychiatrists and laymen by offering data useful to one group as well as intelligible to the other.

In spite of the present unsatisfactory use of psychiatric expert witnesses, there would be an improvement with the introduction of EFA. Even if the defense and prosecution were to insist on having their own psychiatric experts testify, the psychiatrists could be asked to give their reports in the form of EFA. Discrepancies on a graph could then be queried by the judge and jury, who would be in a better position to evaluate the soundness of the expert findings than they would be without this aid. Furthermore, psychiatric testimony would gain credibility and dignity if one could point to such demonstrable factors as episodic loss of impulse control possibly related to signs of minimal brain dysfunction (MBD) or show that a chronic loss of self-boundaries causes confusional states.

It would be equally helpful if two psychiatrists for the defense and two for the prosecution could make an EFA independently (blind) and, it is hoped, produce data with high agreement.

In the legal context, EFA could be used to evaluate a defendant or to allow the psychiatrist to provide testimony that, while not invading the confidentiality of the patient–doctor relationship, would offer precise information that would be helpful in determining the legal responsibility of the individual. Because EFA is useful in determining specific behavioral difficulties that may have existed throughout the life of an individual, this method would obviously be of value in determining legal accountability.

For example, let us say that EFA reveals that throughout his life an individual has demonstrated that he is more or less normal in terms of his reality testing and judgment but has, at the same time, exhibited a marked inability to control his impulses. This finding would then indicate a further medical-psychiatric workup to determine the cause of the poor impulse control. It should be determined, for example, whether the patient is suffering from minimal brain dysfunction, some form of temporal lobe epilepsy, and so on. The presence or absence of an organic or neurological deficit would obviously be important in terms of the individual's legal responsibility, since accountability has to do with a person's ability to control his behavior. Similarly, if EFA showed that an individual had, since early childhood, demonstrated abnormal thought processes, an inability to distinguish between inner and outer reality, and other symptoms of schizophrenia or psychosis, these data would be important in determining legal responsibility.

Outside the area of criminal law, accurate psychiatric evaluation is also relevant in deciding such issues as an individual's capacity to enter a legal contract or make a will, since this capacity is dependent on such ego functions as the ability to exercise judgment and anticipate the consequences of actions.

PSRO, Third-Party Funding, and Choice of Treatment Approach

EFA can be used for professional standards review organization (PSRO) and third-party funding since this method of psychiatric evaluation is a valuable aid in making decisions about the advisability of admission to, or discharge from, inpatient facilities. Once the patient has been correctly diagnosed in terms of specific ego strengths and weaknesses, and his or her adaptive capacities have been analyzed, this assessment should have clear consequences in determining the nature and setting of the patient's treatment. For example, if a patient were experiencing an acute psychotic episode that includes impairment of reality testing, thought processes, and judgment, but at the same time has a history that includes a high characteristic level of ego functioning with marked achievement in the area of mastery and competence, he would merit intensive psychotherapy, possibly on an inpatient ward, since his prognosis is relatively good.

A quite different case would be a patient who exhibited the same symptoms, appearing acutely psychotic, but who had a history of low levels of ego functioning since early childhood with relatively poor object relations and little achievement in terms of mastery and competence. This individual would not necessarily warrant the same intensive psychotherapeutic efforts, as the prognosis is poor; he might be better treated with supportive psychotherapy and/or psychopharmacological agents.

The advantage of using EFA as opposed to a more intuitive method to determine issues of admission or discharge is clear. The former provides a reliable scheme for evaluation and observation that can be keyed to hospital policy and clearly communicated to third-party payers, such as insurance companies or government agencies. In the cases just mentioned (two patients who presented with identical symptoms), EFA can be used to justify logically why one patient might require costly hospitalization and intensive treatment whereas the other might not.

Beyond the issue of admission to, or discharge from, an inpatient facility, EFA can be valuable in determining the necessity for ongoing outpatient treatment. This may be relevant in the future when some kind of accurate psychiatric evaluation may be a requirement if third-party payment is involved for continuing psychotherapy or psychoanalysis.

Justification of the duration of therapy should depend on measurements other than symptom relief alone since the presence or absence of manifest symptoms is not sufficient by itself to determine the patient's mental status or psychological health and may be deceptive in terms of evaluating overall ability to function. Sometimes a patient is still in conflict even though symptoms have disappeared. For example, a patient may be relieved of acute depression or anxiety but remain impaired in terms of the quality of his or her object relations. He or she may, therefore, suffer from social isolation, marital maladjustment, and so on. EFA provides a much more reliable method for assessing the necessity for further treatment than does a symptom checklist, which says nothing of the overall quality or character of a person's life.

EFA, Personnel Selection, and Vocational Guidance

To be a file clerk or an electrician, one must have demonstrable skills and sometimes even a license. Almost the only remaining jobs for which no evidence of ability, experience, or training is necessary are surely the most difficult ones: being a parent and serving in government.

Every 4 years the political process brings to light problems concerning some of the candidates for the nation's highest office. Even candidates for elected office below the level of the presidency can present alarming difficulties. [The possibility of using EFA for a double-blind assessment of candidates has been discussed elsewhere by Bellak (1975).] Tape recordings with electronically altered voices could be judged by a panel chosen by lot and findings accepted only if high reliability could be demonstrated for the ratings, that is, a high correlation between several independent raters. To be sure, EFA would only be treated like a medical report or a financial report on a candidate, not as a substitute for the will of the people expressed in the voting booth.

With regard to personnel selection in other areas, the armed forces have reason to want to assign people to atomic submarines, for example, who show that they not only have good impulse control currently, but that the span between highest and lowest ratings is narrow; in other words, impulse control is characteristically good—a matter important for men living in cramped conditions for lengthy periods of time. The expensive pilot training program might also benefit from ego function assessment of applicants.

Corporations have long been in the habit of having their prospective executives examined by vocational psychologists. The psychologists might find EFA useful for themselves and for communicating data to candidates and employers. Similarly, rehabilitation counselors and vocational guidance professionals can often be more effective in determining work and career possibilities for clients when ego function is seriously considered as an important variable.

In summary, EFA, which constitutes a statistically reliable and valid method of evaluating personality and its dysfunctions, is a useful tool not only within the clinical psychiatric setting, but in many arenas outside the field as well.

REFERENCES

Bellak, L. *Psychodiagnostic test report blanks*. Larchmont, N.Y., CPS, 1974.

Bellak, L. *Short form for recording and analyzing Thematic Apperception Test and Children's Apperception Test*. Larchmont, N.Y., CPS, 1974.

Bellak, L. *Overload: The new human condition*. New York: Behavioral Publications, 1975.

Bellak, L., & Sheehy, M. The broad role of ego function assessment. *American Journal of Psychiatry*, 1976, *133*, 1259–1264.

Bellak, L., with Small, L. *Emergency psychotherapy and brief psychotherapy*. New York: Grune & Stratton and CPS, 1978.

Ego Function Assessment Considered in Relation to Current Issues in Psychoanalytic Theory

LISA A. GOLDSMITH

Ego function assessment (EFA) emerged from an effort to give clinical referents to the abstract propositions of psychoanalytic ego psychology. During the past decade, however, there has been considerable debate concerning various aspects of psychoanalytic theory; its methodology and its "metapsychology"—of which ego psychology is a part—have been called into question. In particular, many of the assumptions on which EFA is based are being challenged. Now, with the updating of the volume by Bellak, Hurvich, and Gediman (1973), it seems timely to articulate the nature of the debate, to tease out its impact on the theoretical underpinnings of EFA, and to reevaluate EFA accordingly.

The current controversy in the literature of psychoanalysis has for the most part pitted those who view psychoanalysis as a discipline grounded in the foundation of natural science formulations against those who regard it as a humanistic study of personal meanings, meanings rooted in subjective-intentional formulations. The two camps have decidedly different sets of premises, and critiques of the metapsychology have in some instances reached such a pitch that the very fabric of psychoanalytic theory and discourse has been threatened. Spence (1976) wryly alludes to a "great dismantling" in the field, with such brilliant theoreticians as the late George Klein (1976), Roy Schafer (1976), and Merton Gill (1978) strenuously rejecting the "old scaffolding" of the metapsychology and metatheories of analysis. On yet another front, such writers as Rosenblatt and Thickstun (1977) and Peterfreund (1980) are advocating the use of information models as an alternative and replacement for the old metapsychological models. While in all this literature, as Peterfreund notes, the concept of psychic energy and its biological analogues have taken the brunt of the critique, the structural model and, with it, the ego concept have certainly come in for their share.

Prior to an appraisal of such pertinent issues it seems useful to cite Grolnick's (1982) reminder that the current debate in psychoanalysis is hardly a new or unique one, there having been analogous polarizations throughout Western intellectual history and thought. Renaissance thinkers, for example, emphasized the concepts of self and free will in counterposition to the determinism of the prevailing classical school. Grolnick—cautioning that a certain perspective be preserved in examining the discourse in psychoanalysis—points to the hope that the current debate may yet result in clarifications and the emergence of new synthetic integrations lest there be a recourse to monolithic ideas, closed systems, or a collapse into mystifying confusion.

RELEVANT ISSUES IN THE METAPSYCHOLOGY CRITIQUE

In proposing that there be a distinctively clinical theory, Klein (1976) and Home (1966) were among the early advocates of framing psychoanalytic theory in terms of subjective personal intentions. Klein argued against the coexistence of what he considered to be two incompatible frames of reference in Freudian thought: the clinical theory—which spoke to the elaboration of intentions, ends, purposes, and those inner states that give directionality to behavior—and the metapsychology, with its roots in mechanistic nineteenth-century neurophysiology, the purpose of which was to establish a "mechanistic deterministic natural science model of the human psyche." Portraying the metapsychological approach as a confusing and unnecessary anachronism, Klein argued it should simply be dropped, and with it all reference to instincts, energies, and—of particular interest here—the structural model, with its introduction of "inner entities" and clinically remote formulations.

The implicit danger of the metapsychology, according to Klein, is that unless clinical explanation sustains a close tie with the experiential data obtained within the psychoanalytic setting, psychoanalysis will fall into the precarious position of becoming stagnated in the reductionistic mechanics of energies, forces, and internal agencies—instruments of theory that will only sidetrack the need to unlock and elucidate hidden meaning. Thus, the "core" level of the patient's phenomenology must be the locus of explanation; as Gill (1963) states, whereas metapsychology "sees man as an arrangement for the most rapid discharge of quantities of blind energies," in the clinical theory "man is a creature of intentions who strives after meaningful goals" (p. 99).

To avoid misinterpretation of his proposals, Klein clearly asserted that he was not advocating an atheoretical approach; he was clear on the point that the clinical concepts can be as abstract and theoretical as those of metapsychology. Rather, what Klein was advancing was the elaboration of clinically related generalizations, wherein one abstracts on the basis of motivational meanings and explanations instead of in terms of abstract processes and forces. In other words, while such an "extraphenomenological" generalization as the term *repression* can help to account for experience, it does so on the basis of abstractions elaborated in terms of purpose, function, and intention. Concepts are meant to illuminate the *significance* of experience, and it is the motivational context that gives behavior its patterning and coherence.

Klein singled out for elaboration a number of core systems, or schemata, viewed as underlying psychological functioning—such as the cognitive-emotional, meaning, and self-schemata. Such schemata are considered to emerge out of the resolution of conflict and, in turn, to frame subsequent perceptions, experiences, and activities. Although accepting certain of the tenets that provide us with concepts such as ego development, psychological change, and restructuralization, Klein considered their relevance only in their ability to encompass the structuring and restructuring of aim and motivation. In other words, concepts such as "self-structures" and "meaning schemata" can serve as abstractions while yet remaining close to and capturing the patient's experience.

In a similar spirit, Gill (1977) has taken the position that the metapsychology, and with it the structural model, imposes a natural science framework on what is essentially an introspective psychology. Gill warns that the metapsychological "pseudoexplanations" should not be accepted even in the metaphorical sense, as this only serves to obscure and beguile the fact that at its core the metapsychology is a "theory of the somatic substrate of the mind," rooted in implicit neurological assumptions. With little in the way of equivocation, Gill finds metapsychology encumbering, "irrelevant" to psychoanalysis, and incapable of being pursued as a purely psychological theory.

From a decidedly different perspective, but with the similar intent of eschewing the energic or force concepts of metapsychology as well as any allusion to personified entities, writers such as Rosenblatt and Thickstun (1977) and Peterfreund (1971) have introduced information processing and system theory concepts to replace metapsychology. In the stead of any reference to "hidden executors" in the explanation of psychic activity, these authors propose that one can view the decisions, selections, and organizations of behavior as emerging out of the processing of information as part, so to speak, of the "intrinsic design of the circuitry." One studies the "design" of the system. On the basis of evolutionary and genetic considerations, learning, and the lifetime experience of the person, the model remains free of energic metaphors or any reference to hidden structures. On the other hand, and in contrast to some of the writers previously discussed, these authors do wish to consider principles of control, organization, integration, and adaptation, but do so in terms of attributes of "programs that emerge from optimum learning" and not in terms of, for example, hypothesized ego functions. As Peterfreund (1971) envisions the model, it has the potential of addressing one of psychoanalysis's greatest deficiencies—the absence of a learning theory. The empirical bases of psychoanalysis are accepted while, as an instance, conflict and pathology are understood from the vantage of inadequate or incompatible programming in the face of wished-for goals—a scientifically more respectable position, according to Peterfreund, than that of the "hydrodynamic system" of Freudian metapsychology.

The critique of metapsychology has thus come from many arenas within psychoanalysis itself. Of those who position themselves within this field, however, the most evocative challenge yet has come from Roy Schafer (1976, 1983); it is in his "action language" that the aspect of Klein's attempt to supplant the drive-discharge model with the language of activity, relationships, and meanings seems to have taken full flourish.

In Schafer's (1976) alternative to metapsychology the term *action,* defined broadly as any goal-directed activity of the person, is offered as an alternative to the prevailing conceptualization of human activities in terms of underlying psychic structures or forces. He has clearly stated—and this harkens back to Klein's argument—that Freud's metapsychology, as well as the efforts of Hartmann and others to speak in the language of forces, energies, structures, function, and apparatus, have at their base an adherence to psychoanalysis created along the lines of a physicalistic psychology. Schafer—here again in line with others—maintains that within such a natural science framework it is not really valid to speak of the person who decides, strives, intends, and acts for reasons. What ensues with the introduction of such nouns as *id, ego, superego* and such phrases as "the dynamic unconscious," "autonomous ego functions," or even "an intense emotion" is an inevitable and infinite regress to substantive entities, reified "things," or as Ryle (1949) put it, "ghosts in the machine." Such anthropomorphic constructions and concretistic errors are the consequence and "stuff" of a mechanistic–organic model of psychological function, and the language of nouns inevitably obscures the fact that we are studying continuous mental actions and ongoing processes.

To supplant the "psychochemical and biological modes of psychological thinking," Schafer (1976) suggests that we regard all psychological process, experience, and behavior as some kind of intended activity, as "sets of actions in various modes," thus positing action as paramount among psychological phenomena and as his primary investigative construct. Action is designated by "an active verb stating its nature and by an adverb . . . stating the mode of action (1975, p. 44)," and Schafer delimits the observational base of psychoanalysis to that which can be described in these linguistic terms.

One may indeed go on to group actions through the introduction of higher-order concepts, but what this really entails is a redescription of classes of actions on the basis of observed regularities. Thus, for example, one may describe classes of activities as "defensive actions" and one may speak of repression as an "activity in a certain mode," but this does not require inferring such infrastructures as mental entities, functions, or propulsive agencies. It is sufficient to state what people do, how they do it, and their reasons for doing such. Furthermore, since psychoanalysis is the study of meaningful behavior, in Schafer's view no action—and hence no explanatory postulate—can be located outside the realm of reasons and meanings. We may assume that a person experiencing himself or herself as being in a familiar situation will act in a predictable fashion, but such a postulate (which Schafer himself introduces) defines the sense of familiarity, or sameness, in terms of a sameness of meaning, so that it is again reasons that give coherence to activity. Schafer stands firm that his redefinitions are not intended to wedge analysis into a behavioristic, atomistic, or atheoretical mode, but what is not required for intelligibility in the clinical method is not required for the clinical theory. When one is able to connect the patterns of behavior to the reasons and motives expressed in that behavior, no other order of explanation is needed. Tersely put, for Schafer "description is explanation."

Of critical relevance to EFA is the discussion Schafer (1976) offers of what he considers to be one of the greatest embarrassments of Freudian metapsychology; that is, the need to posit a "mover" of the apparatus, an "I," a self, or an ego. According to Schafer this proliferation of terms is entrenched in mechanistic trappings, mixed modes of discourse, metaphoric allusions, and a confabulation of experiential constructs and abstract postulates of regulatory agencies that direct and prescribe activity. Schafer's position is that the reduction of terms to reifications, anthropomorphisms, or the like—and here he gives ego functions as an instance par excellence—is inevitable when one's language is a natural science language rather than one of personal intention. In adopting a language whereby persons are defined by their actions and choices, there is no need to posit any mover of the apparatus, self, ego, or "thing" stated in the form of something one has; rather, being a person is defined by the kind of actions one performs. To refer to this person Schafer suggests the term *personal agent,* as it is close to common-sense experience and introspective awareness and is but a pointer to the person "as the originator of actions and modes of action." To support his position Schafer reminds the reader that in the analytic setting actions and modes of action, not "persons," are what the analyst interprets.

For Schafer, if one uses the term *ego,* and if that is the term one wishes to use, one is referring to nothing more than a designated class or characteristic mode of action, such as the action to perceive, to remember, to test reality, to defend, and so forth. Freed from the implication of hidden homunculi, the entire tripartite model could be subsumed under different classes of action. Thus, action language can accommodate, in Schafer's (1978) words, "the high degree of consistency with which people perform their primitively wishful actions (the id), their defensive and adaptive actions (the ego), and their moral, self-hating, and self-punishing actions (the superego)," and can do so without recourse to reification, structure, or location.

Action language, Schafer stresses, does not preclude an effort to understand complex actions and can comprehend such factors by elaborating constituent functions, such as families of actions, multiple descriptions of actions from varying points of view, actions described in unconscious as well as conscious modes, and the full scope of clinical phenomena. For instance, if one were to speak of anxiety tolerance, heretofore described as a function of the ego, Schafer (1976) would limit the use of the term to the prediction of a "noteworthy regularity and continuity of actions and modes of action" in situations of danger. Anxiety tolerance is not, for Schafer, a trait, a capacity, or a "something" one has but rather the "continuing to do whatever one is doing despite the fact that one is doing it anxiously"; no references to underlying processes, structures, and hierarchies are required; explanatory comprehension is provided instead by descriptions of the complex rules and priorities that have been set by the person himself or herself.

While willing to accept certain labels of the older metapsychology as long as they are limited to descriptive foci, Schafer hopes that such terms as *id, ego,* and *superego* will eventually be replaced. The emphasis is to be on clinically anchored accounts and descriptions; with the older phraseology there is still a readiness to slip into the mechanistic trappings of metapsychology. Says Schafer, "I am just trying to bring out the human referents of the metapsychological terms . . . to emphasize what one sees when one observes people psychoanalytically. One does not see metapsychological entities; one sees actions being performed in various modes, some in the form of thinking, some in emotional language, some in motor performance, and most of them in complex forms" [1979, p. 871].

As Schafer's position bears on the full range of structural constructs—internalization, ego, character formation, and the like—it calls for reform in the way in which one specifies the consistency and regularity of psychic activity. For Schafer (1979), since consistency in action requires no more than a specification of the psychological circumstances under which one observes the regularity of action, character in turn need simply be defined as "a form of explanation through systematic redescription(s) of action." Character development is not the emergence of a stabilized entity but in action language refers to actions that people "typically perform in the problematic situations that they typically define for themselves."

REACTIONS TO THE CRITIQUE OF METAPSYCHOLOGY: A CRITIQUE OF THE CRITICS

If the amount of response to the critics of metapsychology is any indication of the relevance of their arguments, at the very least one may suppose that these critics have raised significant issues. The proposed revisions of Schafer, Klein, and Gill, as well as the alternatives offered from other quarters, have left many analysts and in fact some philosophers unsettled as to what is the most fitting methodological and theoretical stance for psychoanalysis. Despite the disquiet, one can also see how in these revisions and counterrevisions a process of "working through" of the most basic terms of psychoanalysis has begun to emerge. On the whole, what appears in many of the critiques of Schafer, Klein, and others is an initial captivation with features of the proposed alternatives. But in the end it is the degree to which the Schafer-Klein-Gill arguments are taken—if you will, the infinite regress of the final positions—that generates a large measure of discord.

In Schafer's (1976) challenge of Hartmann, and in Klein's program for a purely psychological psychoanalytic theory, there is a stated conviction that the field must be divorced from its neurophysiological ambitions and roots. A metapsychology wedded in nineteenth-century natural science had as its inevitable consequence a regress to physiology, and an outmoded and irrelevant physiology at that. Daniel Shapiro (1977) and many other writers readily support a disentanglement of psychoanalysis from such quasibiological assumptions yet do not agree that it is to such a set of biological assumptions that the metapsychology—as implicitly treated by Schafer and others—must necessarily be reduced. Arlow (1975) asserts that those who, for example, wish to replace structural theory level their criticisms not against the clinical aspects of the theory but against a biological tradition that may not in fact be relevant to current psychoanalytic usage. Thus there are the rumblings that what has been put forth as critique is really but a straw-man argument—namely, that what is being criticized has already been acknowledged as outdated and that the metapsychological hypotheses are being regarded in an unfairly reductionistic way. There is certainly a biological tradition in the field, and in some circles a wish to articulate psychoanalytic findings in a manner consistent with data from the biological sciences; nevertheless, as Arlow (1975) reports, most who support a clinical structural theory show a definite tendency to eschew biological assumptions and to rely on psychological considerations in their efforts to give coherence to behavior. Wurmser (1977), for instance, challenges Schafer's position that the term *function* is an implicit biologism, pointing to its widespread use in mathematics and throughout the natural sciences, where the term simply refers to a "carrying out."

Schafer's warning against the use of substantives, metaphorical abstractions, and the formulation of structures and processes underlying surface psychological phenomena, however, raises problems more thorny than the caveats directed against biological reductionism. As previously stated, the position taken by Schafer was that the employment of such hypothetical constructs inevitably results in allusions to reified entities, logical inconsistencies, and other forms of metaphoric allusiveness. Again an element of the argument reaches receptive ears. A ready recourse to the use of jargon, a prevalence of murky expository styles, a confounding of different levels of discourse, and a proclivity toward reifications and personifications are considered rife in psychoanalytic writings. While many would agree as to the vast misuse of terms in psychoanalysis [see, for example, Esman's (1979) warnings against the use of "hybrid concepts"], Schafer's argument is more substantive than any objection to literary imprecision. As Gedo (1977) comments, while it is one thing to disdain the "naive abuses of Freud's materialist heritage," it is quite another to regard as illegitimate the use of theoretical constructs, the inferring of enduring predispositions, and the attempts to account for the patterning, regularity, and repeatibility of behavior apart from action terms.

Aversion to the causal and deterministic explanations of which structural concepts are a part is endemic to the philosophical position taken by Schafer, Gill, and others who contrast explanation provided by locating reasons with explanation provided by ascribing causes. Spiro (1979), himself a philosopher, has much to say on the philosophical position taken by this group of analysts. He comments that within the philosophical community itself there is scarcely any consensus as to the importance of making distinctions between explanations as provided by reasons and those as provided by causes; moreover, there is considerable debate on the very issue of intentionality itself. Spiro thus questions whether distinctions on the basis of reasons and causes can serve to support the arguments used in the current theoretical polarizations. In fact, he states that the point at which Schafer moves beyond the suggestion that action language may "best render" psychoanalytic theory—a determination that itself would have to be evaluated on a case-by-case basis—and proposes the rejection of substantives, Schafer assumes a rather old, and what Spiro considers anachronistic, philosophical stance. Spiro holds that Schafer's argument as to the dangers of reification, the use of formulations that specify entities, and the reliance on various other abstractions implies a view of these constructs as being on the order of "physical entities." According to Spiro, Schafer's position is in itself in danger of falling into concretistic error in the way in which substantives, metaphors, and hypothetical constructs are regarded. Spiro holds that the use of nouns and adjectives in psychology requires no unwavering "ontological commitment,'' nor does it in the physical sciences or for that matter in present-day philosophy. A hypothetical construct is not a phenomenon; it is an attempt to find some level of coherence in observed phenomena. Spiro is responsive to the idea of ridding discourse of illegitimate uses of reification and concretistic errors. At the very least, sound thinking requires an acknowledgment of the use of metaphor as such and of its heuristic purposes, but the very use of substantives or structural formulations does not, Spiro reminds us, inevitably lead to reification. (Spiro calls Schafer's position a product of ''reification anxiety.'') Further, Spiro points out, *action* is itself a noun and yet is used by Schafer with no implications of things in the physical sense.

To illustrate his point, Spiro suggests that using a noun in the form of a statement that one ''has a cold'' does not of necessity imply that ''having a cold or fever is . . . to possess a thing-like entity''; to say that one ''has a feeling'' or is in a particular state of mind is empirically valid, in that it is the actuality of an ongoing mental event—and not necessarily any particular physical event—that is being described. Thus, the statement that one has a feeling points to a psychological process or a dynamic state located in ''some way inside the person,'' but it does not in itself require postulating thinglike properties or entities in the materialistic sense. It is interesting in this regard to return to an early paper written by Brierly (1944), in whose work issues relevant to the current critiques of the metapsychology can be found. It was her conviction that metapsychology had to be considered a ''process theory of the mind,'' where ''mind ceases to be thing, or entity, and becomes a nexus of activities, a sequence of adaptive responses.''

Spiro demonstrates from the vantage of postoperationalist positions within philosophy that there is no need to eschew formally the use of substantive and theoretical entities in science and psychology. Substantives can be used in varying and different orders of discourse and have to be evaluated for their empirical and explanatory power; there may be no reason to lose ''feeling'' or the concept of the ego even if ''cathexis loading ideas'' must go.

While Spiro's comments are lively, some of Schafer's considerations as to the use of substantives can be heeded, it would seem, without having to throw out the baby with the bathwater or reinvent the wheel. Schafer (1973) raised strong objection to the use of such terms as *internalization* and, by implication, *structuralization*. He posits that as a construct internalization has no systematic generative power, since it is an inherently pseudo-spatial metaphor, expressive of an introjective fantasy, and is hardly the basis for a ''systematic description of a person acting conflictually.'' That such terms do have dynamic implications and resonances is an observation that many analysts would accept, and it is useful for Schafer to remind us of this, but it is questionable that the existence of dynamic content in an abstraction destroys its usefulness.

Meissner (1979) has given a most elaborate rejoinder to this aspect of

Schafer's (1976) thesis. Again the sentiment seems to be that while starting with a cogent warning about the misuse of concepts, Schafer in his criticism of "internalization" goes too far and himself becomes party to an infinite regress to the concrete. Meissner, as does Spiro, states that confusion as to the spatial metaphors of internalization occurs when what is lost sight of is precisely the fact that it is a metaphor. When one bypasses the metaphorical meaning of structure and reduces it to the level of literal expression, one loses sight of the usage of the term in the systematology. For example, when one attributes concrete status to such terms as *ego functions* or *memory images,* one forgets that one's conceptual position is to find a means of abstracting hypothetical sets of dynamic mental processes. Meissner suggests that a process view of internalization, for example, is needed and explains how the introjective experience itself can be designated as a series of interlocking processes operating within the person, involving a potential array of "perceptual, memory, affective, and other cognitive processes." Further, within the "process" frame of reference one can begin to elucidate how the very experience of personal agency in Schafer's terms could emerge from particular processes and levels of psychic organization. What seems to be essential here, and is a position that will be elaborated when considering EFA in subsequent sections, is that the level of discourse, the frame of reference be preserved—whether one is speaking at the level of fantasy expression or from the vantage of an abstraction of processes.

As for levels of abstraction, while Meissner is hardly proposing a literal and spatial usage of the phrase "in the mind," when one refers to an organization of mental activities one is articulating something real in the sense of the "nonmaterial and nonextended." Meissner makes no pretense of being able to supply the conceptual bases and methodology needed to account for these processes, but to say that such formulations are not currently within our conceptual reach is not to obliterate the usefulness of all structural concepts or to reduce them to spatial designations. Structural conceptualizations such as the ego are systematic elaborations of classes of mental events that are certainly in need of further definition or, if indicated, rejection, but it is on the basis of further research and not solely on the basis of the finding of a misplaced metaphor that such rejections need be made. Meissner asserts that when analysts take recourse to such anthropomorphic phrasing as "the superego punishes the ego," there are few who would presume, as he puts it, that "there is an entity or homunculus called the superego in the head that is somehow beating on another entity or homunculus called the ego." What Meissner considers is that in this context what is being expressed is a dynamic phenomenon and complex forms of human action, expressed in terms that have a heuristic value and that do not require the kind of slippage to the thinglike entities or biological imperatives that Schafer considers inevitable. In other words, the term *internalization,* as process and product, has a legitimate conceptual status as an *abstraction,* to be assessed not on the basis of its concreteness but according to its usefulness in ordering and predicting behavior and mental activity.

In this context, a quote from Loewald (1976) on the place of a process structural view of the concept of ego seems relevant, not merely to Meissner's comments but as a response to some of Schafer's criticisms. Loewald writes: "[T]he ego is, as Freud thought—and I believe this is his deepest insight into its psychology—the precipitate, the internalization, of what goes on between the primitive psyche and its environment; it is an organization of reproductive action on a new stage, the stage of internality. This interplay on the internal stage of action constitutes the process structure of the ego" (p. 323).

Meissner and Spiro are but two of the writers who have taken issue with the structural implications of the critique of metapsychology, for there are many who feel disarmed without a means to account for some order of process at the level of enduring, patterned, and repetitive classes of behavior. The need to generate some useful formulations as a means of referring to the organization that underlies human behavior—and to do so apart from the language of meaning, fantasy, and action—was articulated also in a paper by Rawn (1979). Rawn states outright that one cannot do without some constructions that imply enduring structure, as without such constructions "one can have no laws, no regularities, no prediction, no science, no psychoanalysis. . . ." In an effort to give order, depth, and coherence to psychological phenomena, Rawn questions whether Schafer's radical and exclusionary proscriptions have much generative power of their own. He indeed questions whether a purely phenomenological and linguistic approach could have itself generated an action language.

To the remarks of Rawn, Meissner, and others regarding the literalization of metaphor in Schafer's position may be added those of Ellman and Moskowitz (1980). They depict as restrictive a theoretical stance that requires an acceptance of the physical reality of its terms when these are couched in nominatives and ideas of entity. Like Spiro, Ellman and Moskowitz contrast the "restrictive realistic position" with the modern and postoperationalistic usage of hypothetical constructs in science and philosophy, pointing to the heuristic value and generative power of such constructs in the other sciences. The construct of fourth-dimensional space and gravitational fields, for example, while having spatial connotations, hardly requires a reference to "palpable entities." What gives such constructs leverage is the way in which they fit into a theoretical matrix, and in turn their ability to provide links to observed phenomena and behavior. Theoretical terms can thus gain "independent characterization" and need not be reduced to a mere metaphoric, circular relabeling and renaming of the very phenomena to be explained. Further, when Schafer (1976) asserts that anthropomorphism is inherent in such propositions as those concerning psychic energy, functions of the ego, and so on, Ellman and Moskowitz question whether the explanatory validity of these propositions can be determined on the basis of a delimited number of examples showing what seems to be tautological thinking. Rather, such terms must be assessed as to their usefulness and heuristic power within their theoretical context; a determination cannot be made without reference to the specification of a field of inquiry.

In Holt's (1979) thinking, the claim for a place for theoretical constructs in psychoanalysis, as in any science, has to be justified on the basis of how these constructs relate to our data and problems. Holt recognizes the argument that psychoanalysis is not a natural science and that therefore analogies to the natural sciences are not relevant. However, he would counterargue that even if this were the case, it is not sufficient to render the use of abstract nouns by psychoanalysis "inherently fallacious" or to make it inevitable that abstract nouns succumb "to reification or to a mechanistic-physicalist psychology." In a similar key, Modell (1981) finds Schafer's proscriptions wrenching, believing that they express an "Aristotelian wish to preserve the phenomena at the expense of denying to ourselves the theoretical tools that we require to think about what we have just observed." Modell regards Schafer as in essence failing to acknowledge that learning and thinking themselves entail the constant interplay between observation and theory.

Others who agree that removing metaphor and structural terms would impoverish psychoanalytic understanding do not find, however, that such terms have truly been obliterated; indeed they question whether they can be, the efforts to do so notwithstanding, so that the terms are brought in surreptitiously "through the back door." In this view, Wurmser (1977) speaks directly to the core term of Schafer's action language, namely, that of action itself. He questions what would really ensue if one were to exclude abstractions and stay at the level of description. Wouldn't action then have to be considered simply as an external motor event? Wurmser submits that Schafer clearly extends the usage of the term *action* when he applies it to feelings and thoughts. In so doing Schafer speaks of classes of actions, of actions in variable modes, making what Wurmser considers to be highly abstract statements, since one has to resort to some level of abstraction if one is to think about action in the first place. Calogeras and Alston (1980) also question whether *person* and *action* are free of metaphorical implications. They find these words entering in as abstract nouns while not being acknowledged as such. In other words, isn't the argument against anthropomorphism and the claim to mere description being based, as Meissner suggested, on shifting sand? Is the "personal agent," to which Schafer assigns a catalogue of attributes and intentional, goal-directed activity, not in itself an ultimate abstraction and anthropomophism? Further, can Schafer legitimately introduce dispositional concepts without reintroducing into the theory the idea of endurance, repetition, and—implicitly—that of structure? Friedman (1976) puts the dilemma tersely: "The anomaly of unactualized action and the equivocation between action as concrete and as abstract grow out of the same frustrations: it is the wish to deal always with something concrete in conflict with the recognition that one must abstract from it to think about it" (p. 134).

Perhaps if Schafer had not introduced as pronounced a restriction on the use of such a basic tool of thought—on the use of abstraction—and recognized the need to account for endurance and underlying organization, his "alternative" would not have been treated so harshly. Klein's proposals, for example, while they have come in for their share of criticism (these also around discussions of the concept of structure), have not encountered such sharp disapproval, perhaps because in Klein's work the concept of structure and the need for structure building were not ultimately rejected.

If we are not given sufficient help in advancing psychoanalytic thinking, and hence of understanding psychic functioning through Schafer's work, ultimately, then, neither do Klein's formulations (or those of self-psychologies in general) avoid the so-called pitfalls of the classical metapsychological formulations. It will be recalled that Klein asserted that psychoanalytic theory calls for the formulation of concepts that are both close to clinical referents and couched not in terms of abstract processes or mechanisms but in terms of motivation and meaning. In an effort to account for experience he introduced such constructs as self-schemata, thus taking a step that placed him at least some distance from phenomenology. As Richards (1982) has noted, Klein, in the process of generalizing and abstracting (as, for instance, in trying to delimit the properties of schemata), has placed his terms at a different level of discourse, one at which they cannot simply be reduced to their phenomenological counterparts. When Klein incorporated the term *apparatus* into his definition of the self-schema, he moved beyond the personal quality with which he sought to ground his self-concept. One feels compelled to ask how an abstraction can be personal or impersonal. It is only the referents that can be truly and uniquely clinically grounded. In other words, Klein too invoked abstractions ultimately in ways akin to many hypotheses found in metapsychology; when he tried to imbue concepts with a personal frame of reference he put himself in danger of reifying concepts—the very pitfall he claimed was inherent in the use of the ego concept. As Friedman (1980) comments, when schemata are elaborated in terms of "active but aborted wishes," in terms of "blocked tendencies," is this so different from those statements for which Klein criticized metapsychology?

Problems similar to those raised by Klein's position vis-à-vis the issue of substrate, schema, and structure, are to be found with his overreaching intention to free psychoanalysis from the constraints of natural science and causal analysis. Berger (1978) has noted that here, again, there is a "return," since when one evaluates Klein's alternative from a formal perspective, one sees an effort to account for lawfulness, to provide units of analysis, and to link observational data to theory. Whether one is looking to establish a level of perceived order in terms of nonphysical events, subjective experience, or otherwise (or as Berger puts it, by instituting "humanistic terms and concepts . . . for more obviously mechanistic terms"), we are not speaking of fundamentally different kinds of explanation or science, a position that Brenner (1980) elaborates and that will be addressed in the next section.

If Schafer and Klein have come under heavy fire, the information theorists, with their wholesale alternatives to metapsychology, have not been without their share of critics. Fonagy (1982) asserts that when the effort is to supplant the language of metapsychology with that of information science and neurophysiology, it is not enough to do so on purely theoretical terms. Without a firm empirical base, a blatant rejection of metapsychological hypotheses not only may be premature but may be self-limiting as well, for in the absence of an assessment as to how such a model offers new ways of organizing and generating observational data, one has merely substituted one metaphorical model for another, a criticism that has been leveled also at Schafer.

Sand, cited by Reppen (1981), queries whether it is necessary at all for the psychoanalyst to give up metapsychology before acknowledging the potential contributions of any other model or models. Sand suggests that clinical principles can be illustrated by a number of models that may thus add to our "explanatory repertoire." The information models, for example, may serve as a bridge between psychoanalysis and cognitive psychologies. Further, in addition to the idea of supplementary models, many are of the opinion that the rejection of one model need not require the collapse of either an entire system or of any other model that is found useful. Ellman and Moskowitz (1980), referring to Modell's methodological comments, point to the situation in the advanced sciences such as theoretical physics, where subsets of postulates are constantly being changed and revised without sacrificing the theory as a whole. In this regard, one would have to ask whether psychoanalysis is at this point such a tightly knit and integrated theory that when one part of the theory is challenged a wholesale collapse must by necessity follow.

Noy (1977) speaks directly to the multimodel nature of the theoretical system of psychoanalysis and suggests that it may be the very allowance of multiple models that accounts for the field's endurance and uniqueness. In this regard he contrasts psychoanalytic theory to other contemporary schools in psychology and the behavioral sciences that have at their base one single and uniform model. It is noteworthy that the theoretical positions mentioned up to this point, having as their intent the supplanting of metapsychological hypotheses, come with their own versions of some "model of models," that is, show signs of attempting to unify psychoanalysis within one or another singular explanatory frame of reference. Noy reminds us that it was Freud's intention to keep psychoanalysis open and in certain respects pluralistic—standing on several bases, capable of determining the relevance or irrelevance of a variety of models in terms of the empirical evidence. Interestingly, it was in this spirit that Freud (1923) presented his at that time new theory of the ego; not to be thought of as a monolithic or closed conceptualization, it was intended to serve to facilitate a refinement in the explanation of observed clinical phenomena, and its value was to be determined on that basis alone.

In sum, a unifying factor in the reactions to the alternative models proposed for psychoanalysis and its structural formulations is an attention to the difficulties inherent in attempting to adapt or adhere to a "model of models" for the field. Barrett (1978), for example, wonders how Schafer's focus on the immediacy of the unitary agent can accommodate the idea of any disjunction between "the language of the unconscious and the structure of conscious intentions." Friedman (1980) asks how one ever could have derived such concepts as those of repression given Klein's claim that alternative models are unnecessary for clinical psychoanalysis. In attending to Klein's claim that aims and motives serve as explanatory tools in psychoanalysis, Eagle (1980) questions whether Klein's position could accommodate the explanation of the very phenomena of aims and motives themselves. When one limits one's thinking to such narrow explanatory bases, one must often assume that which one is trying to explain. Kovel (1978) cites aspects of action language in this regard, noting that when Schafer moves away from the immediately observable, he is forced to assume that which he has to explain—for example, human agency itself.

Also addressing the issue of the pitfalls of precluding alternative frames of reference for psychoanalysis, Modell (1981) asserts that when alternatives are precluded, one is in danger of not being able to accommodate developmental and maturational considerations. If, as Schafer argues, intentions cannot have causes within a uniquely psychoanalytic point of view, one must, as Aufhauser (1979) states, "pick up the story later . . . once there are intentions." Within the action language there is no point of discovery as to how meaning, intentionality, or agency emerge; it is as if the "person" must arise de novo. Friedman (1980) puts the matter succinctly when he states, "we cannot study meaning transformation if we take meaning for granted."

Thus, certainly many have raised the objection that any one model of models has as its sequella a closing of doors. At the same time, the singular, holistic alternatives can be seen to cast nets that are too large or, as Eissler (1969) concludes, when scientists propose that their "theoretical armamentarium" is adequate to explain all relevant phenomena in their field, one would assume that the said theories are too "loosely knit." Eissler gives as an example those who insist that the psychoanalytic situation proper is all that is required and relevant for the generation of psychoanalytic data. Eagle (1980), in his remarks on Klein, and Ellman and Moskowitz (1980), in their critique of Schafer, question why psychoanalysis is not free to borrow terms and contributions from other sciences or to use other methodologies, and to do so in whatever manner might be useful. Eagle predicts that the overconcern with "what is distinctively psychoanalytic" may lead to a stagnation—

that is, to itself an unproductive orthodoxy—where questions such as, "Is it there?" and, "Is it deeply and freely explanatory?" become replaced with, "Is it distinctively psychoanalytic?"

Richards (1982) has criticized many of the current self theories for a kind of "humanistic holism" that places psychoanalysis in the "false position" of having to understand the whole person before one has explained any of the details of the person's thought, behavior, and adaptive functioning. In a statement that has a bearing on Schafer's unitary agent, Richards points out that when the focus of one's inquiry is, for example, on "idealizing and mirror transference formations," one precludes inquiry into layers of latent material or into the underlying organizational principles out of which such content emerges. Here it may be fitting to recall one of Rapaport's (1960) tenets: He asserted that "no content yields its full meaning unless its formal characteristics . . . are taken into consideration." Content can itself serve as a guide to a network of formal relationships and, by implications from Richard's comments, so can latent content.

Before going on to offer some synthetic formulations, two significant issues concerning the current status of metapsychology need emphasis. One is that with all its admitted difficulties and ambiguities, metapsychology is still, as Noy pointed out, an open system that does not require premature closure of one's conceptual and methodological base. The generative power of metapsychology remains, and one might wonder, along with Calogeras and Alston (1980), for example, whether the contributions of Kohut, Mahler, Erikson, and others could have emerged on the basis of action language, information theory, or any other singular model.

On the other hand, it would seem unfortunate to turn away completely from some of the revisions suggested by Klein, Schafer, and others. Their calls for clarity of expression, for the weeding out of contaminated levels of discourse and the deflating of overblown metaphors, and their efforts to free psychological explanation from "quasi-psychobiological obscurity" (Rawn, 1979) seem well worth heeding. Schafer's focus on subjectivity, psychic reality, and meaningful activity is in its own way a reattending to one of Freud's most essential clinical contributions, and it speaks to a fundamental point of view of psychoanalytic interpretation. Schafer's ideas, as Meissner (1979) suggests, keep one ever alert to the "action in apparent inaction," and such an observation can be put to use in the clinical situation. To use such an observation is not the same, however, as imposing a particular language or frame of reference on the patient.

The second issue is that a successful rethinking of psychoanalytic concepts requires a return to the data and a ferreting out of the confusions in our observational and theoretical languages. It is at this descriptive level that one may find a genuine consonance of action language with the methodological position of EFA. To be ever open to rearticulating one's "description of classes of mental events" is very much in the spirit of EFA. With the introduction of the ego-psychological approach, as Bibring (1954) stated, there has emerged a focus on the broadest "phenomenological exploration of behavior." The exploration has resulted in a most careful and systematic description of patterned activity, and the study of patterns has become a pathway to an understanding of a full array of psychic determinants. Although at this level of descriptive elucidation EFA and action language have a commonality, the point to which Schafer takes his action language and the exclusionary premises on which action language is based are not consonant with the principles of EFA. As Spiro (1979) suggested, however, if one considers the rather "respectable" methodological position taken by action language and does not insist on any singular replacement for psychoanalytic theory or move into the embarrassing metaphysical position of positing events that exist nowhere, then there is something of great utility being said. To determine empirically whether a concept contributes to our systematic understanding and predictions is critical. Nevertheless, to rule out structural concepts and all efforts at explanatory formulations and to limit one's descriptive analysis to one and only one frame of reference are quite another matter.

THOUGHTS ON A "PARADOXICAL" SYNTHESIS: A DUAL FRAME OF REFERENCE

To take stock of these differing theoretical and methodological positions and to do so in a manner that can enrich our thinking about EFA, the contributions of Brenner (1980), Wallerstein (1976), and Grossman and Simon (1969) will be drawn upon.

Brenner, in his 1980 paper "Metapsychology and Psychoanalytic Theory," reviews the entire metapsychology controversy, tracing the evolution of the term *metapsychology* in the progression of Freud's thinking. As Brenner states, Freud initially used the term to encompass the study of unconscious mental processes and thereby to distinguish psychoanalysis from those theories that considered what was mental to be by definition that which was conscious. Brenner himself, along with others, considers that the term can be used broadly to refer to whatever is the prevailing psychoanalytic theory. Given the recognition now granted to unconscious mentation and the fact of the frequent misuse of *metapsychology* as a term, Brenner questions whether the term, although not the concepts it encompasses, may have outlived its usefulness. Specific ways in which the term has been used may in fact lead to a closing off of inquiry. Rapaport and Gill (1959), for example, have used the term to denote a set of postulates, assumptions, or "a priori proposition," on the basis of which psychoanalytic theory rests. In so doing they may forestall consideration of the theory as a revisable body of assumptions, sensitive to the current array of observational data. Waelder

(1962) takes metapsychology to mean that which is at the most abstract end of psychoanalytic hypotheses. Brenner argues that the simplest observations can involve ideas of the most abstract order.

What is relevant to Brenner in evaluating concepts of a metapsychological order, and here he sees himself to be in line with Freud (1915), is not the level of abstraction or concreteness in theoretical discourse (e.g., how "close" it is to the clinical data and to subjective experience) but the degree to which the theory is supported by relevant data. It is on this basis that the usefulness, dependability, and explanatory potential of a theory can be gauged. Metapsychology is not equivalent to any biological or neurobiological explanatory framework, nor is it a direct bridge to phenomenological experience. What it is is a heuristic device, an "auxiliary tool," in Freud's words "an intellectual scaffolding." Brenner gives as an example the critique leveled at drive theory, commenting that drive theory is a theoretical model and as such has to be evaluated as to its usefulness in ordering data and giving data meaning within a matrix of hypotheses. In a similar vein, Noy (1977) pointed to the absurdity in stating that one believes or fails to believe in the truthfulness of the libido concept. One does not "believe" in the truth or falsity of a hypothetical construct; rather, one finds constructs such as those of the structural model useful or of little use in ordering and giving coherence to clinical observations. If otherwise, one is dealing along the dimension of "fictions" or doctrines. In sum, if we are to follow Brenner's suggestions vis-à-vis the current controversy, the proposed alternatives will not stand or fall on the basis of philosophical argument but on the basis of their power to organize data as coherently and simply as possible.

This tenet as to the utility of constructs has direct relevance to EFA, for the issue here is not whether the EFA model is replete with hypothetical abstractions (for how can a methodology be devoid of such abstractions?); rather, it is a question of the utility of the EFA concept in generating and guiding research. The evaluation of EFA's utility is the raison d'être of this entire volume, and hence the research papers presented here seek to examine whether EFA has proved useful in the explanation, description, and prediction of clinical data. To the extent that EFA keeps its grounding in clinical source material, it can, it is hoped, avoid the dangers of empty theorizing, unheeded reifications, and unrecognized tautologies of which the critics have warned. Mayman (1976) has suggested that in essence we are begging the question when we put our efforts into attacking metapsychology. What we should be attacking is the job of systematizing our clinical data, and this is the job that the work on EFA—in this instance through the study of the empirical bearing of structural theory—is attempting. Metaphor, when present here, may be provisional, but it may alert us to those areas in which our descriptions of psychological processes are in need of still further data; metaphor here may thus have a built-in utility that Fonagy (1982), for one, strongly defends. The real issue is not whether our concepts are experience-distant but whether they take us back again to experience and lead to the elucidation and elaboration of phenomena.

The data of psychoanalysis are unique and hence different from those of any other science. This, as Brenner (1980) tells us, should be little cause for difficulty, for if there were no uniqueness to the data, psychoanalysis would not constitute a "branch of science." Science, moreover (as Brenner reminds us), is not "nominal"; it is "adjectival," and here again the critical dimension resides in an empirical attitude toward one's observations. When analysts generate lawful relations on the basis of observational data and make inferences as to the emergence of wishes, symptoms, or classes of behavior, they are functioning, in principle, as any scientist does. Similarly, as Holt (1972) submits, science is not defined by its subject matter but by its method, and in this regard we are in no way enjoined as analysts from dealing with meanings, qualities, or the uniqueness of individuals.

These statements of Brenner's as to the position of psychoanalysis as a natural science bring us full face with the discrepant views of the natural science and subjective-intentional positions discussed at such length in the previous section. As Modell (1978) and others have suggested, the scientism–humanism distinction articulates two "fundamentally different categories of human knowledge." On the one hand, there is historical knowledge, where the observer imaginatively enters into the world of the subject and observes phenomena "from the inside"; on the other, there is the objective orientation of the observer—a view from without—with the delineation of repeated configurations and generalizations of patterned activity. There is in some circles a felt incompatibility between psychoanalysis as the interpretative study of meaning and psychoanalysis as an observational science, rooted in causal analysis (Meissner, 1981).

Grossman and Simon (1969), well before the full emergence of the current controversy, highlighted the double usage, the dual frame of reference, that has permeated every level of psychoanalytic theory. Whether it be the distinction drawn between intentionality and causality, person and organism, phenomenology and system, empathy and cause, or subject and object, there has always been a double registration in psychoanalytic discourse. Again, whether the distinction be between the subjective and the objective, the nomothetic and the ideographic, the "experiential and the nonexperiential" (Sandler and Joffe, 1969), we are speaking of different positions of the observer. In Grossman's (1967) words, at issue is whether the "one who formulates takes the point of view of a spectator or the point of view of the subject." In our clinical work (and here Grossman's choice of terms has a certain irony and farsightedness), it is the patient's viewpoint and reasons for behaving that are of concern—the patient's "behavioral events as actions"—which the analyst and the patient endeavor to make intelligible. We are not discussing "laws of behavior" but the "rules the patient follows for classifying experience."

It may be noted here that while not explicit in interpretative activity, both spectator and observer modes of knowledge are active in the analytic encounter. Modell (1981) describes the analyst and patient as in an "I–Thou" relationship that shifts and oscillates for the analyst into an "I–it" position. The analyst moves, and not necessarily defensively, into the position of an observer when there is an effort to crystallize and identify recurring configurations and to give coherence to the "buzzing confusion of immediate clinical experience." Meissner (1979) also has made reference to the analytic task itself as being neither exclusively experiential nor exclusively observational but a constant alternation and interplay between "empathic experiencing with the patient and the objectivizing observation and formulating of process." It may be added that this process in the analyst not only has its counterpart in the patient but, as Kris (1952) asserts in his description of the biphasic nature of controlled regression, is endemic to creative and many other forms of thought. As is being suggested here, such a process may in addition be an essential characteristic of theoretical and analytic understanding. As part of his crystallization of the concept "Regression in the Service of the Ego," Kris pointed to an "inspirational" (empathetic?) and "elaborational" (explanatory?) phase to such integrative activity. Lichtenstein (1976, cited by Rawn, 1979) spoke of the "Januslike quality of human experience." This shifting back and forth between levels of experience and reflection may be so much a given in both our theorizing and the way in which we ordinarily think that when a theorist like Schafer requires us to attend to our ideas in the way he does, many experience a vague disorientation. What seems critical for psychoanalytic theorizing is not to lop off one frame of reference for the integrity of the other but to acknowledge the level of discourse at which one happens to be.

McIntosh (1979) speaks of this split between subjectivism and objectivism and the current "revisionary" trend to push psychoanalysis in the direction of purely interpretive subjectivism and away from natural science objectivism. He asserts that the trend runs counter to the fact that it was Freud, more than any other modern thinker, who cut across this schism and envisioned psychoanalysis as a unique discipline that would endeavor to encompass both forms of knowledge. It is this coexistence of two forms of knowledge within psychoanalysis that Modell purports to be one of the central paradoxes of the field's epistemology. While one of its thornier problems, this "double vision" lends psychoanalysis its greatest strength and power; it is this "double vision" that enables psychoanalysis to describe phenomena that are unique and at the same time to observe repeated configurations reflective of enduring structures. Such is what imparts to psychoanalysis its uniqueness as a science and, as suggested by Modell, precludes its fitting into a "ready-made epistemology."

Several of the writers who hold firm to the position that psychoanalysis must encompass both forms of reference take heed in Ricoeur's (1977) shift away from his heretofore exclusively hermeneutic, phenomenological position. Modell (1981) cites how Ricoeur has had to acknowledge that in order to understand levels and transformations of meaning one cannot study meaning apart from an examination of the nature, structure, organization, and manner of functioning of the mind. Draenos (1982) refers to Ricoeur's need to come to terms with the "mixed discourse" of psychoanalysis, where the means of proof reside in an articulation of the entire network of theory, hermeneutics, therapeutics, and narration. Ricoeur (1977) has indeed questioned whether in order to explain the vicissitudes and the emergence of meaning one may have to insert several steps of causal explanation into the "process of self-understanding in narrative terms." To sum up, here again is Meissner's (1981) position: To limit psychoanalysis in the way recently promulgated can lead one into the awkward position of either speaking of "sterile abstractions" or, at the other extreme, using "disembodied significances." In Friedman's (1976) terms, we would be left in the absurd position of an "individuality without features" or of "features without individuality."

Psychoanalysis qua psychoanalysis requires both meaning and structure, both reasons and causes, both understanding and explanation. Throughout this dialectic of models a number of critical features have been brought into relief. Renewed focus and articulation have been given to the "tension" in psychoanalytic theory and to the challenges that go with—as Barratt (1978) put it—the coexistence of the first- and third-person perspectives. Many have stated that there cannot be an "either–or" resolution, and as Goldberg (1975) suggests, the field requires this very integration of "the observer's ability to understand through introspection with the theorist's ability to conceptualize . . . data at higher levels of abstraction." For Meissner (1980) the organization of the self can be integrated with those "relatively autonomous aspects of ego functioning (that) give rise to a sense of self-as-agency."

Schafer tried to keep the nature of the psychoanalytic subject in mind by doing away with dialectical tensions, and for this his alternative has been criticized. However, what Schafer and others have done is not only to realert us to differing perspectives but to indicate the difficulties that emerge when distinctions become murky. While different frames of reference may be relevant to each other, they cannot be directly reduced to one another without resulting in confusion of languages, mixed frames of reference, and recourse to differing levels of abstraction. It is in this situation that the real theoretical and methodological dangers emerge—the pernicious reifications, unrecognized anthropomorphisms, and confusions of subjective experience and theoretical postulation.

Hartmann forewarned in 1956 that when one has worked with a given set of assumptions and hypotheses for a long time they begin to "interpenetrate with fact finding," and do so in such a way that one loses sight of their hypothetical character. When highly abstract concepts begin to merge with descriptive statements, we lose a clarity of thought and we gloss over what may be significant gaps in our understanding. And yet to keep levels of conceptualization distinct is not to rule out abstraction and explanation. As Schlessinger (1975) notes, one cannot bypass Freud's ingenious use of metaphor, and while it may be instrumental to generate explanations by a creative use of "primary process modes of thought," it does not follow that such modes of thought must become a "pervasive trend in communication."

Schafer (1976) has himself made such critical comments on the issue of conceptual level and he criticizes Kohut for the use of mixed (as opposed to multiple) modes of discourse. When Kohut, for example, writes of the "narcissistic self " (or for that matter, one might add, when Klein writes of a "self-schema"), there is a confounding of a phenomenological, experiential concept with a structural-energic frame of reference. Within the broad literature on "the self" and "the ego" one is in the first instance referring to a substantialization and concretization of an experiential referent, while in the second instance one is personifying a series of hypothetical constructs. Again we are back to the issue of a confusion of languages, which in turn has direct impact on our discussions of the ego as an abiding configuration of mental activities.

Here Peterfreund's (1971) distinctions can be used as a barometer throughout our discussions of EFA. While we may, for example, acknowledge a need for theories about thinking, we cannot say that a "theoretical concept referring to thinking can think." Thus, what seems convincing is that the critical problems of "hybrid" conceptualizations (Esman, 1979), the regression of concepts to spatial locations, and the recourse to reified entities may be, in part, a product of this loss of conceptual focus. The effort within psychoanalysis and, in particular, within psychoanalytic ego psychology to describe and account for the stability and transformations of processes and forms of mental activities need not, by definition, hold to an "infinite regress" of one's mode of discourse. While such efforts are responsive to creative modes of thought, there has to be a "return," if you will, to the levels of thinking of secondary process distinctions.

The emphasis given here to distinctions as to vantage points still leaves us with the question of how the two levels of discourse can be bridged. In this regard Wallerstein's (1976) suggestions are relevant. He asserts that each level must be given its due and that in this regard, we are met with a three-fold task. One aspect of the task is the systematic clinical examination of experience—"the experiential realm" of mental contents and events. Here would be placed the exploration of subjective meanings, ideas, fantasies, feelings, and strivings—the "why" questions of clinical evidence and interpretive fit that Schafer, Klein, and others have considered the appropriate domain of psychoanalysis. A companion task is the contemporaneous investigation and elaboration of the "nonexperiential realm"—the conceptual substrate, the ordering principles that address the regularity, expectability, and commonalities of process, organization, and structure. This domain refers to those hypothetical constructs that address the *how* questions, how the mind works. Succinctly, a full psychoanalytic study must pursue both the lawful regularities of human psychological functioning and, as Wallerstein (1976) states, "the idiosyncratic genetic unfolding of the succession of meanings and reason, overt and covert, that the individual lives by and imposes upon his being in the world."

Gill (1963) has stated that what one is conscious of is "the 'outcome' of the working of the mind . . . not of the working itself." In this context can be added the distinction Hartmann drew, and Rapaport (1957) came to insist on, between the "inner" and "internal worlds": The inner world consists of the "intrapsychic cognitive map," mental contents, fantasies, perceptions, and so on; the internal world comprises the organization and integration of intrapsychic structures, defense organizations, identifications, and so on. Loewald (1973, 1976) places his conceptualizations of internalization and its structural resultants within this latter domain, distinguishing this realm from those functions made possible by the creation of the "internal world." These distinctions between content and organization are repeatedly alluded to and seem to crystallize in Grossman's (1982) effort to distinguish, as an instance, the *self*—a term of ordinary personal reference—from the *ego*—a technical term of classification.

However, questions as to complex interaction remain, and here Wallerstein reaches the third task. While both realms of discourse must be kept conceptually distinct, there must also be a way to see them in their interrelatedness. Although Rapaport (1957) firmly stated how the inner world is, as it were, "in the force-field of the organization of the internal world," the question remains as to how one studies this. Here Wallerstein (1976) speaks to the need to delineate linkages, rules, and canons of correspondence between the two realms, an inquiry that he considers one of the prime and future tasks of psychoanalysis. It is through the simultaneous inquiry into both realms and the use of the full variety of research methodologies, be it the case study or more formal study, that the hardly begun task of specification and systematization can be pursued. Wallerstein concedes that the establishment of rules of correspondence and regularity will occur at varying levels of construction and inference. Such rules are not meant to collapse the two modes of discourse—the two "languages" into one. As Grossman and Simon (1969) have asserted, the only way to coordinate two "logically independent models of explanation" is to coordinate them in their application to the "empirical unity" of the phenomena under investigation. They analogize to psychophysical research where one works with covariants so as to establish a concordance that will ultimately reveal correlations. There is as yet, as Meissner (1980) has reminded us, no "superordinate framework" that can resolve the contradictions or reduce each perspective to an instance of some "general, all-encompassing view." At present, we need to recognize both perspectives, keep their language distinct and unconfounded, and continue to place our theory in a proper relationship with the evidence obtained.

Holt (1981) has submitted that in practice theories in all sciences grow in a more or less oscillating fashion. Hypothetical constructions, be they "gravitational fields" or the structural theory of psychoanalysis, are introduced when they serve to organize data; a variety of research methodologies may be employed in the manner and to the degree that they prove useful. What is critical is the effort to render our abstractions testable via sets of correspondence rules, which give empirical bearing to our critical concepts, and it is here that EFA as a methodology has pertinence. It is one response to this need to correlate and integrate the constructs of structural theory with the data of observation. In other words, EFA is a methodology that could accommodate the dual perspectives without a premature confounding of the two. First, however, it might be useful to take another look at certain structural conceptions and theoretical underpinnings from which EFA emerged, as it is these concepts against which so many current writers have inveighed.

A REAPPRAISAL OF CERTAIN STRUCTURAL CONCEPTS

In terms of the structural theory as a whole Glover (1956) reminds us that it was in the context of presenting the tripartite model that Freud warned against seeing the mental systems as "armed camps." Rather, these mental systems were presented as psychic systematizations that represent a codification of clinical observations. What the current debate has alerted us to is that when we say as an instance that the "ego tests reality," what we are speaking of is a class of psychic processes—as Schafer (1976) might say, a "class of mental events." Such formulations are systematic statements at the level of theoretical abstractions, and this is in contrast to references to some entity, something given by nature, or some hidden executor. The formulations are conceptual groupings, ordering abstractions, that in their turn refer to characteristics of behavior. The terms *ego, superego,* and *id* are theoretical devices used to classify data. Such statements as "taken into the ego" or "present in the ego" are shorthand for an ego function or process.

Several principles of classification have been considered by various authors and the principles along which psychic processes are sorted into structural units can be varying and complex. In Rapaport's writings (1951) the ego as a concept that refers to aspects of behavior that are delayable, bring about delay, or are themselves "products of delay" has been given emphasis. It is in no way contradictory that processes have also been classified and grouped according to their "alignment in conflict and adaptation" (Beres, 1965). The observation of the ubiquity of conflict in the psyche led to a conceptualization of the psyche as structurally divided. Behavior was to be thought of as a resultant of the interaction of functional units that have a degree of stability and coherence. The theory, Meissner (1981) reminds us, went beyond modes of conceptualization needed to explain symptoms or conflicts and endeavored to encompass those characteristics reflected in "abiding configurations and patterns of organization." As Pine (1983) describes the evolution of psychoanalytic concepts, "conceptual bridges" were established between a focus on drive psychology, unconscious fantasy, and processes of learning, perception, memory, and the like.

Despite the varying systems of classification employed by structural theory, the ego as a concept seemed to survive. What is critical in the present context is that whether one speaks of stability of modes of function, the pervasiveness of psychic conflict, slow rates of change, or centers of psychic function, our conceptualizations need not be reduced to spatial locations, a "prime mover," or the like. In designating the ego concept as a coordinate that expresses a relationship of processes we are not designating a "thing."

Another conceptual question has been raised in terms of the teleological use of the term *ego:* the ego defined as a "problem-solving agent," a "central steering agency" (Waelder, 1930), or the agent that "tests reality." Here again if levels of discourse are clearly articulated there is less risk of circular and tautological reasoning. Waelder (1960), for example, wrote of two ways in which teleological concepts can be used: one at the level of description and one at the level of explanation. He asserted that teleological concepts should remain at the descriptive level in psychoanalysis. The adaptiveness, directedness, or survival value of a process may be described, and such descriptions may serve as an aid to fruitful discovery and an understanding of process, but this is not the same as *explaining* the process. Designations can be made at different levels of inference, and while it is one thing to note the functionality of a psychic process, it is another to conceptualize at the level, for example, of how organized processes and structures come into being.

Distinctions between structure and function also have their history in psychoanalytic discourse. Here we go back to Beres' (1965) program to equate structure and function. To stave off any indictment as to anthropomorphism, Beres asserted that one can restrict one's definitions of structure to a series of summary statements about psychic functions. Wilson (1973) and Kaplan (1977) feel that such a clinging to empirical dogma is outdated and unnecessary. As was previously discussed, the philosophy of science has gone beyond the narrow empiricist requirement of having to reduce all one's theoretical terms to empirical fact. This is a call not for a concretization of our hypothetical constructs but for an evaluation of them on the basis of their systematic relevance, range, and capacity to enlarge our observational base.

Structures refer to different levels of organization, patterning, and interpretation that can help to explain the presence of functions such as impulse control, self-esteem maintenance, the ability to self-signal, and so on. We are thus using the term *structure* in a general sense in the way of Rapaport's (1960) concept of structures as "abiding determiners" of behavior that are characterized by permanence and invariance, or at least a "relatively slow rate of change." When behavior displays qualities of coherence, organization, and endurance, the existence of structure is inferred. Structural determinants, according to Rapaport (1967), can account for the observation that motivations do not determine behavior in any one-to-one fashion. Further, Schafer (1958) once wrote of how similar motives operating under different structural conditions are experienced differently, with different consequences and different manifestations. *Structure,* therefore, refers to stable components of the nonexperiential realm. As Sandler and Joffe (1969) have suggested, the concept of structure is a very broad one, able to encompass certain inborn biological structures but also able to include those relatively permanent levels of organization that are created "during the course of development as a consequence of adaptation."

Structures are implied in functional concepts. Holt claims that it is impossible to imagine how an inner order could be achieved and maintained "without enduring structural means." We do not have to assume a direct correspondence between a nameable function or particular type of product, "for a function can be represented by relationships among many activated structures." Nor need we, in Holt's terms, "postulate a personified structure within the model . . . prime mover . . . to whom all information . . . must be reported . . ." (1967, p. 359). What is being suggested, and here Schafer's work becomes pertinent, is the emergence of behavioral contingencies, "rules of action" (Schwartz, 1981), that reflect a level of organization that is not in itself directly observable.

There are varying models offered to describe how structures are formed; one or another principle becomes pertinent to the degree that it is heuristic. One problem is to show, for example, how an "object representation is translated from its representational (cognitive) status as a mental content to a form of internalized (and correspondingly structuralized) part of the psychic apparatus" (Meissner, 1979), and this process is barely understood. Some of the work that has a bearing in this process was done by Spitz (1959). From his infant observational studies he was able to distinguish a shift from a period of nonspecific, undirected random activity in the young infant to a mental organization manifested by the appearance of the smiling response. Spitz observed that it was as if a structural pattern had emerged that had not existed before, "as if a number of functions had been brought into relation with each other and linked into a coherent unit" (Spitz, 1959). This was the emergence of a new organizational unit, an organization that could be seen in a variety of sectors of function, be they perceptual, cognitive, or volitional.

Different theoretical models have been and continue to be offered to account for structure formation. Rapaport (1967) hypothesized that structures derive from drive energies and the transformations of these energies. Starting from the idea of innate thresholds in the discharge pathway, he spoke of how energies pitted against each other become solidified. Other writers, such as Schwartz (1981) and Parkin (1983), accept traditional definitions of psychic structure but without recourse to transformation of energy concepts or physicalistic notions of force and counterforce. Shevrin (Chattah, 1983) writes of structure formation as a process of increasing organization where one can describe the transformation of, for example, affect discharge into signal affect as "an increase in organization to the point at which the affect is readily recognized and responded to. . . . The higher the order of organization, the more constrained and less random the operation of its constituent parts, the more it approaches the status of a signal" (p. 694).

Greenspan (1979), in an effort to integrate Piagetian concepts of cognitive structure with structural concepts within psychoanalysis, highlights, as did Rapaport (1960), that Piaget's concepts assume a hierarchical layering of progressively differentiated structures. While Piaget's interest was in the underlying organization of intellectual operations that make possible characteristic patterns of response, he assumed different structural properties existing at different stages of mental organization. The way in which internal structure is formed through the interaction of the organism and the environment has always been rather vague in psychoanalysis. Greenspan points out how Piaget's concepts of assimilation and accommodation could offer psychoanalytic theory a rather specific hypothesis as to certain aspects of structure formation. To consider the level of structural organization and integration at each phase of development may have great pertinence for psychoanalysis in such areas as learning processes, establishment of object constancy, and identity formation.

Pine (1970) conceptualizes the process of structuralization as the "emergence of order and permanence in psychic life." Drawing on Waelder's (1930) idea of multiple function—that psychic activity serves diverse requirements and thus is multiply determined—Pine asserts that any psychic act that successfully meets such a "diverse set of requirements" is likely to achieve a degree of permanence and stability, in the way of "structuralized drive–defense relationships." In other words, what is "a multiply functional psychic act from one point of view can be seen as a structuralized arrangement from another." This consistent, repeatable, and regularized patterning of behavior not only implies structuralization in the way of a stabilized inner arrangement of forces that meets multiple demands, but also implies that the patterning is actively produced by the person. Within Pine's assertions there seems to be no need to take recourse in Waelder's ideas of a "central steering agent." What Pine does is to use the hypothesis of multiple function as one way of understanding how certain characteristic and dynamic functional units develop. In this way he adds a dynamic and motivational aspect to the development of semipermanent structures, and by so doing takes structure formation far from the realm of any "mindless growth of complexity" (Pine, 1970).

Coming from a slightly different vantage point but in no way reducing the significance of the motivational variables, Moses (1968) asserts that it was from psychoanalytic ego psychology that we became alerted to the significance of the formal, stylistic aspects of expressive behavior. With this added focus another dimension of psychoanalytic understanding was introduced, and stylistic aspects of functioning—such as the nature of the thought process or the differential handling of affects—could be clarified and used to map out certain axes along which structure formation and differentiation occur. Further, Moses stated that all that is recognized as "a process giving form and shape to psychic material" could be regarded as falling within the rubric of ego activity. In fact, the vast research literature on cognitive styles represents a body of work that tries to map out consistency in the realm of formal properties of thinking and perceiving, while at the same time attempting to forge some level of correspondence between these higher-order categories and empirical referents.

Gardner et al. (1960), in summarizing their research on cognitive controls, elaborated how structural concepts proved of great utility in their work. They observed that such control principles seemed to be in operation in a variety of areas of individual functioning and that these control principles seemed to become relatively stable and enduring attributes of cognitive organization over the developmental course. Furthermore, what was also conceptualized by the cognitive style theorists was an array of behaviors of the order of secondary adaptations to enduring arrangements of processes, which in turn gave new coherence to what had previously been discrete terms of data. While principally speaking of conceptual and perceptual variables, Gardner et al. asserted that structural patterns could also be discerned in characteristic styles in the channeling of drives, the patterning of interpersonal relationships, and so on.

David Shapiro (1965) extended the study of cognitive styles to broad areas of structure and functioning, including the means by which styles give shape to emotional experience, to aspects of symptom formation, and to defensive operations. Such broad patterns of mental activity did not seem attributable to manifestations of any specific defense or drive derivative but rather seemed to reflect a fluid, dynamic, and complex configuration of psychological organization. Like Gardner et al., Shapiro used the style construct in two ways: to refer to a formal consistency in thought, experience, and action and, in turn, to conceptualize functioning as a form-giving structure itself.

Shapiro (1970) also has written of the role of style features in the construction and reconstruction of meaning and motivated actions, and it is here that his ideas can be brought into some direct relation with those of Schafer. Shapiro encourages the "phenomenological description of details of the mental superficies" that might otherwise be overlooked. However, he asserts too that in regard to action, choice, and what he calls "volitional action" it is impossible to come to a full understanding of these subjective states without reaching some degree of clarification as to the psychological processes that give shape to intentionality and meaning. Knowledge of the more stable forms of thinking and attitude adds a dimension to the understanding of ways in which meaning and choice come to be experienced.

On the other hand, Shapiro asserts, à la Schafer, that the neurotic person, for example, does not "suffer neurosis"; rather, he actively participates in it and functions according to it. In other words, the neurotic problem "is the person." Neurosis, according to Shapiro, consists not of a constellation of internal forces and agencies operating on the individual, in the way of the older "marionette conception," but comprises "certain subjectively restrictive, often extremely uncomfortable . . . self-maintained ways" that reflect the way the individual is organized. Such subjectively restrictive factors are an inevitable product of what the person is—the person's attitudes, points of view, modes of thought, and so forth. Activity can therefore be assessed along the dimensions of consciousness, attention, thinking, and the like— mediational processes that give shape to subjective, intentional experiences of choice, conscious motive, and the experience of "impulse." This structural analysis of the volitional process in no way obviates the role of intrapsychic conflict, of psychic reality, or of unconscious need, but attempts to spell out those processes, as Shapiro asserts, "by which the impetus to action is generated." Unconscious need does not move the person like "a marionette" but affects action as it affects the various stages of volitional processes. Decisions follow from a state of mind, a mode of thought that affects the very experience of, for instance, "coming to a decision."

Shapiro's (1965) discussion on the impulsive style and on the nature of impulsive action merits particular mention at this point, because it relates so clearly to the way action terms can themselves be enhanced by the addition of a "nonexperiential" level of explanation. On the impulsive character Shapiro writes that despite the diversity within this group "a general mode of action in common" can be discerned. It is a mode that can be described as a relatively concrete and impressionistic cognitive style, and associated with this style is a characteristic and distinctive way of experiencing action and the motivation to action. What one observes in the subjective experience of these people is an impairment of the normal feelings of deliberateness and intention. The experience of choice and intention, while certainly reflecting defensive processes or—as Schafer might say—a "disclaiming of action," itself follows from the attenuation of the volitional process. Characteristic of this style is a "short-circuiting of integrative process" that might otherwise lead to a crystallization of stable and long-range anticipations. There is a premature crystallization of vague intentions. The experience of "giving in to impulse" is not merely due to the person's incapacity to help himself or to assume responsibility but results from a loss of interest at some critical point in "wanting to help himself." According to Shapiro, this kind of individual characteristically acts too immediately to feel himself wanting, considering, deciding, and so on. What can be taken from this is that the idea of purposeful action is useful and should not be discarded, although it does need to be "fleshed out" and given greater articulation—and not exclusively from one single frame of reference, however significant the frame of reference might be. The processes involved in the phenomenological transformations themselves have to be articulated, and it would seem that a structural understanding of action could give our clinical observations greater specificity and, in the end, greater meaning.

This section will close with reference to an article by Allport (1955). He wrote that one of the most striking features of behavior is the marked variation in time and place in which events can occur and "still leave the *pattern* of the events." In this patterning, this structuring, of mental events one does not find "agencies" or "entities" or "particle-elements," but rather, according to Allport, "cyclical-ongoings . . . a geometrical format of continuances connected by events." Allport urges that we leave aside linear or molar-agency explanations of perceptual structures and in their place attempt to discern and articulate relatively enduring and myriad structures of "ongoings and events." Further, if one is looking for some principle of aggregation, or structure formation, one cannot approach the study globally; one must map out "elements" in relation to each other, and when this is done the "agent" disappears.

THE UTILITY OF EGO FUNCTION ASSESSMENT

Bellak, Hurvich, and Gediman's (1973) extensive work on EFA emerged from a number of theoretical and methodological considerations and is in a line with those features of the tradition of psychoanalytic ego psychology that have been discussed in this paper. With an eye to the current controversy within psychoanalysis, in the very process of constructing the EFA scales, the requirements for the ratings of clinical judges, and the instrumentation of the profile, an effort was made to put the explanatory power of the structural model to an empirical test, and to do so with a replacement of global terms by detailed descriptive statements.

From the start, Bellak (1958) asserted that there was nothing sacrosanct about the tripartite model but rather that it was to be considered as one that had utility and breadth as a series of working hypotheses. Bellak et al. (1973) found the ego model to be a useful one in that particular process variables could be delineated, broken down into "more or less arbitrary subdivisions," and used to refer to adaptively relevant actions and reactions of the person. From a conceptual position, function became one way to study structure. However, while EFA clearly grew out of the larger dynamic conceptual scheme of structural theory, the authors asserted that one could make use of the methodology without committing oneself to any particular stand on energy concepts, instinct theory, or the like. The critical criterion was to be an empirical one, that is, the degree to which the methodology served to order and codify meaningful categories in the assessment of clinical data.

Bellak et al. (1973) explored the empirical referents of ego processes in such a way that the methodological requirements of a clear definition of terms, interrater reliability, and criteria of cross-validation could be met. To this effect component factors of each area of functioning were delineated and organized into ordinal scales keyed to interview questions and capable of being rated along a dimension of adaptiveness–maladaptiveness. Each area and component factor thus had to be articulated in such a way that reliable judgments by independent clinical judges could be made.

EFA was designed to find some concordance among measurable areas of function, patients' self-observations, and judgments made by clinicians. Each area was to be viewed critically in the light of the other and an effort made to form some sort of concordance. The principles of organization used by the raters in making their clinical judgments were of an order that entailed just that oscillation between an inside and outside view posited in this paper as critical to a conceptualization of psychoanalytic data, a process that parallels the shifts in the work of the psychoanalytic clinician. What EFA adds as a research instrument is a way to home in on those variables from the nonexperiential and experiential realm that emerges as "correspondences" in the inference processes of the clinician—processes that are themselves organized and guided according to certain articulated procedures. The model requires no introduction of a "mover of the apparatus," relying instead on a series of theoretical abstractions with a clinical counterpart in manifestations of specific actions, thoughts, and affects, and on the integrative activities of the clinician.

Certainly questions could be raised as to the nature of the EFA profile. One could question the very process of codifying functions and component factors. In this regard Bellak has always acknowledged that such classifications are in ways arbitrary but yet flexible and open to change. They do derive from clinical material and may be considered capable of encompassing the major dimensions of behavior as currently recognized. A more basic question can also be raised, namely, why codify or label areas of functioning as discrete in the first place? Here some of Rangell's (1982) comments seem pertinent. Rangell pointed out how it was at the level of the global and the "whole" that Freud started, and that it was Freud's breakthrough to dissect the whole into its parts and to assign each a coherent role. As Rangell states, "while we have learned that analogizing to somatic processes has its limitations, the organism does not perform its functions, somatic or mental, as a unit without parts" (1982, p. 869). In terms of the arguments raised by those who sponsor a "holistic" model, Rangell asserts that by abandoning our knowledge of internal structure, of the ways in which specific and composite actions are derived, we would be returning to a "psychology of the composite whole," which he asserts would be in the way of a "scientific regression." It seems worth commenting here that it is in particular when we begin to speak of the "ego" as a totality that we seem to start speaking of a "mover of the apparatus," an anthropomorphic executor, and the like.

While such areas of function as perception, thinking, and defense share certain features, variations among them are sufficient to require a differential approach. Beres (1956) was continuously impressed by the variant anomalies of different ego function patterns in patients, and it may be recalled that one of Hartmann's essential contributions was in the area of the intrasystemic analysis of the ego construct. On the other hand, there has been no presumption here—or on the part of other writers—that these areas of function are independent and unrelated; clearly, there is overlap. Nevertheless, and as Rapaport (1950, 1954) asserted, it is the patterning of areas of strength and weakness that allows for inferences concerning organization. For Bellak the question of overlap can only be addressed once one is clear as to one's definitional terms. Although processes are clearly multidetermined, what EFA endeavors to do as a first critical step is to replace such global terms as *ego deficit* with specific statements so as to help tease out precise areas of disturbance and strength.

Another question that could be raised is about EFA's isolation as a mode of investigation, in that EFA precludes a consideration of drive, motivation, and other factors in studying levels of personality organization. Bellak has always agreed that there are drive, affect, and ego-adaptive aspects to any given process, and scales have been included in the EFA profile to accommodate such levels of assessment. It remains true, however, that any material can be approached from any number of conceptual paths. As Eissler (1968) has stated, scientists are "forced to cut out of the universe a certain section of it, and to look at that section as if it were indeed self-contained."

Such pitfalls for EFA, while they remain potential, can still be seen from another tradition within psychoanalytic ego psychology. Rapaport (1950, 1954) recognized that psychoanalysis, more than any other theory, provides the means to conceptualize an intimate connection between cognitive and motivational phenomena. In his systematic approach to the structure of though processes he taught how thought organization itself is a key to the specification of personality dynamics. Thus, personality organization expresses itself in various segments of behavior, and it is through a study of the thought processes in particular that one can study the sequella of personality organization in all its multidetermination. What this approach does is to take us far from the notion of a simple taxonomy of functions or faculties— thought processes can open up for study the whole fabric of personality organization. Thus, when Bellak notes how EFA allows for the study of "a final common pathway" for a variety of determinants in the schizophrenias, one might add that EFA also allows us one way of assessing a "final common pathway" of behavior in all its multidetermination.

Continuing with questions as to methodology, the issue may be raised as to why Bellak et al. (1973) started from a theoretically based versus an empirically constructed assessment instrument. The authors addressed this question in the first EFA book, stating that instruments such as EFA can generate a whole network and matrix of interrelations that give order and meaning to observational data. An instrument grounded in psychoanalytic theory can have broad implications for developmental and therapeutic issues, for the area of personality theory, and so on. One would be hard put to approach this level of systematization in a simple search for correlations between behavior measures and isolated test scores.

While certainly this rejoinder has merit, some of Wallerstein's (1975) comments about the feasibility of psychoanalytic research make a further point. Wallerstein wrote of how psychoanalytic theory has at its very base a denial of any "isomorphic relationship between discrete behaviors and intrapsychic states." Rather than take an approach that leads to the formation of complex underlying states by working inductively, within psychoanalysis we can expect to work most fruitfully from the other direction, that is, by starting with a "more overarching concept," then differentiating its components and possible pathways of representation, and next discovering the array of possible empirical referents in the data of observation (Wallerstein, 1975). Further (and again with reference to the idea of dual frames of reference and the establishment of correspondence rules), the inference process itself, the establishment of linkages, must be made as "public" and as objective as possible.

Given the problem of the remoteness of theoretical concepts from observation in psychoanalytic research, Wallerstein and Sampson (1971) offer as one possible paradigm the use of clinical judgments themselves as "data." They posit that through the progressive refinement of those clinical judgments that reach interrater agreement and allow for the derivation of predictions that can be tested empirically there can be a process of "pushing clinical judgments of complex psychological events in the direction of more reliable, hence more measurable, statements." EFA meets such criteria— independent clinical judgments form the base from which predictions are made. EFA, as clearly stated by Bellak et al. (1973), is in no way a questionnaire; it is a framework for the clinician's thinking rendered explicit and anchored at critical points in behavioral data.

Wallerstein and Sampson (1971) are also of the opinion that such research strategies could constitute collaborative adjuncts to the "clinical retrospective method" of the analytic situation. Such collaborative approaches speak to such potential problems as hidden circularity, the need to generate specific clinical predictions, and so on. EFA has the capability of approaching that level of clinical description. Although it approaches such a continuing process of description and redescription from the framework of a dual perspective, EFA has as its further goal to render our abstractions and constructs increasingly articulate.

Nevertheless, where Schafer, Gill, and others wish to focus on what can be gained exclusively from the use of the psychoanalytic method, many remain committed to the use of multiple pathways for the generating of psychoanalytic data. Shevrin (1976), for instance, advocates a convergence of methods. Speaking against what he considers a "methodological monogamy," he asserts that the psychoanalytic situation cannot itself be a "self-contained field," as it is not possible "to use an assumption and demonstrate its validity simultaneously." He feels that the psychoanalytic situation, rather than becoming a "straightjacket" for psychoanalytic research, can only be strengthened by supporting evidence from "far afield and based on totally different methods." Anna Freud (1966), on the other hand, cautioned that such ancillary methods must be understood as providing data that has "a sign- or signal-function" for the observer. That is, the role of alternative methodologies cannot be of the order of an accumulation of discrete behavioral signs, traits, symptoms, and so forth. For such behavioral referents to be useful for psychoanalytic research, they must be synthesized by the analytic observer within a matrix of hypotheses and with a full appreciation of unconscious developments. EFA, as one effort in this tradition, is very much in the spirit of a convergence of methods.

To reiterate: it is in its capacity to generate specific, articulated, and testable hypotheses that the true test of EFA lies, and it was to meet this end that the present volume was designed. Further, it is hoped that the systematic use of EFA will be helpful in establishing the rules of correspondence between concepts of psychic structure and the domain of purposeful action.

REFERENCES

Allport, F. H. *Theories of perception and the concept of structure.* New York: Wiley, 1955.

Arlow, J. A. The structural hypothesis: Theoretical considerations. *Psychoanalytic Quarterly.* 1975, *44,* 509–525.

Aufhauser, M. C. Book review: A New Language in Psychoanalysis, by Roy Schafer. *Journal of the American Psychoanalytic Association,* 1979, *27,* 287–314.

Barratt, B. B. Critical notes on Schafer's "Action Language." *The Annual of Psychoanalysis,* 1978, *VI,* 287–314.

Bellak L. *Schizophrenia: A review of the syndrome.* New York: Logos Press, 1958.

Bellak, L., Hurvich, M., & Gediman, H. *Ego functions in schizophrenics, neurotics, and normals.* New York: Wiley, 1973.

Beres, D. Ego deviation and the concept of schizophrenia. *Psychoanalytic Study of the Child,* 1956, *11,* 164–235.

Beres, D. Structure and function in psychoanalysis. *International Journal of Psychoanalysis,* 1965, *46,* 53–63.

Berger, L. S. Innate constraints of formal theories. *Psychoanalysis and Contemporary Thought,* 1978, *1,* 89–117.

Bibring, E. Psychoanalysis and dynamic psychotherapies. *Journal of the American Psychoanalytic Association,* 1954, *2,* 754–770.

Brenner, C. Metapsychology and psychoanalytic theory. *Psychoanalytic Quarterly,* 1980, *49,* 189–214.

Brierley, M. Notes on metapsychology as a process theory. *International Journal of Psychoanalysis,* 1944, *25,* 97–106.

Calogeras, R. C., & Alston, T. M. On "Action Language" in psychoanalysis. *Psychoanalytic Quarterly,* 1980, *49,* 663–696.

Chattah, L. (Reporter). Metapsychology: cultural and scientific roots. *Journal of the American Psychoanalytic Association,* 1983, *31,* 689–698.

Draenos, S. *Freud's odyssey: psychoanalysis and the end of metaphysics.* New Haven: Yale University Press, 1982.

Eagle, M. George Klein's *Psychoanalytic Theory* in perspective. *Psychoanalytic Review,* 1980, *67*(2), 179–194.

Eissler, K. R. The relation of explaining and understanding in psychoanalysis. *Psychoanalytic Study of the Child,* 1968, *23,* 141–177.

Ellman, S. J., & Moskowitz, M. B. An examination of some recent criticism of psychoanalytic "metapsychology." *Psychoanalytic Quarterly,* 1980, *49,* 631–662.

Esman, A. H. On evidence and inference, or the babel of tongues. *Psychoanalytic Quarterly,* 1979, *49,* 628–630.

Fonagy, P. The integration of psychoanalysis and experimental science: A review. *International Review of Psychoanalysis,* 1982, *9,* 125–145.

Freud, A. Links between Hartmann's ego psychology and the child analyst's thinking. In R. M. Loewenstein, L. M. Newman, M. Schur, & A. J. Solnit (Eds.), *Psychoanalysis—a general psychology: Essays in honor of Heinz Hartmann.* New York: International Universities Press, 1966.

Freud, S. *Instincts and their vicissitudes (standard ed.,* Vol. 14). London: Hogarth Press, 1915.

Freud, S. *The ego and the id (standard ed.,* Vol. 19). London: Hogarth Press.

Friedman, L. Problems of an action theory of the mind. *International Review of Psychoanalysis,* 1976, *3,* 129–138.

Friedman, L. The barren prospect of the representational world. *Psychoanalytic Quarterly,* 1980, *49,* 215–233.

Gardner, R. W., Jackson, D. N., & Messick, S. J. Personality organization in cognitive controls and intellectual abilities. *Psychological Issues,* Vol. II, No. 4. New York: International Universities Press, 1960.

Gedo, J. E. Book review: Psychology versus metapsychology: Psychoanalytic essays in honor of George S. Klein. *Psychoanalytic Quarterly,* 1977, *46,* 319–325.

Gill, M. M. Topography and systems in psychoanalytic theory. *Psychological Issues,* Vol. III, No. 2. New York: International Universities Press, 1963.

Gill, M. M. Psychic energy reconsidered: Discussion. *Journal of the American Psychoanalytic Association,* 1977, *25,* 581–597.

Gill, M. M. Metapsychology is irrelevant to psychoanalysis. In S. Smith (Ed.), *The human mind revisited: Essays in honor of Karl A. Menninger.* New York: International Universities Press, 1978.

Glover, E. *On the early development of mind.* New York: International Universities Press, 1956.

Goldberg, A. I. Book review: *Perception, Motives, and Personality,* George S. Klein. *Journal of the American Psychoanalytic Association,* 1975, *23,* 643–650.

Greenspan, S. I. Intelligence and adaptation. *Psychological Issues,* Vol. XII, No. 3/4. New York: International Universities Press, 1979.

Grolnick, S. A. The current psychoanalytic dialogue: Its counterpart in renaissance philosophy. *Journal of the American Psychoanalytic Association,* 1982, *30,* 679–699.

Grossman, W. I. Reflections on the relationship of introspection to psychoanalysis. *International Journal of Psychoanalysis,* 1967, *48,* 16–31.

Grossman, W. I. The self as fantasy: Fantasy as theory. *Journal of the American Psychoanalytic Association,* 1982, *30,* 919–938.

Grossman, W. I., & Simon, B. Anthropomorphism: Motive, meaning, and causality in psychoanalytic theory. *Psychoanalytic Study of the Child,* 1969, *24,* 79–111.

Hartmann, H. Notes on the reality principle. In H. Hartmann (Ed.), *Essays on ego psychology.* New York: International Universities Press, 1964 (1956), pp. 241–267.

Holt, R. R. The development of the primary process: A structural view. In R. R. Holt (Ed.), *Motives and thought: Psychoanalytic essays in honor of David Rapaport, Psychological Issues,* Vol. V, No. 2/3. New York: International Universities Press, 1967.

Holt, R. R. Freud's mechanistic and humanistic images of man. *Psychoanalysis and Contemporary Science,* Vol. I, pp. 3–24.

Holt, R. R. Book review: *Language and Thought,* Roy Schafer. *Psychoanalytic Quarterly,* 1979, *48,* 496–500.

Holt, R. R. The death and transfiguration of metapsychology. *International Review of Psychoanalysis,* 1981, *8,* 129–143.

Home, H. J. The concept of mind. *International Journal of Psychoanalysis,* 1966, *47,* 43–49.

Kaplan, D. M. Differences in the clinical and academic points of view. *Bulletin of the Menninger Clinic,* 1977, *41,* 207–228.

Klein, G. S. *Psychoanalytic theory: An exploration of essentials.* New York: International Universities Press, 1976.

Kovel, J. Things and words: Metapsychology and the historical point of view. *Psychoanalysis and Contemporary Thought,* 1978, *1,* 21–88.

Kris, E. *Psychoanalytic explorations in art.* New York: International Universities Press, 1952.

Loewald, H. W. On internalization. In *Papers on psychoanalysis.* New Haven, Yale University Press, 1973.

Loewald, H. W. Perspectives on memory. In M. M. Gill and P. S. Holzman (Eds.), *Psychology versus metapsychology: Psychoanalytic essays in memory of George S. Klein. Psychological Issues,* Vol. IX, No. 4. New York: International Universities Press, 1976.

Mayman, M. Psychoanalytic theory in retrospect and prospect. *Bulletin of the Menninger Clinic,* 1976, *40,* 199–210.

McIntosh, D. The empirical bearing of psychoanalytic theory. *International Journal of Psychoanalysis,* 1979, *60,* 405–431.

Meissner, W. W. Methodological critique of action language in psychoanalysis. *Journal of the American Psychoanalytic Association,* 1979, *27,* 79–105.

Meissner, W. W. The problem of internalization and structure formation. *International Journal of Psychoanalysis,* 1980, *61,* 237–248.

Meissner, W. W. Metapsychology—who needs it? *Journal of the American Psychoanalytic Association,* 1981, *29,* 921–938.

Modell, A. H. The nature of psychoanalytic knowledge. *Journal of the American Psychoanalytic Association,* 1978, *26,* 641–658.

Modell, A. H. Does metapsychology still exist? *International Journal of Psychoanalysis,* 1981, *62,* 391–402.

Moses, R. Form and content: An ego-psychological view. *Psychoanalytic Study of the Child,* 1968, *23,* 204–223.

Noy, P. Metapsychology as a multimodel system. *International Review of Psychoanalysis,* 1977, *4,* 1–12.

Parkin, A. Structure formation and alteration. *International Journal of Psychoanalysis,* 1983, *64,* 323–351.

Peterfreund, E. Information, systems and psychoanalysis: An evolutionary, biological approach to psychoanalytic theory. *Psychological Issues,* Vol. VII, No. 1/2. New York: International Universities Press, 1971.

Peterfreund, E. On information and systems for psychoanalysis. *International Review of Psychoanalysis,* 1980, *7,* 327–345.

Pine, F. On the structuralization of drive–defense relationships. *Psychoanalytic Quarterly,* 1970, *39,* 17–37.

Pine, F. The development of ego apparatus and drive: A schematic view. *Contemporary Psychoanalysis,* 1983, *19,* 238–247.

Rangel, L. The self in psychoanalytic theory. *Journal of the American Psychoanalytic Association, 30,* 863–891.

Rapaport, D. The theoretical implications of diagnostic test procedures. In R. P. Knight and C. R. Friedman (Eds.), *Psychoanalytic psychiatry and psychology.* New York: International Universities Press, 1954, pp. 173–195.

Rapaport, D. *Organization and pathology of thought.* New York: Columbia University Press, 1951.

Rapaport, D. A theoretical analysis of the superego concept. In M. M. Gill (Ed.), *The collected papers of David Rapaport.* New York: Basic Books, 1957; 1967.

Rapaport, D. The theory of attention cathexis. In M. M. Gill (Ed.), *The collected papers of David Rapaport.* New York: Basic Books, 1967.

Rapaport, D., & Gill, M. M. The points of view and assumptions of metapsychology. *International Journal of Psychoanalysis,* 1959, *40,* 153–162.

Rawn, M. L. Schafer's "action language": A questionable alternative to metapsychology. *International Journal of Psychoanalysis,* 1979, *60,* 455–465.

Reppen, J. Symposium: Emanuel Peterfreund on information and system theory. *Psychoanalytic Review,* 1981, *68*(2), 159–190.

Richards, A. D. The superordinate self in psychoanalytic theory and in the self psychologies. *Journal of the American Psychoanalytic Association,* 1982, *30,* 939–957.

Ricoeur, P. The questions of proof in Freud's psychoanalytic writings. *Journal of the American Psychoanalytic Association,* 1977, *25,* 835–871.

Rosenblatt, A. D., & Thickstun, J. T. Modern psychoanalytic concepts in a general psychology. *Psychological Issues,* Vol. XI, No. 2/3. New York: International Universities Press.

Ryle, G. *The concept of mind.* New York: Barnes & Noble, 1949; 1965.

Sandler, J., & Joffe, W. G. Towards a basic psychoanalytic model. *International Journal of Psychoanalysis,* 1969, *50,* 79–90.

Schafer, R. Regression in the service of the ego: The relevance of a psychoanalytic concept for personality assessment. In G. Lindzey (Ed.), *Assessment of human motives.* New York: Holt, Rinehart and Winston, 1958, pp. 119–147.

Schafer, R. Psychoanalysis without psychodynamics. *International Journal of Psychoanalysis,* 1975, *56,* 41–55.

Schafer, R. *A new language for psychoanalysis.* New Haven: Yale University Press, 1976.

Schafer, R. *Language and insight.* New Haven: Yale University Press, 1978.

Schafer, R. Character, ego-syntonicity, and character change. *Journal of the American Psychoanalytic Association,* 1979, *27,* 867–891.

Schafer, R. *The analytic attitude.* New York: Basic Books, 1983.

Schlessinger, N. Book review: Nathan Leites: *The new ego: Pitfalls in current thinking about patients in psychoanalysis. Psychoanalytic Quarterly,* 1971, *44,* 659–662.

Schwartz, F. Psychic structure. *International Journal of Psychoanalysis,* 1981, *62,* 61–72.

Shapiro, Daniel. Pruning or uprooting? Reshaping psychoanalytic theory. *Contemporary Psychology,* 1977, *22,* 279–281.

Shapiro, David. *Neurotic styles.* New York: Basic Books, 1965.

Shapiro, David. Motivation and action in psychoanalytic psychiatry. *Psychiatry,* 1970, *33,* 329–343.

Shevrin, H. David Rapaport's contribution to research: A look at the future. *Bulletin of the Menninger Clinic,* 1976, *40,* 211–228.

Spence, D. P. Psychoanalysis in a new key. *Contemporary Psychology,* 1976, *21,* 787–788.

Spiro, A. M. A philosophical appraisal of Roy Schafer's *A new language for psychoanalysis. Psychoanalysis and Contemporary Thought,* 1979, *2,* 253–291.

Spitz, R. A. *A genetic field theory of ego formation.* New York: International Universities Press, 1959.

Waelder, R. The principle of multiple function. *Psychoanalytic Quarterly,* 1930, *15,* (1936), 45–62.

Waelder, R. *Basic theory of psychoanalysis.* New York: International Universities Press, 1960.

Waelder, R. Book review: *Psychoanalysis, scientific method and philosophy:* A symposium edited by Sidney Hook. *Journal of the American Psychoanalytic Association,* 1962, *10,* 617–637.

Wallerstein, R. S. *Psychotherapy and psychoanalysis: Theory, practice, research.* New York: International Universities Press, 1975.

Wallerstein, R. S. Psychoanalysis as a science: Its present status and its future tasks. In M. M. Gill and P. S. Holzman (Eds.), *Psychology versus metapsychology: Psychoanalytic essays in memory of George S. Klein, Psychological Issues,* Vol. IX, No. 4. New York: International Universities Press, 1976.

Wallerstein, R. S., & Sampson, H. Issues in research in the psychoanalytic process. In I. M. Marcus (Ed.), *Currents in psychoanalysis.* New York: International Universities Press, 1971, pp. 265–302.

Wilson, E. The structural hypothesis and psychoanalytic metatheory: An essay on psychoanalysis and contemporary philosophy of science. *Psychoanalysis and Contemporary Science,* 1973, *2,* 304–328.

Wurmser, L. Metapsychology—eagle or dodo? *Journal of Nervous and Mental Disease,* 1977, *164*(5), 362–368.

PART TWO

EFA as a Research Tool in Therapy

CHAPTER FIVE

Ego Functions and Clinical Outcome in Schizophrenia

JOHN P. DOCHERTY AND SUSAN FIESTER

Psychiatric thought and practice have historically been characterized by several approaches to understanding psychopathology. Descriptive psychiatry and dynamic psychiatry represent two approaches that have tended to develop in parallel and have remained remarkably unintegrated. As a result, we have not benefited from the potential complementarity of these two approaches. A conceptual overview of descriptive and psychodynamic psychiatry suggests that these two approaches might function in a manner analogous to the interaction of anatomy and physiology in the biological sciences. The task of descriptive psychiatry is a progressive refinement and articulation of the phenomenological features of psychiatric disorder while dynamic psychiatry addresses a progressive understanding of the processes that underlie and determine those features.

Recent methodological advances in both descriptive and dynamic psychiatry have now made this integration a possibility. An accumulating body of descriptive research in schizophrenia has resulted in a novel concept referred to as "multidimensionality of outcome." Quite simply, this concept encompasses a view of outcome as a complex construct composed of relatively independent outcome axes. Recent cross-sectional studies (Schwartz et al., 1975; Strauss and Carpenter, 1972, 1974; Gittleman-Klein and Klein,

1969; Keniston et al., 1971; May and Tuma, 1964; Ellsworth and Clayton, 1959; Erikson, 1975) have suggested that the outcome dimensions of hospitalization, symptomatology, social functioning, and work functioning have only moderate degrees of intercorrelation. Additionally, Fontana & Dowds (1975) have demonstrated that these outcome dimensions, when they are traced from admission through year-long follow-up, show as many patterns as there are dimensions; that is, the pattern of the waxing and waning of each of these dimensions is unique. This means that an individual patient might be doing well or poorly on all outcome dimensions, or well in some areas and poorly in others.

In the area of dynamic psychiatry, ego impairments consistently have been implicated as a major source of the diverse symptomatology of schizophrenia (Federn, 1952; Freeman et al., 1966; Hartmann, 1964). However, there have been few empirical investigations attempting to document in a specific and reliable fashion the particular ego deficits in schizophrenic patients. Further, the relationship of specific ego deficits to clinical course and outcome has not previously been articulated. Bellak and his colleagues (1973) have developed a reliable method for assessing ego functions, using a semistructured interview. This type of instrument has great potential for integrating descriptive and psychodynamic research.

These developments offer the possibility for a much more comprehensive understanding and monitoring of the course and outcome of schizophrenic disorders. The descriptive research we have cited has provided a dissection of the major structures of course and outcome—symptoms, work, social performance, and hospitalization. Concurrent systematic assessment of ego functioning and of each outcome dimension in a group of schizophrenic patients provides us with a possibility of linking underlying psychological process to the functional status in a much more meaningful way.

The aim of this study is to determine the relationship between ego functioning and specific aspects of outcome in schizophrenia.

METHODOLOGY

Subjects

The population consisted of patients currently being followed in the Continuing Care Division (CCD) of the West Haven Veterans Administration Hospital.

The patient group was selected on the basis of the following criteria:

1. Current clinical diagnosis of schizophrenia
2. Followed continuously in the CCD for more than 5 years
3. Age 20–59
4. Not currently hospitalized
5. Adequate records of hospitalization dates, treatment and follow-up

The charts of 47 patients meeting the study criteria were randomly selected from a population of 223 eligible patient subjects.

Procedure: Chart Review

Subjects' inpatient medical–psychiatric records and their outpatient psychiatric charts were reviewed. Comprehensive information on each psychiatric hospitalization—including dates and location, symptomatology, diagnosis, type of treatment, and hospital course—was recorded.

Three sets of diagnostic criteria were applied to material from the chart: the International Pilot Study of Schizophrenia Flexible System of Diagnosis (IPSS) (Carpenter et al., 1973), the Research Diagnostic Criteria (RDC) (Spitzer et al., 1978), and the New Haven Schizophrenia Index (NHSI) (Astrachan et al., 1972). The NHSI was scored for symptoms noted during *any* episode of psychiatric hospitalization while the IPSS and the RDC were applied to the initial episode of hospitalization. A symptom was scored as positive if it was described in the admission examination, progress notes, or discharge summary.

In addition, patients were rated on three measures of onset of illness—age of first social incapacitation, age of first psychiatric symptoms but no treatment, and age of first psychiatric treatment.

Procedure: Interview

After giving written informed consent, patients were interviewed with standardized interview formations. Of the 47 patients whose records were reviewed, 32 were available for interview.

Five major dimensions of outcome were evaluated using the following measures:

Dimension	Measure	Source
1. Rehospitalization	Hospitalization indices*	Record
2. Symptomatology	BPRS (Overall & Gorham, 1962)	Interview
3. Occupational Functioning	Employment history— standard rating scales	Record– interview
4. Social Adjustment	Social Adjustment Scale (Weissman & Paykel, 1974)	Self-rating
5. Global Functioning	Global Assessment Scale (Endicott et al., 1976)	Interview

* Several measures were devised to quantify the data on hospitalization in a more meaningful way. Three dimensions were felt to be critical:

1. Frequency: $\dfrac{\text{total number of hospitalizations}}{\text{duration of illness (years)}}$

Footnote continued on page 74.

Ego functions were evaluated by semistructured interview using the Bellak Ego Function Scale. Patients were rated on a 13-point scale for each of the 12 ego functions and their major components, included in Bellak et al. (1973). Interrater reliability for this scale was assessed by percentage of rater agreement. Based on two raters' independent ratings of 17 patients, an overall agreement of 90.06% was obtained. The percentage agreement obtained for each of the 12 subscales ranged from 84.03 to 98.62.

RESULTS

Sociodemographic Characteristics

The characteristics of this population with respect to age, social class, and marital status were tabulated. Average age of patients in this sample is 41, with a range of 28–58. There is a loading of patients in the lower social classes, with 82.5% in classes IV and V and only 5% in classes I and II. Only 29.8% of the patients are currently married, with 14.9% separated or divorced. By far the greatest number have remained single (55.3%).

History of Illness Characteristics

The average age at first psychiatric hospitalization was 24.6, with a range of 18–44 years. The mean duration of psychiatric illness for these patients was approximately 17 years.

Diagnostic Characteristics

All the patients scored positive for schizophrenia on the NHSI, and 94% scored positive on the IPSS when a cut-off of five or more symptoms was used. By RDC criteria, 77% of the patients were diagnosed as schizophrenic, while 23% were schizoaffective.

---

2. Severity: per episode $= \dfrac{\text{total in-hospital days}}{\text{total number of hospitalizations}}$ per year

$= \dfrac{\text{total in-hospital days}}{\text{duration of illness (years)}}$ per year

$= \dfrac{\text{total out-of-hospital weeks}}{\text{duration of illness (years)}}$

3. Latency: per episode $= \dfrac{\text{total out-of-hospital weeks}}{\text{total number of hospitalizations}}$

Ego Function

Results for ratings of ego functioning are shown in Table 5.1 and Figure 5.1. On the Bellak Ego Functions Assessment Scales, mean score for all functions is 7.0. This is the midpoint on a 1–13 rating scale, with 13 representing most adaptive and 1 most maladaptive. This population scored best on judgment and synthetic integrative functioning and poorest on regulation of drives and adaptive regression in the service of the ego (ARISE).

These data can be compared to that of Bellak et al. for the schizophrenic population used in standardizing the scale (1973). Although those investigators used acute schizophrenic inpatients, half of whom were females, the age, education, IQ, and social class of his sample are comparable to the one in this study. Bellak's schizophrenics had a mean score of 5.86, considerably lower than this sample. Bellak et al.'s sample of neurotics had a mean score

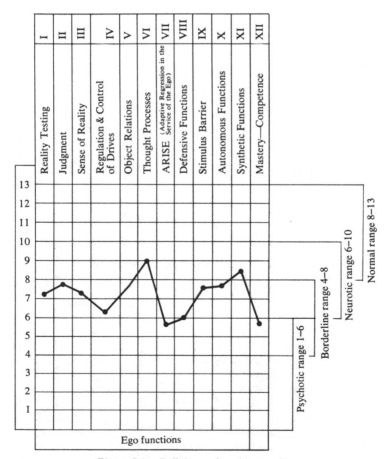

Figure 5.1.   Bellak ego functions profile.

Table 5.1. Ego Functions—General Results

	Mean	SD	Range
Total	7.0	.35	5.6–7.8
Reality Testing	7.3	.42	3–11
Judgment	7.8	.34	4–11
Sense of Reality	7.3	.40	3–11
Regulation of Drives	6.3	.36	3–11
Object Relations	6.5	.30	3–11
Thought Processes	6.9	.33	4–11
ARISE	5.6	.20	3–9
Defensive Functioning	6.5	.30	4–10
Stimulus Barrier	7.5	.33	3–10
Autonomous Functioning	7.6	.29	5–11
Synthetic–Integrative Functioning	7.8	.32	3–11
Mastery–Competence: Actual	6.8	.38	1–10

of 7.42 and that of normals, a score of 9.08. Thus, our population of chronic patients came close to the level of ego functioning of a group of neurotics. This somewhat surprising finding is probably the result of comparing a group of well-medicated schizophrenics with a group of acutely disturbed nonmedicated neurotics. However, it should be noted that the range of each ego function assessed in the schizophrenic sample was extremely broad (e.g., from 1 to 10 on Mastery–Competence), and here may lie a significant difference from the neurotic sample, namely, variability in the profile itself may be diagnostic.

Table 5.2. Intercorrelations of Total Ego Function with the Outcome Dimensions

	Ego Functioning
Rehospitalization:	
Rate	−.24
Severity per episode	.23
Severity per year	.09
Symptomatology	−.72***
Occupational Functioning	−.41*
Social Adjustment	−.56*
Global Functioning	+.36*

Note: * $p < .05$, *** $p < .001$.

Table 5.3A. *Variables Correlated with Individual Ego Functions: Ego Functions 1-6*

Area	Reality Testing	Judgment	Sense of Reality	Regulation of Drives	Object Relations	Thought Processes
Rehospitalization						
Rehospitalization rate	-.36*					
Total in-hospital days	.42*					
Severity per episode	.42*		.36*			
Symptomatology						
BPRS—total	.58***	-.46**	-.54**	-.52**	-.66***	-.43*
Work						
Before first hospitalization						
Since first hospitalization						
Current						
Overall						
Social Adjustment						
Social Adjustment Scale					-.48*	

Note: $* p < .05, ** p < .01, *** p < .001.$

Table 5.3B. *Variables Correlated with Individual Ego Functions: Ego Functions 7–12*

Area	ARISE	Defensive Functioning	Stimulus Barrier	Autonomous Functioning	Synthetic–Integrative Functioning	Mastery–Competence: Actual
Rehospitalization						
Rehospitalization rate						
Total in-hospital days						
Severity per episode						
Symptomatology						
BPRS—total	−.36*	−.59***	−.45*	−.38*	−.56***	−.50**
Work						
Before first hospitalization		.48**			.43*	
Since first hospitalization		.52**		.38*	.42*	.42*
Current		.48**		.50*	.39*	.46**
Overall		.63***		.40*	.46**	.48**
Social Adjustment						
Social Adjustment Scale	−.49**		−.51**			−.61***

Note: * $p < .05$, ** $p < .01$, *** $p < .001$.

78

Correlation of Total Ego Function with the Major Outcome Dimensions

Correlation of total ego functioning score with the major outcome dimensions is shown in Table 5.2. Total ego function correlates best with symptomatology but also correlates moderately well with overall occupational history, including both quantity and quality of lifetime work. Good ego functioning is also significantly associated with good social adjustment and global functioning. Total ego functioning did not correlate significantly with any of the rehospitalization measures.

Correlation of Specific Ego Functions with Other Variables

Tables 5.3 A–B present the correlation of each of the 12 ego functions with each major outcome dimension. For rehospitalization indices, severity per episode is positively correlated with a sense of reality. The only function that correlates with a number of indices is reality testing. Patients with good reality testing tend to have had lower rates of rehospitalization but have greater total days in the hospital and longer episodes of hospitalization.

For symptomatology, each of the ego functions is highly negatively correlated with total BPRS score, suggesting that absence of symptoms or mild symptomatology is strongly associated with good ego functioning.

In the area of occupational functioning it appears that good defensive functioning, autonomous functioning, synthetic–integrative functioning, and mastery–competence are highly positively correlated with quantity of work both in the premorbid period and after the onset of illness as well as with overall lifetime quantity and quality of work.

Good social functioning is positively correlated with good object relations, ability to regress adaptively, high stimulus barrier, and actual mastery–competence.

DISCUSSION

As dynamic theory would predict, we found that total ego function correlated significantly with every major dimension of outcome except rehospitalization. On closer examination we found that rehospitalization correlated significantly with only one specific ego function, reality testing.

The other main dimensions of outcome varied in the degree to which they were correlated with ego function. Symptomatology was most highly related to ego functioning. Social adjustment was next, followed by occupational functioning; rehospitalization was last. This finding may reflect the degree to which a particular outcome dimension is related to intrapsychic as well as other factors, such as competency training or the social environment.

The strong correlation between the specific ego functions and symptomatology may be understood from the following perspective. Symptoms are sensitive reflections of the functional integrity of the individual. To the extent that integrity is impaired, symptoms will appear. On the other hand, work function is not an especially sensitive indication of overall psychological integrity. Work function can at times reflect particular component functions rather than depend on the integrity of the ego as a whole. This is similarly true for certain minimal adaptations in the area of social function.

These data lead us to ask why certain ego functions are especially connected with specific outcome dimensions. Social functioning's correlation with object relations is expected and self-explanatory. The other three ego functions correlated with social function may all be regarded as supporting the critical task of being able truly to listen to the other person. Adaptive regression may indicate empathy and defensive flexibility. High stimulus barrier reflects tolerance for confusing and high-quantity information input, and mastery–competence reflects the self-esteem and task proficiency that are essential to tolerating the potential threat to the self encountered in any social interaction.

Work is most closely related to defensive functioning, autonomous functioning, synthetic–integrative functioning, and mastery–competence. Defensive functioning is important for work because good defenses minimize anxiety, which at high levels has a disruptive effect on task performance. Autonomous functioning and synthetic–integrative function are ego functions traditionally regarded as existing in the "conflict-free" sphere of the ego and associated with such aptitudes as occupational proficiency. Mastery–competence is both a direct assessment of task proficiency by definition and a reflection of a measure of self-esteem perhaps mirroring the "can-do-it" attitude traditionally associated with good work performance.

An understanding of the particular ego deficits that accompany specific functional deficits may have important implications for effective treatment planning. Delineation of these ego functioning disturbances might be used to design more rationally based and specific treatment programs for chronic patients. Causal inference cannot be made from the correlational type of data presented in this report. We might, however, speculate that specific types of therapy can be developed and directed toward improving specific aspects of functioning. For example, a treatment program might be designed that was oriented not toward simply teaching chronic patients to work, but rather toward improving those specific deficits that might bring about greatest improvement in work functioning. This type of approach would allow for an integrated treatment program simultaneously informed and guided by both descriptive and dynamic psychiatry.

ACKNOWLEDGMENTS

We would like to express our deep appreciation to Dr. Myrna Weissman for her advice and consultation, and to Mrs. Jane E. Rowell for her expert secretarial assistance.

REFERENCES

Astrachan, B. M., Harrow, M., Adler, D., et al. A check list for the diagnosis of schizophrenia. *British Journal of Psychiatry,* 1972, *121,* 529–539.

Bellak, L., Hurvich, M., & Gediman, H. K. *Ego functions in schizophrenia, neurotics, and normals: A systematic study of conceptual, diagnostic and therapeutic aspects.* New York: Wiley, 1973.

Brown, G., Birley, J., & Wing, J. Influence of family life on the course of acute schizophrenia: A replication. *British Journal of Psychiatry,* 1972, *121,* 241–258.

Carpenter, W. T., Straus, J., & Bartko, J. Flexible system for the diagnosis of schizophrenia: report from the WHO International Pilot Study of Schizophrenia. *Science,* 1973, *182,* 1275–1278.

Ellsworth, R. B., & Clayton, W. H. Measurement of improvement in mental illness. *Journal of Consulting Psychology,* 1959, *23,* 15–20.

Endicott, J., Spitzer, R. L., Fliss, J., & Cohen, J. The global assessment scale: A procedure for measuring overall severity of psychiatric disturbance. *Archives of General Psychiatry,* 1976, *33,* 766–771.

Erikson, R. C. Outcome studies in mental hospitals: A review. *Psychological Bulletin,* 1975, *82,* 519–540.

Federn, P. In E. Weiss (Ed.), *Ego psychology and the psychoses.* New York: Basic Books, 1952.

Fontana, A. F., & Dowds, B. N. Assessing treatment outcome. I. Adjustment in the community. *Journal of Nervous and Mental Disease,* 1975, *161,* 221–230.

Freeman, T., Cameron, J., & McGhie, A. *Studies on psychosis.* New York: International Universities Press, 1966.

Gittlemen-Klein, R., & Klein, D. Premorbid asocial adjustment and prognosis in schizophrenia. *Journal of Psychiatric Research,* 1969, *7,* 35–53.

Hartmann, H. *Essays on ego psychology.* New York: International Universities Press, 1964.

Keniston, K., Boltax, S., & Almond, R. Multiple criteria of treatment outcome. *Journal of Psychiatric Research,* 1971, *8,* 107–118.

May, P. R. A., & Tuma, H. Choice of criteria for the assessment of treatment outcome. *Journal of Psychiatric Research,* 1964, *2,* 199–209.

Overall, J. E., & Gorham, D. R. The Brief Psychiatric Rating Scale. *Psychological Report,* 1962, *10,* 799.

Schwartz, C., Myers, J., & Astrachan, B. Concordance of multiple assessments of the outcome of schizophrenia. *Archives of General Psychiatry,* 1975, *32,* 1221–1227.

Spitzer, R. L., Endicott, J., & Robins, E. Research diagnostic criteria: Rationale and reliability. *Archives of General Psychiatry,* 1978, *35,* 773–782.

Strauss, J., & Carpenter, W. The prediction of outcome in schizophrenia. I. Characteristics of outcome. *Archives of General Psychiatry,* 1972, *27,* 739–746.

Strauss, J., & Carpenter, W. The prediction of outcome in schizophrenia. II. Relationships between predictor and outcome variables: A report from the WHO International Pilot Study of Schizophrenia. *Archives of General Psychiatry,* 1974, *31,* 37–42.

Weissman, M. M., & Paykel, E. S. *A study of social relationships.* Chicago: University of Chicago Press, 1974.

CHAPTER SIX

Ego Function Assessment—Its Relationship to Psychiatric Hospital Treatment Outcome and Follow-up Adjustment: The Factor Analytic Study

LOLAFAYE COYNE, PATRICIA J. SCHRODER,
SIEBOLT FRIESWYK, MARY CERNEY,
GAVIN NEWSOM, AND PETER NOVOTNY

The Patient Profile Study, an aspect of which is described in this chapter, was an outgrowth of a collaborative length-of-stay study group comprising five private psychiatric hospitals that, in response to PSRO legislation, attempted to find predictors of length of inpatient hospital stay. Later, the Menninger Patient Profile Study Group was formed to investigate the predictability of length of stay and *treatment outcome* from profiles of initial patient characteristics. This chapter describes scales that were developed or whose assessment was modified in order to provide this profile of initial patient characteristics on the basis of which homogeneous patient groups could be derived for which length of stay and treatment outcome could be more effectively predicted. The patients involved were inpatients at the C. F. Menninger Memorial Hospital, a hospital with a strong tradition of long-term psychodynamically oriented treatment. Therefore, it was conceptually important to include in this profile the patient's characteristic ways of evaluating reality, delaying impulses, and organizing work; the patient's manner of internalizing relationships with others; and the character, quality, and tone of the patient in dealing with emotions. To answer these needs we chose the Bellak scales of ego functioning but modified their method of assessment, and two sets* of multi-item scales were developed, the first to assess dimensions of Quality of Object Relations and the second to assess dimensions of Capacity for Emotions. Sets of developmental variables for childhood, latency, adolescence, young adulthood, and adulthood were also selected, and methods of quantification were devised.

THE STUDY PROPER

Subjects

The goal of the study proper was to determine homogeneous groups of patients based on the profile of initial characteristics whose measures were selected after three reliability studies and, for these homogeneous groups, to ascertain the effectiveness of prediction of outcome† and length of stay. The final set of variables was collected for 300 patients discharged from the long-term units of the C. F. Menninger Memorial Hospital between 1973 and 1976 whose records contained adequate information. Table 6.1 presents a summary of the characteristics for these 300 cases.

SCALE DEVELOPMENT

Rating Procedures

A pair of raters rated each of the 300 cases. Although it would have been desirable to have the same pair of raters rate the entire 300 cases, the amount of time required to read the relevant case material and make the ratings was prohibitive. Hence, pairs of raters were chosen from among experienced

---

* These sets of scales are to be reported in a separate paper.
† Findings for a subsample of 78 patients are reported in Chapter 8 in this book.

Table 6.1. Summary of Characteristics of First 150 Cases, Second 150 Cases, and Total Sample

	First 150	Second 150	Total
Admission age			
16–25	88	102	190
26–35	23	24	47
36–45	20	12	32
46–55	13	8	21
56–65	5	4	9
Over 65	1	0	1
Sex			
Male	74	83	157
Female	76	67	143
Adopted	12	17	29
Readmissions	30	30	60
Prior hospitalizations (elsewhere)			
0	34	39	73
1	9	8	17
2	72	57	129
3	21	24	45
4	14	20	34
Over 4	0	2	2
Admission diagnosis (DSM-II)			
Schizophrenia	65	60	125
Major affective disorders	7	6	13
Paranoid states	2	0	2
Other psychoses	3	3	6
Neuroses	25	24	49
Personality disorders	42	52	94
Sexual deviations	1	0	1
Alcoholism	1	2	3
Drug dependence	2	1	3
Special symptoms	1	0	1
Transient situational disturbances	1	2	3
Borderline mental retardation	0	1	1
Discharge diagnosis (DSM-II)			
Senile and presenile dementia	1	1	2
Alcoholic psychosis	0	1	1
Psychosis associated with other cerebral condition	2	1	3
Psychosis associated with other physical condition	0	1	1
Schizophrenia	54	56	110
Major affective disorders	9	6	15
Paranoid states	2	0	2
Other psychoses	1	2	3

Table 6.1.   (Continued)

	First 150	Second 150	Total
Neuroses	18	20	38
Personality disorders	62	62	124
Drug dependence	1	0	1
Length of stay			
3 months or less	32	34	66
3–6 months	34	27	61
6–9 months	19	11	30
9–12 months	11	17	28
12–18 months	22	21	43
18–24 months	15	18	33
24–30 months	9	8	17
30–36 months	3	6	9
More than 36 months	5	8	13
Discharge type			
Straight	106	107	113
Without consent	10	8	18
AMA	34	35	69
Finances involved in discharge	46	49	95
Further treatment			
Here	59	59	118
Elsewhere	41	54	95

clinicians; each pair rated 10 or 20 cases selected in a quasi-random fashion. All raters participated in group rating training sessions. Each pair was then individually supervised by a member of the core group in rating one or more practice cases. The raters completed their ratings separately,* then met and made consensus ratings for the variables on which they were discrepant. In this study *discrepant* was defined as more than one point difference on the five-point scales, more than 10 points difference on the 100-point example-anchored scales, and more than 1 point on the Bellak scales of ego functioning.

Measures

The Bellak scales of ego functioning were designed to be used in conjunction with a clinical interview, but in our study cases they were rated on the basis of medical record data only; we rated only the characteristic level of

* For 13 of the rater pairs, the separate ratings were available and reliability estimates were computed. These are presented for the Bellak scales in Table 6.2.

functioning. Although we did the ratings for the global scales as well as the subscales, we focused on and analyzed only the subscale ratings. Our feeling was that this provided additional information beyond that of Bellak et al. (1973) in *Ego Functions in Schizophrenics, Neurotics, and Normals* about the reliability and the structure of the component parts (the subscales) that make up the global ego function scales. Differences in reliability or differences in factor structure among the subscales point to problems with the use of the global scales alone.

The set of scales constructed to assess dimensions of *Quality of Object Relations* consisted of 54 multi-item scales rated on a five-point Likert-type scale ranging from "no evidence for the behavior" to "extreme evidence of such behavior." The set of *Capacity for Emotion Scales* consisted of 33 multi-item scales rated on the same five-point Likert-type scale. *Developmental variables* were grouped into five different age ranges: *childhood, latency, adolescence, young adulthood,* and *adulthood.* Ratings were done on the basis of clinical inference using five-point example-anchored scales that were specially developed in an attempt to enhance reliability.

Reliability Studies

Three pilot reliability studies were conducted to select variables with adequate reliability. Only the third study is reported. Two groups of raters rated the case summary and social work history and, for certain variables, the discharge summary. The 15 cases that were rated by each group included five diagnoses of schizophrenia, four of neurosis, and six of personality disorders. One group of raters consisted of five experienced clinicians who had helped construct or rate these scales in previous reliability studies; the second group consisted of four experienced clinicians who had not worked with these rating scales previously but who had used rating scales before.

The statistical method used was Spearman–Brown corrected intraclass correlations, which give the estimated reliability of an *average* rating. We chose these because average ratings were to be used in the study proper. Reliabilities were categorized as negative, low (below .50), moderate (between .50 and .70), and high (.70 or above).

Eighteen* of the 34 Bellak scales were rated with moderate or better reliability by both groups of raters. We found that variation in experience in using these scales did not affect the reliability, nor did discipline differences, as long as the raters were experienced clinicians in our setting, familiar with our treatment philosophy and medical records. Table 6.2 gives reliabilities of an average rating for the 34 Bellak scales. Four Bellak scales [Sense of

---

* When reliabilities were recalculated because of an earlier error, the two subscales of Autonomous Functioning no longer met the criterion for adequate reliability. They were retained, however.

Table 6.2. Reliabilities: Bellak Scales

Scales	Five Raters, r_{av}	Four Raters, r_{av}	Mean, r_{av}	Study Proper Mean r_{av}[b]
Reality Testing				
Inner and Outer	.71	.71	.71	.87
Accuracy of Perception	.74	.79	.76	.81
Reflective Awareness—Inner	.47	.64	.56	
Judgment				
Anticipation of Consequences	.61	.69	.65	.71
Manifest in Behavior	.70	.75	.72	.77
Emotional Appropriateness	.79	.67	.73	.76
Sense of Reality				
Extent of Derealization	.24	.70	.47	
Extent of Depersonalization	.32	.61	.46	
Self-Identity and Self-Esteem	.24	.73	.48	
Boundaries—Self and World	.31	.38	.34	
Regulation and Control of Drives, Impulses, and Affects				
Directness of Impulse Expression	.78	.85	.82	.71
Effectiveness of Delay Mechanisms	.56	.83	.70	.77
Object Relations				
Degree and Kind of Relatedness	.57	.72	.64	.74
Primitivity–Maturity	.61	.48	.54	
Others Perceived Independently	.61	.42	.52	
Object Constancy	.68	.68	.68	.56
Thought Processes				
Memory, Concentration, Attention	.43	.57	.50	
Ability to Conceptualize	.64	.72	.68	.84
Primary–Secondary Process	.85	.69	.77	.82
Adaptive Regression in the Service of the Ego				
Regressive Relaxation of Acuity	.01	.45	.23	
New Configurations	.21	.63	.42	
Defensive Functioning				
Presence of Defensive Indicators	.62	.40	.51	
Success and Failure of Defenses	.53	.46	.50	
Stimulus Barrier				
Threshold for Stimuli	− .62	.25	− .18	
Coping Success	− .42	.61	.10	

Table 6.2.   (*Continued*)

Scales	Five Raters, r_{av}	Four Raters, r_{av}	Mean, r_{av}	Study Proper Mean $r_{av}[b]$
Autonomous Functioning				
Freedom of Impairment—Primary	.44	.51	.48[a]	.85
Freedom of Impairment—Secondary	.45	.50	.48[a]	.78
Synthetic–Integrative Functioning				
Reconciliation of Incongruities	.72	.73	.72	.84
Active Relating Together of Events	.63	.72	.68	.75
Mastery–Competence				
Actual Competence	.69	.69	.69	.79
Sense of Competence	.35	.16	.26	
Discrepancy—Performance and Self-Feeling	.35	.16	.26	
Superego Scale				
Guilt	.75	.70	.72	.68
Ego Ideal	.74	.71	.72	.67
Mean of 18 retained:			.69	.76

[a] Included because of an earlier error.

[b] Mean of Spearman–Brown-corrected product-moment correlations between members of a rater pair for 13 rater pairs.

Reality, Adaptive Regression in the Service of the Ego (ARISE), Defensive Functioning, and Stimulus Barrier] were dropped from the project, having no subscales that achieved adequate reliability. Mastery–Competence was represented by only one subscale, Actual Competence. From Reality Testing and Thought Processes one subscale was dropped because of inadequate reliability, and from Object Relations two subscales were dropped. Only the global scales of Judgment; Regulation and Control of Drives, Impulses, and Affects; Autonomous Functioning; Synthetic–Integrative Functioning; and Superego Adaptation had all subscales retained. This may have had implications for the factor analyses to be described later.

Twenty-five of the 54 Quality of Object Relations items achieved moderate to high reliabilities,* as did 16 of the 33 Capacity for Emotion items. Twenty of the 22 Developmental Variables rated on the basis of clinical inference on example-anchored scales achieved at least moderate reliability. The set of Developmental scales was revised one final time, and in spite of our concerns about the sparseness of developmental data in the medical

* These reliabilities may be obtained from the authors.

record, this set was included. The 25 Quality of Object Relations items, the 16 Capacity for Emotions items, and 19 Developmental Variables were retained.

Sampling Strategies

Since the number of variables in the study proper was large, strategies were devised to guard against interpretation of chance relationships in the statistical analyses. One such strategy was to divide the sample of 300 patients randomly into an initial sample of 150 and a replication sample of 150. These samples were found to be remarkably similar on length of stay, type of discharge, and proportions of our two predominant diagnoses, schizophrenia and personality disorder. Table 6.1 also gives the sample characteristics for the first and second random samples of 150 cases.

Statistical Analysis

There was a need for basic (and independent) dimensions within the broad areas of structure, ego functioning, object relations, ways of dealing with emotions, and development that would aid in the interpretation of future findings in addition to being interpretable on their own. Hence, factor analyses of the sets of variables included in the profile of initial patient characteristics were conducted using principal components analysis and rotation to the normal varimax criterion.* The dimensions that emerged (i.e., the rotated factors) were examined for clinical interpretability and then independent (uncorrelated) factor scores were calculated for each of these dimensions. These factor scores represent the original variables but are fewer in number and on a conceptually higher level. They were used for the Bellak scales, Quality of Object Relation scales, Capacity for Emotion scales, and Developmental variables in further statistical analyses.

Following the determination that the factor solutions were indeed clinically interpretable, the factor analyses were then repeated for the second (replication) sample of 150 cases. These two factor structures were compared by the Kaiser Factor Matching Method (Kaiser, 1960) to see how well the factor structure from the first sample was replicated by that from the second sample. In most cases they were found to be comparable. Then the factor structure obtained from the initial sample was used to calculate factor scores† for the second sample.

The final analysis to be reported is the intercorrelation of factor scores from different content areas. This procedure enabled us to look for possible overlap among the factors obtained from different sets of variables but repre-

---

* Those factors with eigenvalues of 1 or greater were rotated.
† Not necessarily uncorrelated when calculated in this manner.

Table 6.3. Normal Varimax Rotated Factor Loadings, Bellak Scales

Scales	Factor I: Freedom from Thought Disorder			Factor II: Judgment and Impulse Control			Factor III: Superego Functioning		
	1st 150	2nd 150	Comp.	1st 150	2nd 150	Comp.	1st 150	2nd 150	Comp.
Reality Testing									
Inner and Outer	.805	.810	.791	—	—	—	—	—	—
Accuracy of Perception	.781	.834	.814	—	—	—	—	—	—
Judgment									
Judgment–Anticipation– Consequence	—	—	—	.803	.809	.849	—	—	—
Manifest in Behavior	—	—	—	.818	.852	.884	—	—	—
Emotional Appropriateness	—	.558	.522	.779	.555	.615	—	—	—
Impulse Control									
Regulation and Control of Drives—Impulse Expression	—	—		.663	.757	.791	.502	—	—
Delay Mechanisms	—	—		.723	.686	.722	—	—	—
Object Relations									
Object Relations–Degree Relatedness	—	—		—	—	—	—	.637	.586
Object Constancy	—	—		—	—	—	—	.538	—

	C1	C2	C3	C4	C5	C6
Thought Processes						
Thought Processes–Ability to Conceptualize	.818	.845	.842	—	—	—
Primary–Secondary Process	.875	.874	.873	—	—	—
Autonomous Functioning						
Freedom Impairment						
Primary	.835	.843	.838	—	—	—
Secondary Autonomy	.726	.721	.721	—	—	—
Synthetic–Integrative Functioning						
Reconciliation of Incongruity	.596	.629	.628	—	.564	—
Relating Together of Events	.624	.650	.667	—	.568	—
Mastery–Competence						
Actual Competence	.599	.494	.522	—	—	.510
Superego						
Guilt	—	—	—	.810	.795	.767
Ego ideal	—	—	—	.782	.846	.818
Percent of total variance	32.88	33.62	24.22	19.27	15.89	20.54

91

senting conceptually similar content. Examination of factors obtained from the sets of variables prompted the hypothesis that certain factors from the Quality of Object Relations Scales and the Capacity for Emotion Scales should be correlated with certain factors from the Bellak scales of ego functioning and with each other and these hypotheses were explored in the last preliminary analysis.

Factor Analyses of the Bellak Ego Function Scales

Initial Factor Analysis. The dimensions that emerged from the first set of factor analyses were clinically interpretable, comprehensive, and represented basic dimensions from which it should be possible to predict outcome and length of stay. In addition, the number of variables to be analyzed was appropriately reduced.

Table 6.3 gives the normal varimax rotated solutions for the two samples together with the composite solution. Table 6.4 gives the comparison of the initial and replication factor structures.

Examination of the Bellak factor structures for the initial sample revealed that three factors were sufficient to account for 73% of the total variance; this is most of the reliable variance common to the 18 original scales. The first factor of the unrotated solution was examined to see if it could be interpreted as a general factor.* For the initial sample this verged on being a general factor. It accounted for 58% of the variance and had loadings of .60 or above on all of the 18 subscales. If this general factor were to be used as the one basic dimension representing the 18 Bellak subscales, it could be conceptualized as a general ego strength factor or, perhaps more generally, as a health–sickness factor. Since we wanted to have more differentiated dimensions representing the areas of ego functioning assessed by the Bellak scales, we utilized the rotated solution for the study. All three factors were quite large and were interpreted.

Factor I had defining loadings on all the subscales of Reality Testing, Thought Processes, and Autonomous Functioning. Smaller loadings were present for the two subscales of Synthetic–Integrative Functioning and the one subscale remaining from Mastery–Competence. It was not a general factor and was named "Freedom from Thought Disorder." The dimension defined by this factor deals essentially with structural considerations rather than relationships. The factor was described as representing the degree of freedom from impairment of the major ego functions, including thought, reality testing, and memory.

The second factor had defining loadings on all the subscales for Judgment and Regulation and Control of Drives, Impulses, and Affects and was entitled "Judgment and Impulse Control." It represents the ability of the patient

---

* A special kind of factor accounting for a very large proportion of the total variance and with defining loadings (.60 or above in this chapter) on all variables.

Table 6.4.   Relate: Cosines Among Factor Axes, Bellak Ego Functions Scales

	Second Sample		
First Sample	Factor I	Factor II	Factor III
Factor I	.9922	.0844	−.9020
Factor II	.0867	.0635	.9942
Factor III	−.0897	.9944	−.0557

to evaluate the appropriateness and consequences of his social behavior in conjunction with the ability to contain or express behavior that is in keeping with that evaluation.

The third factor had only two defining loadings (the two subscales of the Superego scale) and hence was entitled "Superego Functioning." A problem with the use of the subscales of the Superego scale is that a high rating might reflect opposite clinical findings; that is, it might mean either an over- or underfunctioning of the superego. There is some question as to the clinical usefulness of the factor in view of this ambiguity. We decided to keep this factor but hoped that other measures would help us interpret what a high score on this factor might mean.

An unexpected finding in the initial sample was that the two subscales of Object Relations did not have defining loadings on any of the three factors. Although the emergence of a separate common factor is somewhat limited with only two subscales, it was difficult to understand why these two subscales were not sufficiently correlated with other subscales so that they loaded on one of the other factors.

Replication Factor Analysis. The factor structure for the Bellak scales from the second sample replicated that of the first quite well. Table 6.4 indicates the matches among the factors.

Table 6.3 also gives the composite factor structure for the Bellak scales of ego functioning. This was considered as an alternative choice for the definition of Bellak factors; however, we used the initial factor solution, in part, because this facilitated calculation of uncorrelated factor scores.

Factor Analyses of the Quality of Object Relations (QOR) Scales*

Initial Factor Analysis. The factor analyses of the QOR Scales for the initial sample yielded four factors that cumulatively accounted for 67.4% of

* These factor analytic results may be requested from the authors.

the total variance. Factor I had seven defining loadings—Indiscriminately Hostile, Tyrannizing, Angry Outbursts, Demanding, Contempt, Extreme Contradictory Reactions, and Exploitative—and was entitled "Infantile Demandingness."

Factor II had four defining loadings—Fantasy Withdrawal, Estranged, Psychotic Confusion, and Confused—and was named "Ego Regression and Isolation."

Factor III had three defining loadings—Gentle, Remorseful, and Cooperative—and was called "Capacity for Concern." It was the one QOR factor that we positively oriented.

The fourth factor had only three defining loadings—Sexually Exploitative, Indiscriminate Relationships, and Perverse—and was entitled "Sexual Exploitativeness."

Replication Factor Analysis. The first two factors of the initial factor solution were almost perfectly replicated in the second solution. Factor III was replicated less well. The fourth factor was replicated. The composite solution represented equally well either of the two separate solutions.

Factor Analyses of the Capacity for Emotion (CFE) Scales*

Initial Factor Analysis. The factor analysis of the CFE scales for the initial sample yielded four factors cumulatively accounting for 68.2% of the total variance.

The first factor had six defining loadings—Discharge Frustration, Angry Outbursts, Acts on Rage Verbally, Sadistic and Hostile, Experiences Rage, Expresses Feelings Wildly, and Acts on Rage Physically. The key concept underlying this factor was aggression and it was entitled "Hostility and Rage."

Factor II had four defining loadings—Acts Impulsively, Feelings Changeable, Driven or Frenzied, and Relationships Willy-Nilly. It dealt with changeability, impulsivity, and the need to reduce tensions and was named "Tension Discharge."

Factor III had three defining loadings: Confuses Feelings with What Others Feel, Loses Ability to Think Clearly, and Arbitrary and Contrary. It reflected the amount of ego regression in the face of strong affect and was called "Psychotic Vulnerability."

Factor IV also had three defining loadings—Shares Emotional Experiences, Exaggerates Feelings, and Mood Elevated. It dealt with affect arousal and was called "Emotional Variability."

Replication Factor Analysis. The first factor was almost identically replicated. Factor II, however, was not replicated. Factor III was almost com-

---

* These factor analytic results may be requested from the authors.

pletely replicated. The fourth factor was somewhat less completely replicated. The matches for this set of scales were somewhat poorer than those
for the Bellak and QOR scales.

Factor Analyses of the Developmental Variables*

Initial Factor Analysis.   Data in the medical record available to make
the required inferences on developmental variables were more sparse than
those for the other ratings. The level of the intercorrelations for this set of
variables was considerably lower than that of any of the other correlation
matrices. This implied that the developmental variables were much more
differentiated than the previous content areas and this was borne out by the
factor solution in which six factors cumulatively accounted for 71% of the
total variance.

The first rotated factor had four defining loadings—Interpersonal Style
and Development, Latency; Interpersonal Style and Development, Childhood; Psychologically Symptomatic, Childhood; and Peer Relations, Latency—and was named "(Poor) Social Adaptation in Childhood and Latency."

The second factor had three defining loadings—Drug and Alcohol Abuse,
Behavior, and Symptoms (all three for adolescence)—and was entitled
"Acting Out."

Factor III had three defining loadings—Learning Difficulties, Symptoms,
and Behavior, all for latency. Hence, this factor was named "School Difficulty." This interpretation was further supported by a smaller (but nondefin-
ing) loading on Learning Difficulties, Adolescence.

Factor IV had three defining loadings—Special Skills, Childhood, Latency, and Adolescence. This factor was quite specific and was called "Special Skills." Although small, it was of interest because it was positively
oriented and represented an assessment of patient assets at admission that
have been considered to be predictive of good outcome.

Factor V had only two defining loadings—Sexual Interest and Interpersonal Style and Development, both for adolescence. It was difficult to find a
common conceptual thread that linked these two loadings; hence, the fifth
factor was not named or interpreted further.

The sixth factor had three defining loadings—Motor Disturbance, Somatic Complaints, and Speech Disturbance, all at childhood. This factor was
named "Organicity."

Replication Factor Analysis.   The first factor was replicated but the second factor was not replicated very well, while factor III was not replicated at
all. Factors IV and VI were partially replicated, while factor V was not
replicated. This poor matching cast doubt on the further usefulness of the

---

* These factor analytic results may be requested from the authors.

Table 6.5. *Intercorrelations of Bellak Ego Functions, Quality of Object Relations, Capacity for Emotions, and Developmental Variables Factors—First Sample*

	Bellak			Quality of Object Relations				Capacity for Emotions			
Scales	F-I	F-II	F-III	F-I	F-II	F-III	F-IV	F-I	F-II	F-III	F-IV
Quality of Object Relations											
Factor I: Infantile Demandingness	−.029	−.453***	−.111								
Factor II: Ego Regression and Isolation	−.765***	−.138	−.140								
Factor III: Capacity for Concern	−.002	.324***	.283***								
Factor IV: Sexual Exploitativeness	.030	−.219**	.126								
Capacity for Emotions											
Factor I: Hostility and Rage	−.055	−.370***	−.258***	.721***	.076	−.252**	−.205				
Factor II: Tension Discharge	.131	−.368***	−.058	.406***	−.027	−.146	.368***				

Factor III: Psychotic Vulnerability	-.726***	-.172*	-.052	.132	.839***	.104	.052				
Factor IV: Emotional Variability	.038	-.050	.278***	.188*	-.125	.371***	.258**				
Developmental Variables											
Factor I: Social Adaptation in Childhood (Poor)	.064	-.080	-.183*	.154	.038	-.026	-.145	.156*	.031	-.073	-.083
Factor II: Acting Out	.117	-.306***	-.035	.174*	-.065	-.121	.293***	.163*	.307***	-.068	.017
Factor III: School Difficulty	-.150	-.158*	-.055	.154	.088	-.116	.027	.141	-.003	.092	.023
Factor IV: Special Skills	-.015	.154	.000	.015	.024	-.002	.003	.031	-.051	-.049	-.015
Factor V	-.221**	-.092	-.067	-.039	.313***	-.139	-.095	.060	-.046	.165*	-.096
Factor VI: Organicity	.012	.040	.045	-.032	.025	.137	-.009	-.052	-.063	.019	-.037

Note: $*p < .05, **p < .01, ***p < .001$.

Developmental Variables factor scores and perhaps even of the Developmental Variables themselves.

Relationships Among Factor Solutions from Different Sets of Scales

Two hypotheses about possible relationships among factor solutions from different sets of scales* were generated on the basis of common theoretical elements in their definitions. These hypothesized relationships were that: (1) Bellak Factor I, "Freedom from Thought Disorder," QOR Factor II, "Ego Regression and Isolation," and CFE Factor III, "Psychotic Vulnerability," should be highly correlated, and (2) QOR Factor I, "Infantile Demandingness," and CFE Factor I, "Hostility and Rage," should be correlated.

Table 6.5 presents the correlation matrix that summarizes the relationships among all the factor scores from the first sample factor solution. Although there were a number of significant correlations among the factor scores from the various content areas, the four highest correlations in the matrix, all above .70,† were the correlations hypothesized earlier. The three factors—Bellak Factor I, "Freedom from Thought Disorder"; QOR Factor II, "Ego Regression and Isolation"; and CFE Factor III, "Psychotic Vulnerability"—were highly, and very significantly, intercorrelated. Similarly, QOR Factor I, Infantile Demandingness," and CFE I, "Hostility and Rage," were highly and very significantly correlated. This may be taken as evidence of construct validity for these factors.

It was observed that one factor from the Developmental Variables was also significantly correlated with each of the three factor scores of hypothesis (1), Bellak Factor I, QOR Factor II, and CFE Factor III. This was Developmental Factor V, the factor that had only two defining loadings, Sexual Interest and Interpersonal Style and Development, both at adolescence, and that had not been named or interpreted. This relationship was puzzling although consistent and significant.

A number of other significant but only moderate-sized correlations were found. Bellak Factor II, "Judgment and Impulse Control," was significantly correlated with a number of factors in the other content areas (see Table 6.5). It was apparent that the factors that related to Judgment and Impulse Control were factors dealing with more specific ways in which poor judgment and/or poor impulse control could be exhibited, or in the case of the one positive factor, a way in which good judgment and/or good impulse control could be demonstrated.

---

* Although factor scores from a given set of scales were calculated so that they would be uncorrelated, as were the factor dimensions, there was no implication that factor scores coming from different sets of scales would be uncorrelated.

† Thus accounting for more than 50% common variance between the two factor scores being correlated.

Bellak Factor III, "Superego Functioning," was highly significantly correlated with several other factors. For the most part, these correlations also made sense, indicating ways in which good or poor "Superego Functioning" could be demonstrated. The one relationship that was difficult to understand was the positive correlation between Superego Functioning and Emotional Variability.

QOR and CFE factors also had several significant interrelationships. QOR Factor III, Capacity for Concern, was significantly related positively to CFE Factor IV, Emotional Variability, which was difficult to understand. CFE factors were also related to several Developmental factors in sensible ways.

The interpretability of the correlations among the various sets of factor scores gives a kind of construct validity to the various factors that have behaved as they could be expected to do on the basis of their definition.

DISCUSSION

If the Patient Profile Study reliabilities for the separate subscales are averaged, some assessment of comparability of reliabilities with those found by Bellak et al. can be made. Several of the global scales in our study were represented by fewer subscales than Bellak intended because they were dropped for reasons of poor reliability based on our own pilot work. Both studies obtained moderately good reliabilities for the following scales: Reality Testing, Thought Processes, Regulation and Control of Drives, and Synthetic–Integrative Functioning. For both studies the reliabilities for Sense of Reality, Defensive Functioning, and Stimulus Barrier were poor: Bellak et al. noted problems with the reliability of ARISE; this too was one of the set of subscales with poor reliability for the Patient Profile Study. The only striking differences between the Bellak et al. reliabilities and the Patient Profile reliabilities were (1) on the global scale of Judgment, for which the Patient Profile reliabilities were considerably higher, and (2) on the global scale of Affective Functioning, for which the Bellak et al. reliability was considerably higher. In general, the results from the two studies parallel each other rather closely; this is of particular interest, since the ratings for the Patient Profile reliability study were done retrospectively on the basis of medical record data while those for the Bellak et al. study were done on the basis of a structured interview designed to assess the ego function scales.

It can be speculated that there is an inherent unreliability in the four global scales that were problematic for both studies, Stimulus Barrier, Defensive Functioning, Sense of Reality, and ARISE. Bellak et al. commented that Stimulus Barrier and ARISE were the two global scales that they had most trouble dimensionalizing. This may call into question the idea that these scales are unidimensional, and lack of unidimensionality is a major source of unreliability.

It was our consensus that at least moderate reliabilities for 16 of the 34 subscales rated retrospectively from medical record data was an achievement not only for our raters but for the Bellak scales, which proved robust when rated from a different, albeit high-quality, data base. We also felt that the set of scales that had adequate reliability made possible a rather complete description of intrapsychic functioning. This was borne out in the factor analyses and their interrelationships and in the findings from the Pilot Study and the Follow-up Outcome Study reported in Chapters 10 and 11 in this book. We concluded that although the reliabilities were not strikingly high, many were acceptable for research purposes and for clinical use as well. The reliabilities obtained in the study proper maintained the suitably high level. Relationships with other variables seemed not to be limited.

Turning to a comparison of the results of the Patient Profile Study and the Bellak et al. factor analyses, the factoring in these two studies was done on an entirely different basis. The Patient Profile Study used *subscales,* which gave a global scale a chance to emerge as a factor. The Bellak et al. study, on the other hand, used *global* scales, which meant that *combinations* of global scales would probably be the factors. Hence, it is difficult to know what the lack of comparability between the solutions means.

The fact that in our study all of the subscales of a particular global scale loaded on each of the three Patient Profile factors has added strength to the original concepts of the global scales whose subscales were devised on the basis of theory rather than empirical data. Our empirical data support, to a degree, their "belongingness."

In part, the validity of the factor solutions can be examined in terms of their clinical interpretability and their usefulness in predicting outcome criteria. We felt that the factor analyses were meaningful clinically. The three factors obtained ("Freedom from Thought Disorder," "Judgment and Impulse Control," and "Superego Functioning") make a rather complete description of intrapsychic functioning. The one puzzling finding was the absence of a factor or a defining loading for the Bellak Object Relations subscales. For the Patient Profile Study, the QOR scales had been devised especially to tap dimensions of Object Relations, and the QOR factors were indeed related to the Bellak factors in meaningful ways. Similarly, the CFE factors were related to the Bellak factors in clinically interpretable ways. The sets of Bellak Ego Function Scales, QOR Scales, and CFE Scales, when factored, seem to yield a set of dimensions that reinforce and supplement each other in the description of the intrapsychic functioning of long-term hospitalized chronically ill patients. It should be noted that this could, at least in part, be due to the cognitive structure relating these concepts in our raters' minds. The concepts implied by the Developmental Variables are also important for our understanding of such patients, but the problems of sparse, inadequately remembered and in other ways problematic developmental data in the medical record had led to assessment difficulties for the Developmental Variables that we have not as yet overcome.

The predictive power of the Bellak factors was tested and is described in Chapters 7 and 8 in this book. In both cases initial assessments of the 18 Bellak subscales factored into the three dimensions described in this chapter were able to predict outcome in clinically meaningful and expectable ways. When follow-up has been completed for all 300 cases of the study proper, the predictive power and the analysis of change provided by the Bellak scales will be further tested with a larger sample size and an opportunity for replication.

REFERENCES

Bellak, L., Hurvich, M., & Gediman, H. K. *Ego functions in schizophrenics, neurotics, and normals: A systematic study of conceptual, diagnostic, and therapeutic aspects.* New York: Wiley, 1973.

Kaiser, H. F. *Relating factors between studies based upon different individuals.* Unpublished, University of Illinois, 1960.

Veldman, Donald J. *Fortran programming for the behavioral sciences.* New York: Holt, Rinehart and Winston, 1967, pp. 238–244.

Ego Function Assessment—Its Relationship to Psychiatric Hospital Treatment Outcome and Follow-up Adjustment: A Pilot Study

SIEBOLT FRIESWYK, PATRICIA J. SCHRODER,
LOLAFAYE COYNE, MARY CERNEY,
GAVIN NEWSOM, AND PETER NOVOTNY

Over the last decade a group of research investigators at the Menninger Foundation's C. F. Menninger Memorial Hospital conducted an extensive investigation of patient characteristics most relevant to treatment planning. Chapter 6 describes the instrument development phase of the project, and this and the following chapters describe our efforts to study increasingly large samples of patients treated at the institution who were followed after hospital discharge to assess the long-range impact of the treatment process. Ours was a project initiated by Peter Novotny, a psychiatrist and psychoanalyst whose principal conviction was that the standard nosology of American psychiatry, *The Diagnostic and Statistical Manual,* was of little relevance to treatment planning. It was a nosology that scarcely began to organize systematically the complex array of interpersonal and intrapsychic factors that appeared to be of major import in assessing the suitability and effectiveness of our treatment approaches. Purely descriptive and phenomenological approaches also had failed to generate the kinds of meaningful groupings of patients that would help us to evaluate the impact of treatment. The publication of Leopold Bellak's seminal contribution *Ego Functions in Schizophrenics, Neurotics, and Normals* (1973) offered a framework that was at once compatible with our basic commitment to a psychoanalytic point of view and that at the same time opened the possibility to quantify observations, develop meaningful groupings of patients independent of the standard nosology, and compare treatment-related change over time within relatively homogeneous groups. It was a fortunate wedding of our interests and a new and exciting methodology. It was a methodology that would allow us to pursue our principal aim.

The aim of our research was to define and quantify patient characteristics predictive of long-term psychiatric hospital treatment outcome and follow-up adjustment. Our primary data were everyday clinical documents. In approaching these data we were guided by two complementary measurement strategies. First, we devised measurement techniques to organize observational data reported by staff at a descriptive level. Second, we employed raters with clinical and theoretical sophistication who shared our psychodynamic frame of reference. We asked these raters to rate patient behavior directly observed by staff and reported descriptively in the clinical documents. We also asked them to rate more abstract, less directly observable ego psychological variables on instruments requiring clinical reference. We pursued this strategy because the descriptive and theoretical frameworks were congenial to our setting and our raters. Our intent was to translate the results of our work into the language and practice of our colleagues to enhance their efforts to understand (1) what makes it possible for a patient to participate in the treatment process, (2) what impediments stand in the way, and (3) what treatment efforts for what groups of patients are most effective.

The data used by the raters in our study were obtained from clinical records of patients discharged within a 4-year period from a long-term psychiatric hospital setting (the psychiatrist's case summary and the social worker's family study). Data from psychological test reports were *excluded* so that the clinical data could serve as external validity criteria for subsequent assessments of quantified test-based measures. The clinical records were, of course, written in a special context, which needs to be described in order to understand more accurately the nature of the data. The hospital is predominantly psychoanalytically oriented, although recent developments in psychopharmacology and the biochemical bases of behavior have been introduced and influence diagnostic appraisals and treatment planning. Historical and psychological data are organized around psychodynamic inferences, family interactions, and an object relations view of the patient's interactions with others in the hospital setting. Each patient has an inpatient evaluation lasting approximately 6–8 weeks, during which time the patient is seen daily for half-hour interviews with the evaluating psychiatrist. The patient is also actively involved with various patient and staff groups, that is, intensive family group meetings, small patient groups organized around therapeutic community principles, patient government groups, and a variety of scheduled activities, including programs of physical exercise and creative crafts. The observations are abundant and must be distilled and integrated by the evaluating psychiatrist. The psychiatrist's case summary thus reflects a mixture of first-level observations, second-hand reports, and psychodynamic inferences.

These complex data need to be evaluated by someone intimately familiar with the setting, its personnel, their theoretical and practical biases, and the evocative and provocative character of the patients' psychopathology. In approaching these data it is imperative for the rater to avoid a kind of naive blindness to the variety of factors influencing the information reported in the clinical documents. Even in making ratings on scales that simply and explicitly describe behavior, the rater must sort out as well as reorganize the data in a disciplined and judicious manner. In other words, it requires as much or perhaps more clinical inference on the part of the sophisticated clinical rater to make ratings on behaviorally anchored scales than it does in making judgments on more inferentially based, abstract, ego psychological variables. The quantitative ratings can thus be considered to be the final end product of multiple layers of patient behavior, staff observation and interaction, and clinical inference.

In our efforts to extract from these extensive clinical data a set of quantitative research measures that would help us to evaluate relevant patient dimensions, we engaged in an extensive process of scale development. The final set of measures included (1) ego function assessment measures (EFA) that were adopted to assess more inferentially based organizing factors in the patient's behavior, and (2) behavioral measures, designed to assess quality of relationships, emotional responsiveness, and developmental characteristics. These latter measures were developed "in-house" and were targeted at behavioral descriptions available in the clinical records. In what follows we will introduce you to these measures.

1. *Bellak Scales (EFA)*.   The Bellak EFA technique (Bellak, Hurvich, & Gediman, 1973) originally was designed to be applied to a semistructured interview conducted along lines suggested in an interview manual. In our application we shifted the data base for the ratings from the semistructured interview to clinical documents and we engaged in an extensive process of scale selection and factor analyses to distill the Bellak measures into a group of scales representing each of three factors: Thought Disorder, Judgment and Impulse Control, and Superego Functioning. Chapter 6 describes that

factor analytic work. The descriptions we evolved for each of the levels on these factors appear in Table 7.1.

2. *Behavioral Measures.* While the Bellak scales are designed to assess important dimensions of object relations (closeness versus distance, primitivity versus maturity, extent of differentiation from self, object constancy versus inconstancy), they do so at a level of clinical inference somewhat removed from the data of observation. Thus, we developed a set of descriptors that characterize commonly observed clinical behaviors. We chose descriptions that would be of interest to us both clinically and theoretically. The scales were designed to be applied to both clinical documents and direct clinical observation and thus could serve as a bridge between information gathered from clinical records and information derived from raters' direct observations of relevant behaviors.

Two sets of measures were developed. The first assessed Quality of Relations (QOR) and the second assessed Capacity for Emotion (CFE). The names of the factors and their descriptions appear in Table 7.2 along with a set of developmental factors. Briefly, the developmental factors were aimed at assessing motor and speech development, somatic complaints, psychological symptoms, peer relationships, special talents, learning difficulties, drug and alcohol abuse, and sexual interests.

SUBJECTS

The subjects for this study were drawn from two research projects in which the senior author either was a coinvestigator or held responsibility for instrument development. The first, a treatment evaluation and follow-up project (see Harty et al., 1981), included the usual diagnostic range of patients treated within the hospital setting in which the research was conducted. The second was a more specialized project focusing on the treatment of schizophrenic patients (see Chapter 9). The total number of subjects included in this study was 32. They ranged in age from 19 to 47 and were hospitalized an average of 649.81 days, with a range of 51 days to 3933 days. There were 17 men and 15 women. The DSM-II diagnoses included in the sample were 24 schizophrenics, 1 other psychosis, 5 personality disorders, and 2 neuroses. All patients in the sample remained in the hospital treatment process long enough at least to complete an inpatient evaluation. Eight patients were discharged against medical advice and three committed suicide after completing inpatient hospitalization.

CLUSTER ANALYSIS

Since the aim of our research was to develop profiles of patient functioning that would be related systematically to outcome, we adopted a special

Table 7.1. Factor Level Composite Descriptions

Level	Factor I: Thought Disorder	Factor II: Judgment and Impulse Control	Factor III: Superego Functioning
1	Little ability to function in a secondary process manner or even to communicate reasonably with others.	Major failures in judgment. Little awareness of consequences. Might take extreme risks that endanger life, limb, and property. Highly inappropriate social behavior. Extreme sexual acting out. Very little impulse control. Chronic self-destructive behavior.	Unrealistic guilt. Extreme self-criticism and self-punishment, including severe depression and suicide.
2	Severe hallucinations, delusions, disorientation, feelings of confusion. Inability to distinguish fantasy from reality on a continuing basis.	Inappropriate judgment. Might actually engage in significantly disruptive social behavior, assaultive acts. Violent behavior either self or other directed. Rapid, extreme mood swings. Physical constraint may be necessary to control behavior. Poor frustration tolerance.	Self-mutilation, delusional guilt, unrealistic standards. Very poor sense of self-worth. Virtual absence of conscious guilt feelings. Psychopathic or extreme impulsivity. Indifference to own performance.
3	Delusions and distortions of reality are mostly stress related. A mixture of delusions and need-determined perceptions.	Sporadic expression of impulse urges, temper tantrums. Might be seen as overly excitable. Either completely controlled or episodically discontrolled.	Rigid authoritarian attitudes about sex and aggression. Strives to avoid blame and criticism. Severely self-critical. Hypercritical of others. Lax, self-indulgent, careless evaluations of self and others. More evidence of shame than guilt.
4	Stress-related disturbances in thinking involving concrete-	Episodic moderate failures in judgment. Hidden chronic	Puritanical, perfectionistic. Glib, happy-go-lucky, casual.

Table 7.1. (*Continued*)

Level	Factor I: Thought Disorder	Factor II: Judgment and Impulse Control	Factor III: Superego Functioning
	ness and failures in logic with some impairment in conceptualization. Occasional peculiar ideas and other minor difficulties. Need-determined projection of inner states onto external reality.	characterological problems in judgment but they are within a broad range. May have poor judgment in social situations but not severe enough to cause major problems in and of themselves. Some failures in judgment and not a great deal of awareness of why such failures occur. Aggression is more likely to be verbal than physical or could be disguised in occupational activity. Fairly excitable with not very flexible control over behavior. Likely to respond to external guidance and instruction.	
5	Minor failures of conceptualization. Occasional vagueness. Occasional peculiarities, personalized associations. Somewhat overly rigid or loose. Minor perceptual inaccuracies.	Minor defects in judging own or other's intentions. Some impulsivity of a mild sort. Some effort is required to control behavior when stressed.	Some tolerance for guilt. Occasional defensiveness, somewhat perfectionistic. Suffers low self-esteem in failure to meet self or others' expectations.
6	No detectable significant distortions in thinking and reality testing. May be egocentric.	Few errors in anticipation of consequences. Past errors in judgment only occasionally repeated. In tune with others except in new situations.	No cases at this level.

Table 7.2. Factor Definitions for Quality of Relations, Capacity for Emotion, and Developmental Factors

Factor Labels	Definition
Quality of Relations (QOR)	
I: Infantile Demandingness	Encompasses behavior described as indiscriminately hostile and includes the following kinds of behaviors: angry outbursts; tyrannizing, demanding, contemptuous, and exploitative behavior.
II: Ego Regression and Isolation	Encompasses behavior described as withdrawn, estranged, and psychotically confused.
III: Capacity for Concern	Encompasses behavior described as gentle, remorseful, and cooperative.
IV: Sexual Exploitation	Encompasses behavior described as sexually exploitative, as may be seen in indiscriminate and perverse relationships.
Capacity for Emotion (CFE)	
I: Hostility and Rage	Encompasses behavior described as hostile, angry, and sadistic in both its verbal and physical expression.
II: Tension Discharge	Encompasses behavior described as impulsive, changeable, and frenzied, as seen at times in fleeting relationships.
III: Psychotic Vulnerability	Encompasses behavior that suggests that emotional arousal leads to disorganized thinking and the progressive inability to distinguish one's thoughts from other's thoughts.
IV: Emotional Lability	Encompasses behavior described as emotionally expansive and exaggerated.
Developmental Factors (DEV)	
I: Interpersonal Problems (Ages 0–12)	
II: Acting Out (Ages 12–18)	
III: Symptom Development (ages 5–12)	
IV: Special Skills	
V: Interpersonal Problems (ages 12–18)	
VI: Organicity	

statistical technique that allowed us to group patients together according to individual profiles and then relate these groups to outcome criteria. The technique we employed for developing these clusters was Ward's Hierarchical Grouping Analysis,* a form of cluster analysis that uses a profile of variables for each patient as data.

OUTCOME CRITERIA

The treatment outcome criteria that we utilized from the two treatment evaluation projects were developed in the Hospital Treatment Evaluation and Follow-up Project conducted by Harty et al. (1981). The data base for these studies included the type of clinical documents described earlier. In addition, discharge summaries and follow-up face-to-face interviews were included for ratings of outcome and follow-up adjustment. The raters conducted their ratings blind to the measures of patient functioning at the beginning of treatment. The outcome measures† were example-anchored assessments of patient functioning, including Motivation for Treatment, Help–Rejection, Self-observation, Impulsivity, Abstract and Conceptual Thinking, Primary-Process Communication, Quality of Object Relations, Global Improvement, assessments of family functioning, and characteristics of the treatment, including Patient–Staff Alliance. As outcome criteria we selected the following marker variables to represent selected aspects of outcome: discharge ratings of Global Improvement, two measures of Ego Integration (Abstract and Conceptual Thinking, Attention and Concentration), two measures of Patient–Staff Alliance (Patient–Staff Alliance, Help–Rejection), and a global measure of Follow-up Adjustment.

Our next step was to determine the relationship between these outcome criteria and the basic dimensions for patient functioning that we had generated in our project.

RESULTS

We will present the results from three perspectives: (1) the cluster analyses, (2) the clinical weightings of prediction variables and their predictive

---

* Each grouping was examined for homogeneity among its members. If it was adequate, the mean profile of the group was examined for its clinical meaningfulness. Grouping solutions across different sets of variables were compared to see what different constellations of patient patterns emerged and how much group overlap there was. The effectiveness of the prediction of outcome criteria by a grouping solution can be ascertained by analyses of variance that assess the significance of the difference among groups on a profile of variables. Discriminant function coefficients as well as univariate analysis of variance significance levels are used to determine those criterion variables that are more effectively discriminated by the groups.

† For descriptions of the scales and their reliabilities please refer to Harty et al. (1981).

.success, and (3) the relationship of the empirical clusters to DSM-II diagnoses given this group of patients.

Cluster Analyses

Our primary interest was to determine what factors in what clusters at the time of the diagnostic evaluation at the beginning of treatment would successfully differentiate the groups at the time of discharge from hospital treatment and subsequently in a period of follow-up adjustment. We selected the cluster solutions on the basis of three criteria: clinical interpretability, major shifts in error variance, and meaningful separations between profiles.

Table 7.3 presents the results of the analyses of variance for each of several groupings of factors. The table compares the results for the Bellak EFA factors considered in isolation and then the behaviorally anchored factors assessing quality of relationships (QOR) and capacity for emotion (CFE) and then the developmental factors (DEV) considered in isolation. These grouping solutions are followed by grouping solutions using all sets of factors (All PPF) and then two grouping solutions with the developmental factors omitted (All PPF-No DEV). We used the groupings without developmental factors because of the scanty information about developmental processes, the relatively lower reliabilities of the scales used to assess the dimensions we did extract, and our clinical judgment that the more important features of patient functioning as currently assessed would have greater predictive value.

The most successful grouping solution was the Bellak nine-group solution, EFA (9 G).* The EFA (9 G) was successful in discriminating the groups in terms of termination ratings of Global Improvement, Abstract and Conceptual Thinking, Attention and Concentration, and Patient–Staff Alliance. Most important, EFA (9 G) was the only solution to discriminate successfully among the groups at an acceptable p value at the time of Follow-up Adjustment.

To understand the clinical relevance of these findings it is necessary to reconstruct the descriptions of each of the nine groups along the dimensions involved in the EFA profile by referring to the level descriptions for each factor in Table 7.1. To illustrate this process let us choose Group 8, which was rated to have improved least at termination and continued to do poorly following hospital discharge at the time of follow-up adjustment. The level description for factor I, Thought Disorder, is "Stress-related disturbances in thinking, involving concreteness and failures in logic with some impairment in conceptualization; occasional peculiar ideas and other minor difficulties; need-determined projection of inner states onto external reality." The level of this group on the second EFA factor, Judgment and Impulse Control, falls

---

* EFA factors are derived from assessments at the *beginning* of treatment and the outcome criteria are based on ratings at the termination of treatment.

Table 7.3. PPF Groupings Differentiating Outcome Criteria: Probability Levels for Single Analyses of Variance

PPF Groupings	Global Improvement	Abstract and Conceptual Thinking	Attention and Concentration	Patient–Staff Alliance	Help–Rejection	Follow-up Adjustment
			Outcome Criteria			
EFA (9 G[a])	.04[b]	.0002[b]	.015[b]	.0118[b]	.24	.016[b]
QOR (6 G)	.07[c]	.0025[b]	.0089[b]	.0828[c]	.1147	.113
CFE (8 G)	.05[b]	.16	.0019[b]	.14	.24	.21
CFE (12 G)	—	.02[b]	.05[b]	.0094[b]	.21	—
DEV (7 G)	.20	—	—	—	.23	—
All PPF (8 G)	.04[b]	.04[b]	.0249[b]	.0503[b]	.24	—
All PPF (11 G)	.10[c]	.07[c]	.07[c]	.14	—	—
All PPF-No DEV (7 G)	.10[c]	.0017[b]	.0036[b]	.05[b]	.14	—
All PPF-No DEV (10 G)	.09[c]	.01[b]	.02[b]	.06[c]	.21	—

[a] (G), description of number of groups for each grouping solution.

[b] Acceptable probability levels.

[c] Marginally acceptable probability levels.

between 2 and 3. Thus, the reader will need to extrapolate the midpoint between levels 2 and 3 as they are next described. The level 2 description is "Inappropriate judgment; might actually engage in significantly disruptive social behavior; assaultive acts; violent behavior either self or other directed; rapid extreme mood swings; physical constraint may be necessary to control behavior; poor frustration tolerance." The description for level 3 is: "Sporadic expression of impulse; temper tantrums; might be seen as overly excitable; either completely controlled or episodically discontrolled." Finally, on the third EFA factor, Superego Functioning, the patients fall approximately at level 2. The description of level 2 for this factor is "Self-mutilation; delusional guilt; unrealistic standards; very poor sense of self-worth or virtual absence of conscious guilt feelings, or, psychopathic or extreme impulsivity; indifference to own performance." To summarize the profile, then, the patients in this group experienced major problems in behavior and impulse control as well as an excessive degree of self-directed aggression, which so often undermines patients' capacity to respond to the treatment process. With this translation of the profile, the group's poor treatment response and follow-up adjustment became more understandable.

By contrast, Group 7 was rated as most improved at the time of termination of hospital treatment, was rated relatively high on the Ego Integration factors and Patient–Staff Alliance, and also achieved nearly the highest level of functioning at the time of follow-up adjustment. At the beginning of treatment the major difference between Group 7 and Group 8 occurred on factor II, Judgment and Impulse Control. The two groups are otherwise identical with regard to the other two factors, Thought Disorder and Superego Functioning. It is of great interest to note that with the difference on this crucial factor the groups were widely different at both the time of termination of hospital treatment and at follow-up adjustment (see Table 7.1 for actual discharge ratings). Thus, the difference on factor II appears all the more significant. The level of Group 7 on EFA factor II, Judgment and Impulse Control, is close to the level 4 description, which is: "Episodic, moderate failures in judgment; hidden chronic characterological problems in judgment but within a broad range; may have poor judgment in social situations but not severe enough to cause major problems in and of themselves; some failures in judgment and not a great deal of awareness of why such failures occur; aggression is more likely to be verbal than physical or could be disguised in occupational activity; fairly excitable but not very flexible control over behavior; likely to respond to external guidance and instruction." The comparison across the two groups on this crucial variable thus suggests that the capacity of the group, with the higher level on factor II, to respond to the treatment process and to continue to do well following discharge from hospital treatment was a better capacity to contain destructive impulses and to exercise better judgment. The group also appeared to be able to respond to external guidance and instruction.

The Developmental Variables (DEV) did not discriminate the group on any outcome criteria. Interestingly enough, however, our behavioral measures of Quality of Relations (QOR) and Capacity for Emotion (CFE) both discriminated the groups on several outcome criteria. When these various sources of information were combined, the degree of success approached the success of the EFA (9 G) solution, as can be seen in the results for both the 8- and 11-group solution utilizing all factor scores, All PPF (8 G) and All PPF (11 G), respectively. Elimination of the Developmental Variables appeared to diminish the power of the combined Bellak (EFA), Quality of Relations (QOR), and Capacity for Emotion (CFE) grouping solutions—All PPF-No DEV (10 G) and All PPF-No DEV (7 G). Thus, the Developmental Variables appear to have made some contribution. Clearly, however, none of these additional sources of information improved the power of the EFA profile.

Clinical Predictions

In addition to assessing the empirical relationships emerging between our cluster profiles and outcome criteria, we were also interested in evaluating how the profiles could be used by *clinical* raters to predict the same outcome criteria. To test this we asked clinical judges to make treatment outcome predictions; we also requested them to report their differential weighting of each of the variables in the patient profile according to the specific outcome criteria being predicted. The results of the judges' predictions are presented in two ways: first, the correlation of the judges' predicted rank orders with the actual rank orders of the groups on the outcome criteria and, second, the contrast of the judges' weighting of each of the factors with the actual differential weighting determined by multiple correlational analysis.

Two judges with extensive clinical experience in the setting were asked to review each of the grouping solutions and predict the outcome criteria. The interrater reliabilities appear in Table 7.4. Most of those values were in the mid-.70s to mid-.90s range. It is interesting to note that the most reliably rated profiles for the EFA-9-group solution and the All-No DEV 10-group solution were also the solutions that most successfully differentiated the outcome criteria in the cluster analyses of variance and were most successfully employed by the clinical judges in predicting outcome. The results of the predictions for each of the grouping solutions appear in Table 7.5. For purposes of this study the outcome criteria were collapsed for the judges as follows: Abstract and Conceptual Thinking was combined with Attention and Concentration under the rubric Ego Integration. Patient–Staff Alliance was similarly combined with Help–Rejection as overall Patient–Staff Alliance. We did so because the clinical judges felt they could not meaningfully discriminate between the members of the pairs. The predictions are reported, however, as separate predictions of each of the outcome criteria. There may be some confusion in reading the table insofar as the probability values change according to the size of the grouping solution. For example,

Table 7.4.   *Interrater Reliability (Two Judges) Using PPF Cluster Solutions to Predict Outcome Criteria*

Cluster Solution	Outcome Criteria			
	Global Improvement	Ego Integration	Patient–Staff Alliance	Follow-up Adjustment
EFA (9 G)	.97***	1.00****	.98****	.98****
QOR (6 G)	.89*	.94**	.94**	.94**
CFE (8 G)	.83**	.88***	.98****	.79*
CFE (12 G)	.76***	.50ⁿˢ	.90****	.83***
DEV (7 G)	.75⁺	.71⁺	.68ⁿˢ	.89**
All (8 G)	.88***	1.00****	.48ⁿˢ	.86**
All (11 G)	.88***	.96****	.67*	—
All-No DEV (7 G)	.79*	1.00****	.07ⁿˢ	1.00****
All-No DEV (10 G)	.99****	.99****	.89***	.96****

Note: ns, not significant; $^+ p < .10$; $^* p < .05$; $^{**} p < .02$; $^{***} p < .01$; $^{****} p < .001$.

even though the relationship of the judges' prediction of Patient–Staff Alliance to the actual outcome value using the QOR 6-group solution is .71, that value is nonsignificant because of the small number of groups; whereas the prediction of Abstract and Conceptual Thinking using the CFE 12-group solution is .64 and is significant at the .05 level.

It is quickly apparent that the most easily predicted outcome criteria are aspects of Ego Integration at the time of termination, as one can see from the sizable values for both Abstract and Conceptual Thinking and Attention and Concentration. The Patient–Staff Alliance was difficult to predict. Not one of the grouping solutions was useful to the judges in making that assessment, with the exception of the scales assessing Quality of Relations (QOR). Because of the previously mentioned statistical problem, however, that relationship did not reach an acceptable level of statistical significance. The judges also found it difficult to make successful predictions regarding Global Improvement unless they took all the factors into account with the exception of the developmental factors. Follow-up Adjustment was most successfully predicted with the same group of factors. Thus, the most important finding from this analysis appears to be that the judges were better able to make accurate predictions of outcome for all criteria when utilizing a *combination* of the EFA, QOR, and CFE factors, as can be seen in the comparative degree of success of the All-No DEV (10 G) solution. The rank order correlations for this solution with actual treatment outcome ranged from the mid-.60s to the mid-.90s.

Our first attempt to apply the profile methodology in the absence of empirically established predictive guidelines was encouraging. The clinical judges had considerably exceeded the predictive value achieved with both canoni-

Table 7.5. Clinical Predictions of Treatment Outcome and Follow-up Adjustment Using PPF: Correlation Coefficients

PPF Groupings	Global Improvement	Abstract and Conceptual Thinking	Attention and Concentration	Patient–Staff Alliance	Help–Rejection	Follow-up Adjustment
			Outcome Criteria			
EFA (9 G)	—	.72*	.83*	—	.65$^+$	.62$^+$
QOR (6 G)	—	1.00***	.94**	.71^{ns}	.77^{ns}	.71^{ns}
CFE (8 G)	—					
CFE (12 G)	—	.64*	.66*			.52$^+$
DEV (7 G)	—	.71$^+$	.82*			
All PPF (8 G)	—	.74*	.83**			
All PPF (11 G)	—	.88**	.93****	.68*		
All PPF-No DEV (7 G)	—	.82*	.89***	.68^{ns}		.93***
All PPF-No DEV (10 G)	.68*	.94***	.94****	.62$^+$		.88***

Note: $^+$ p < .10; * p < .05; ** p < .02; *** p < .01; **** p < .001; ns, not significant.

cal and multiple correlational techniques. The success of the All PPF-No DEV (10 G) solution was a result in part because the clinical judges became increasingly familiar and comfortable with the PPF profiles. This solution was the last to be ranked on the outcome criteria and thus followed extensive discussions and practice. The subtle differences between groups based on the *combination* and *interaction* of the PPF factors were recognized. The fact that the predictions of outcome were done totally blind to the actual results and thus relied on clinical inference based only on clinical experience held exciting implications for us. It indeed seemed possible to generate a profile of patient functioning that could be used by experienced clinicians to forecast important treatment developments. It demonstrated the effectiveness of a clinical inference process exercised by clinical judges. Finally, it strongly reinforced the initial motivation of the study, that is, to translate our clinical frame of reference into quantitative terms that would permit confirmation–disconfirmation and that would generate a deepened understanding of what patient characteristics are associated with what treatment response and outcome. Our follow-up evaluation of our entire sample of 300 cases will enable us to apply the differential weightings derived from the multiple correlational analysis as well as the experience of success and failure with the predictive use of the profiles. Knowledge also of the patterning of outcome criteria should enhance the clinical judges' ability to utilize differentially the profile information.

Comparisons with DSM-II Diagnosis

The major assumption underlying our study was that a differentiated profile of patient functioning would help us to anticipate treatment response accurately and to discriminate the effects of treatment on groups of patients systematically differentiated along relevant treatment dimensions. The standard nosological framework in use at the time we conducted the study was

Table 7.6. Interrelationships of Predictions of Treatment Outcome Criteria All-No DEV (10 G)

Outcome Criteria Predictions	Outcome Criteria Predictions		
	Global Improvement	Ego Integration	Patient–Staff Alliance
Global Improvement			
Ego Integration	.99		
Patient–Staff Alliance	.90	.85	
Follow-up Adjustment	.99	.98	.87

Table 7.7. Interrelationship of Actual Outcomes for Treatment Outcome Criteria for All PPF-No DEV (10 G)

Actual Outcomes	Actual Outcomes				
	Global Improvement	Abstract and Conceptual Thinking	Attention and Concentration	Patient–Staff Alliance	Help–Rejection
Global Improvement					
Abstract and Conceptual Thinking	.47				
Attention and Concentration	.50	.98			
Patient–Staff Alliance	.14	.64	.64		
Help–Rejection	.40	.89	.93	.67	
Follow-up Adjustment	.45	.80	.83	.58	.81

the Diagnostic and Statistical Manual, DSM-II, developed by the American Psychiatric Association. As a regular part of clinical workups, each patient was assigned an appropriate DSM-II diagnostic label. We were thus able to determine the diagnostic classification of each of the patients in each of the grouping solutions. We were then able to compare a presumed treatment outcome based on the DSM-II classification versus the outcome predicted from membership in the profiles of patient functioning. There are few specific hypotheses regarding prognosis associated with each of the DSM-II diagnostic categories (schizophrenic, other psychoses, personality disorder, and neuroses). Certainly every clinician recognizes that more detailed information regarding prior and current treatment response, current clinical behavior, ongoing relationships with staff, symptomatology, motivation, character style, current life adjustment and relationships, family constellation, genetic loadings, and neurological and biomedical dysfunction can all prove useful in further refining the general diagnostic and prognostic framework afforded by DSM-II. The question is how much more is required beyond the general diagnostic label to forecast treatment response adequately. Our methodology helped us to approach a partial answer. We assumed an invariant order of outcome on each of the outcome variables according to the diagnostic label, neuroses → personality disorder → other psychosis → schizophrenia. The basic assumption in this order is, of course, that the more healthy the patient, the better able he is to respond to treatment and that this overall dimension of health–sickness is reflected in the general diagnostic classifications. The first comparison of interest to us is that of the diagnostic groupings versus the EFA 9-group solution. The diagnoses of each of the patients is listed according to group membership in Table 7.6. The actual outcome ratings for each of the EFA groups is listed in Table 7.7.

Table 7.8. DSM-II Diagnostic Labels for Patients in the EFA (9 G) Solution

| EFA (9 G) Group | Number of Patients in Each Group According to DSM-II Diagnoses | | | |
	Schizophrenia	Other Psychoses	Personality Disorder	Neuroses
1	10			
2	4		1	
3	4			
4	3			
5			1	1
6	1			
7	1		1	1
8			2	
9	1	1		

Table 7.9. *Actual Treatment Outcomes for the EFA (9 G) Solution*

Global Improvement		Abstract and Conceptual Thinking		Attention and Concentration		Patient–Staff Alliance		Help–Rejection		Follow-up Adjustment	
Group	Mean	Group	Mean	Group	Mean	Group	Mean	Group	Mean	Group	Mean
7	62.5	5	65	5	73.4	5	68.9	[3]	60.9	[9]	7.5
[1][a]	56	7	64.7	[9]	64.2	[6]	65.7	[4]	59.4	7	6.2
[2]	55.5	[9]	60.9	7	60.8	[9]	64.7	[1]	59.3	[2]	6.0
5	52.5	[2]	50.2	[2]	54.7	7	61.5	8	57.5	5	5.3
[9]	44.7	[6]	43.3	[1]	49.0	[2]	59.3	[6]	45	[6]	5.2
[6]	38.7	[1]	39.3	[6]	49.3	[4]	57.1	5	43.4	[4]	4.2
[4]	38.2	8	38.3	8	45.0	8	51.2	7	42.5	[1]	3.6
[3]	29.9	[4]	27.7	[3]	34.6	[1]	47.0	[2]	40.8	8	3.3
8	28.4	[3]	23.9	[4]	31.9	[3]	43.0	[9]	30.0	[3]	2.8

[a] Brackets indicate groups with either exclusively or predominantly schizophrenic patients.

As one can see from inspection of the tables, the patients diagnosed as schizophrenic belong to groups whose outcomes are highly variable; they are not consistently the worse nor the best. Conversely, those patients with personality diagnoses and diagnoses of neurotic disorders also are spread across the spectrum of outcomes. Thus, the invariant order of the more healthy patient responding better to treatment than the less healthy patient is not supported by these findings. Rather, the patient's outcome appears to be more related to the interaction of the treatment and specific characteristics evaluated by the patient profile factors. The same conclusions can be drawn from an inspection of the tables reporting the same type of information for the All-No Developmental 10-group solution, where it is possible to see even more dramatically that the patients who have been diagnosed as schizophrenic according to the DSM-II criteria have highly variable outcomes. Specifically, patients diagnosed as schizophrenic were found in groups 1, 2, 3, 4, 5, and 10 in this grouping solution. One would thus expect these six groups to do most poorly consistently on all the outcome criteria and not to be essentially differentiated one from the other. However, there is a wide range of outcomes for each of these groups and their order is not invariant. Some clearly do very well in the treatment process and at the time of follow-up adjustment. Some do very poorly. The profile of patient functioning encompassing the assessment of the broad range of characteristics developed in the study clearly helps to differentiate those who respond well to treatment and those who do not. This discrimination is not possibly based solely on the initial diagnostic level. Thus, the most important clinical implication of this study is that a careful assessment of ego functions as described by Bellak et al. (1973) is of great help in assessing prognosis.

REFERENCES

Bellak, L., Hurvich, M., & Gediman, H. K. *Ego functions in schizophrenics, neurotics, and normals: A systematic study of conceptual, diagnostic, and therapeutic aspects.* New York: Wiley, 1973.

Harty, M., Cerney, M., Colson, D., Coyne, L., Frieswyk, S., Johnson, S. B., & Mortimer, R. Correlates of change and long-term outcome: An exploratory study of intensively treated hospital patients. *Bulletin of the Menninger Clinic,* 1981, *45*(3), 209–228.

CHAPTER EIGHT

Ego Function Assessment—Its Relationship to Psychiatric Hospital Treatment Outcome and Follow-up Adjustment: The Follow-up Study

MARY CERNEY, PATRICIA J. SCHRODER, LOLAFAYE COYNE, SIEBOLT FRIESWYK, GAVIN NEWSOM, AND PETER NOVOTNY

INTRODUCTION

One of the most compelling problems facing American psychiatry today is finding a diagnostic scheme that has direct implications for treatment and prognosis. Of the many frustrations with the diagnostic and statistical manual (APA, 1968, 1980) that has served as the major nosological framework for American psychiatry is its lack of clear-cut implications for treatment planning and its lack of empirically demonstrated relationship to treatment response and outcome. Out of this frustration, like the mythical Phoenix of old, emerged a group effort to define patient populations more predictively.* We are now in the most interesting phase of this work, examining the outcome of the patient population we have been studying. Although our data are as yet incomplete we are beginning to see some relationship between initial profiles and outcome. We are paying close attention to our findings as certain trends are beginning to emerge that may have clinically useful implications.

This chapter is one of three describing the Patient Profile Study (PPS), a study of 300 patients discharged within a 4-year period (1973–1976) from the C. F. Menninger Memorial Hospital. For methodological reasons, this 300-member sample was divided into two randomly selected replication samples of 150 patients each after initial ratings were completed.† This chapter will focus on follow-up outcome data obtained from 78 patients from one of the two 150-member samples. The special emphasis will be on the analysis of outcome using the Bellak Ego Function Scales. In this chapter we will first discuss the procedures used in obtaining and rating follow-up information from the 78 patient interviews completed. We will then present hypotheses generated by the PPS Core Group. In our analysis, we report first on how much the 78-member sample changed between the initial rating and follow-up rating on the Bellak Ego Function Scales. Then we assess change by dividing the sample into a High, Middle, and Low Group based on the initial health–sickness rating. Next, we study patterns of change within two diagnostic groups: Schizophrenic and Borderline, the only diagnostic categories with groups large enough to test. Finally, we conclude by examining the hypotheses generated by the PPS Core Group.

INSTRUMENTS AND RATING METHODS

Initially, the PPS Core Group planned to use discharge data as the criteria for treatment outcome. Discharge summaries limited to information about disposition and the physician's statement, however, could not answer the PPS Core Group's questions about treatment outcome, particularly, "Do patients who have similar patient profiles at admission have similar outcomes?"

To answer that question and related questions, the PPS Core Group initiated a follow-up study in which initial ratings on the following scales were to be compared with ratings based on a follow-up interview with the same patients in the original sample who were now discharged from the hospital

---

* For a history of the development of the project, see L. Coyne et al., Chapter 6, this book.

† For an in-depth description of the statistical procedures utilized in the PPS and related studies, see Coyne et al., Chapter 6.

for 5 or more years. Some of the follow-up scales selected had been used reliably in a previous study (Harty et al., 1981) and others, in the first phase of the PPS (see Coyne et al., Chapter 6). These scales measured the patient's general adjustment with regard to current level of intrapsychic functioning, management of daily life with emphasis on work and play, and status of interpersonal relationships (see Table 8.1).

Ratings of General Adjustment.   The eight scales included here are from the early phase of the PPS and are part of a much more extended version on which patients were rated at each developmental stage of their life. We experienced difficulty in rating patients on these scales prior to age 12 because of insufficient data in the charts. The later phases of development could be more reliably rated (see Coyne et al., Chapter 6, this book) because the material was current and included as part of the diagnostic summary or family study.

The scales are five-point scales that rate the individual on a continuum from average expectable behavior to severe pathological functioning. Two of the scales "Sexual Interests" and "Interpersonal Relationships" are two-pronged. After the initial anchor point, the scale divides as it progresses toward the pathological end of the continuum measuring extremes in opposite directions. The final two anchors of "Sexual Interests" speak to individuals who are promiscuous, highly active sexually or who have no sexual interest evident. The final two anchors for "Interpersonal Relationships" describe individuals who are essentially isolated or who have tentative, unstable relationships.

Health–Sickness Rating Scale.   The health–sickness scale has been used in many studies in our setting and is frequently cited in the literature. It was developed by Luborsky (1975) and is an example-anchored rating scale assessing global severity of psychopathology. The scale's anchors range from zero ("any condition which, unattended, would quickly result in the patient's death") to 100 ("an ideal state of complete functioning, integration, of resiliency in the face of stress, of happiness and social effectiveness"). This scale was used in the initial phase of the PPS. It is listed under Hospital-wide Follow-up Study (Harty et al., 1981) because it was with the group of scales taken from that study (see Table 8.1).

Hospital-wide Follow-up Study Scales (Harty et al., 1981)

Raters in the Hospital-wide Follow-up Study used these scales for an admission rating and a discharge rating in their study. At admission the reliability of an average rating (corrected intraclass correlation) ranged from .741 to .923 and at discharge from .744 to .921 (Harty et al., 1981). The following scales from this study were selected for use in the PPS Follow-up Study because of their predictive significance as found in that study—and the Schizophrenic Follow-up Study (Cerney et al., in progress).

Table 8.1.   Patient Profile Follow-up Scales

   I. Ratings of General Adjustment (PPS)
- A. Behavior
- B. Symptoms
- C. Drugs and/or Alcohol Abuse
- D. Sexual Interests
- E. Interpersonal Relationships
- F. Work Adjustment
- G. Dependence—Independence
- H. Special Skills

  II. Hospital-wide Follow-up Study Scales (Harty et al., 1981)
- A. Health–Sickness Rating (Luborsky, 1975)
- B. Follow-up Adjustment
- C. Global Improvement
- D. Extent of Separation from the Family of Origin
- E. Abstract and Conceptual Thinking
- F. Quality of Object Relations
- G. Acquisition of Skills and Interests

 III. Bellak Scales (1973)
- A. Reality Testing:
    1. Distinction between inner and outer stimuli
    2. Accuracy of perception
- B. Judgment:
    1. Anticipation of consequences
    2. Manifest in behavior
    3. Emotional appropriateness
- C. Regulation and Control of Drives, Impulses, and Affects:
    1. Direction of impulse expression
    2. Effectiveness of delay mechanisms
- D. Object Relations:
    1. Degree and kind of relatedness
    2. Object constancy
- E. Thought Processes:
    1. Ability to conceptualize
    2. Primary–secondary process
- F. Autonomous Functioning:
    1. Degree of freedom from impairment of primary autonomy apparatuses
    2. Degree of freedom from impairment of secondary autonomy
- G. Synthetic–Integrative Functioning:
    1. Degree of reconciliation of incongruities
    2. Degree of active relating together of events
- H. Mastery–Competence:
    1. Actual competence
- I. Superego Scale:
    1. Guilt (self-directed punishment, unconscious sense of guilt, blame–avoidance, talion principle—desire for revenge)
    2. Ego ideal (self-evaluation, sense of worth, self-esteem regulation)

---

1. *Follow-up Adjustment*—a nine-point scale that describes the patient's follow-up adjustment, ranging from Very Poor ("includes suicides, those who are institutionalized with no apparent prospect of improvement, and those who are living extremely chaotic, antisocial, very withdrawn, or otherwise clearly pathological and unproductive lives with little or no indication of efforts toward greater stability") to Very Good ("The person is maintaining a stable, satisfying life situation, requires no unusual supports from the environment to continue functioning successfully and autonomously, and actively contributes to the well-being of other people and the community").

2. *Global Improvement*—a 100-point scale that describes the overall change in adaptive functioning and intrapsychic organization that has occurred within the patient since the initial assessment. The extreme anchors range from 10 on the low end ("The person's overall condition is much worse than it was initially. There has been a substantial deterioration in his ability to meet the demands of life, and there is no evidence of positive changes that might compensate for the decline") to 90 on the high end ("There is a marked change for the better in adaptive functioning, reflecting significant intrapsychic changes in the direction of conflict resolution and ego strengthening. It is likely that these gains will be maintained or further built upon after the end of treatment").

3. *Extent of Separation from the Family of Origin*—a nine-point scale that describes individuals who range from 1 ("totally surrounded by family of origin, living at home, making no occupational or educational progress toward independence, and with little or no interaction with persons outside his family") to individuals who are rated 9 ("fully independent from family of origin with no more ties to remain other than the ordinary ones of friendship and fondness").

4. *Abstract and Conceptual Thinking*—a 100-point scale that emphasizes the patient's ability to use abstract thinking for *adaptive* purposes. Abstract ability that is used in rigidly maladaptive ways (to produce inappropriate generalizations, to escape from important aspects of concrete reality, etc.) should not elevate this rating. As much as possible this rating is independent of other aspects of cognitive functioning, such as memory, concentration, and so on. This rating measures the degree to which the person can employ abstract or concrete modes of thinking in a way that is flexibly adapted to the requirements of the situation facing him. Its anchors range from 5 ("rarely, if ever, can the person perform tasks calling for abstraction or conceptualization. Thinking is extremely concrete or extremely overinclusive; there is no comprehension of metaphors, similes, or proverbs, and no distinction is made between objects and the symbols for them verbal or otherwise") to 95 ("conceptual thinking is highly developed; there is an appropriate and effortless shifting between abstract and concrete modes of thought as the situation requires").

5. *Quality of Object Relations*—a scale that examines the extent to

which the individual can experience stable, enduring relationships, in which the expression and gratification of individual needs does not compromise the person's empathy and respect for the other. The anchors range from 5 ("virtually no capacity of relatedness to people which recognizes their independent existence or their difference from inanimate objects; others are treated with ruthless, indiscriminate, aggressive exploitation, or are responded to in completely autistic and undifferentiated ways. There is little recognition of, or concession to, even the most basic of social conventions") to 100 ("the person's relationships are stable, mature, and well-differentiated. He understands and empathizes with others but does not confuse their needs with his; tolerates differences without loss of regard for others; is genuinely concerned for the well-being of others; feels gratified by his relationship without feeling guilt").

6. *Acquisition of Skills and Interests*—a nine-point scale with anchors ranging from 1 ("the development of no skills which could help the individual strain himself, develop friendships, or gratify curiosities and interests. There are no indications of either occupational endeavors or hobbies") to 9 ("the patient is working at an occupation—or preparing himself for an occupation in which he is interested and in which he sees a future. In addition, he is following some avocational interest or interests"). If the occupational interests seemed complete, but there was no avocational pursuit, the individual would be ranked at 8 instead of 9.

7. *Bellak's Ego Functions Scales* (*Bellak et al., 1973*).   The same Bellak scales used in making the initial ratings were also used in rating ego functions at follow-up (see Coyne et al., Chapter 6, this book), and are listed in Table 8.1 (see Table 8.1). This paper will deal primarily with this set of scales.

Interview Procedure and Raters

The senior author (M. C.) with experience from two previous follow-up studies (Hospital-wide Follow-up Study, Harty et al., 1981; and Schizophrenic Follow-up Study, Cerney et al., in progress) conducted all follow-up interviews reported in this chapter. Since the patient population being studied is so widely distributed geographically, the PPS Core Study group decided to use telephone interviews where face-to-face interviews were impossible because of the time and expense involved. Only 15 of the 78 follow-up interviews reported in this chapter were face-to-face interviews. All others were telephone interviews.

The interview follows a detailed format developed during the Hospital-wide Follow-up Study (Harty et al., 1981). The interview format covers the patient's present life, his life since he was discharged from the hospital, a review of his treatment in the hospital and how he feels about being interviewed. On completion of the interview, the interviewer dictates, using the outline for the interview, a detailed almost verbatim summary made from the notes taken during the interview proper.

Table 8.2.   Follow-up Data Form Variables

  I. Demographic data
      A. Present area of residence
      B. Type of residence
      C. Sources of financial support, not including treatment expense
      D. Present marital status
      E. Present household composition
      F. Number of changes of residence since discharge
      G. Present education
      H. Present occupation
      I. Present socioeconomic status
      J. Number of changes of employment since discharge
 II. Treatment since discharge
      A. General type of aftercare
      B. Specific aftercare modalities
      C. Rehospitalizations
      D. Formal individual or group therapy since discharge
      E. Medication currently being taken
      F. Medication prescribed by
      G. Frequency of medication
      H. Source of financial support for treatment

After completing the interview, the interviewer (M. C.) rates the patient using the set of scales described earlier and completes a special follow-up data form developed during the Hospital-wide Follow-up Study (Harty et al., 1981). This form contains basic demographic and treatment data (see Table 8.2). The typed summary of the interview and discharge material, to give a baseline for rating, are then sent to two other raters, senior clinicians and members of the PPS Core Group,* who independently rate each patient. If the two raters disagree more than five points on 100-point scales and more than one point on other scales, they meet to make a consensus rating. This procedure was developed earlier in the PPS and is discussed by Coyne et al., Chapter 6.

Predictors of Follow-up Adjustment

The initial ratings in the PPS were used to predict follow-up ratings. As a first step in this process the initial ratings of the Bellak scales were factor-analyzed† for the two 150-member samples and the 78-member subsample. All emerged with basically the same three factors (see Table 8.3). Factor I, labeled Freedom from Thought Disorder, deals primarily with the individ-

---

* Patricia Schroder rated all of the 78 interviews; Gavin Newsom and Siebolt Frieswyk rated approximately 39 each.
† For details concerning the factor analysis, see Coyne et al., Chapter 6.

Table 8.3. *Factor Loadings on the Bellak Scales Sample (N = 150) and Subsample (N = 78)*

Scales	Factor I: Freedom from Thought Disorder		Factor II: Judgment and Impulse Control		Factor III: Superego Functioning	
	N = 150	N = 78	N = 150	N = 78	N = 150	N = 78
Reality Testing						
1. Distinction between inner and outer	.805	.722				
2. Accuracy of perception	.781	.720				
Judgment						
3. Anticipation of consequences			.803	.788		
4. Manifest in behavior			.818	.837		
5. Emotional appropriateness			.779	.791		
Regulation and Control of Drives, Impulses, and Affects						
6. Directness of impulse expression			.663	.587	.502	
7. Effectiveness of delay mechanisms			.723	.697		.557

Object Relations		
8. Degree and kind of relatedness		
9. Object constancy		
Thought Processes		
10. Ability to conceptualize	.818	.823
11. Primary–secondary process	.875	.849
Autonomous Functioning		
12. Freedom from impairment—primary autonomy	.835	.884
13. Freedom from impairment—secondary autonomy	.726	.759
Synthetic–Integrative Functioning		
14. Reconciliation of incongruities	.596	.688
15. Relating together of events	.624	.672
Mastery–Competence		
16. Actual competence	.599	.638
Superego Scale		
17. Guilt	.810	.797
18. Ego ideal	.782	.830

ual's ability to evaluate what is real and what is not, what is inner and what is outer, and to use whatever information may be available to validate the process. A second component of this factor reflects the extent to which language and thought is infiltrated with the thought process. In other words, is primary process thought or secondary process thought evident in the individual's thinking and communication? This factor deals with essentially structured considerations embedded in how well organized the patient's capacity is to structure and organize thought, evaluate reality, and maintain autonomous functioning.

Factor II, Judgment and Impulse Control, reflects the ability of the person to evaluate the appropriateness and consequences of his behavior in conjunction with his ability to contain or express himself in keeping with that evaluation.

Factor III, Superego Functioning, deals with an individual's experience of guilt and blame in regard to aggressive and libidinal drive experience, the transformations and displacements of this experience and how reality-based they are. In addition, it taps into an individual's sense of worth, self-esteem regulation, and how realistic his ego goals and strivings are.

HYPOTHESES AND RATIONALE

Prior to making the follow-up ratings the PPS Core Group made predictions as to which of their PPS Follow-up Scales would relate to each of the three pretreatment Bellak factors. These they outlined with their rationale as follows:

Factor I: Freedom from Thought Disorder should be correlated with:

I.   Ratings of General Adjustment
   *B.   Symptoms: The presence or absence of a thought disorder is one of the major symptoms considered in the diagnosis of patients.
II.   Ratings from Hospital-wide Follow-up Scales (Harty et al., 1981)
   A.   Health–Sickness (Luborsky, 1975): The presence or absence of a thought disorder is one of the major components of health–sickness.
   B.   Abstract and Conceptual Thinking: The quality of one's thinking is one of the considerations in making a diagnosis of the presence or absence of a thought disorder.
   F.   Quality of Object Relations: To a great extent the quality of one's object relations is influenced by how one thinks.

Factor II: Judgment and Impulse Control should be correlated with:

I.   Ratings of General Adjustment
   A.   Behavior: Behavior is the result of one's judgment and the amount of control one has over one's impulses, affects, and drives.

* Ordering is according to PPS Follow-up Study Manual (see Table 8.1).

C. Drugs and/or Alcohol Abuse: Drugs and/or alcohol abuse is a form of acting out that results from faulty judgment and impulse control.

F. Work Adjustment: The possibility of correlation was questioned but included because to a certain extent one's ability not only to choose appropriate work but also to remain with it is related to judgment and impulse control.

II. Ratings from the Hospital-wide Follow-up Scales (Harty et al., 1981)

A. Health–Sickness (Luborsky, 1975): Another important component of health–sickness is one's ability (1) to make appropriate judgments, (2) to control one's impulses, and (3) to be aware of the consequences of one's behavior.

B. Follow-up Adjustment: An individual's adjustment is predicated on his behavior, which is influenced by his judgment and impulse control.

G. Acquisition of Skills and Interests: In order to develop a skill and maintain interest one must make appropriate judgments and exercise reasonable control over one's impulses.

Factor III: Superego Functioning should be correlated with:

I. Ratings of General Adjustment

A. Behavior: Behavior is influenced by the strictness or laxity of one's superego.

B. Symptoms: The strictness or laxity of an individual's superego is one of the more debilitating symptoms.

E. Interpersonal Relationships: How one judges oneself is reflected in one's interaction with others.

II. Ratings from the Hospital-wide Follow-up Study Scales (Harty et al., 1981)

D. Extent of Separation from Family of Origin: The possibility of correlation was questioned but included because one must be able to deal with one's own sense of guilt and blame in order to separate from one's family of origin.

F. Quality of Object Relations: The quality of one's object relations is influenced by one's own sense of guilt and blame.

ANALYSIS OF DATA

Overview

In this section (1) we examined the data by comparing initial ratings of patients with their follow-up ratings on the Bellak scales. Differences between initial ratings and follow-up ratings were required to reach a $p < .01$ level of confidence to be considered significant. Then (2) by dividing the data into three groups—High, Middle, and Low—based on their initial Health–Sickness rating, we determined if our study follows the trend seen in other studies where the "rich get richer" phenomenon prevailed. Our next step involved (3) an examination of initial and follow-up data to find within which diagnostic category the greatest difference occurs and the direction of that difference. Then (4) we compared the factor structures of the initial and follow-up ratings on the Bellak scales as well as relating each initial rating to the corresponding follow-up ratings. Finally, (5) we tested the hypotheses that were generated by the PPS Core Group prior to rating the follow-up interviews.

Methods

We examined the data and tested the hypotheses by means of the following analyses. We compared the initial and follow-up factor analytic solutions. If the factor structure had remained the same, the tests of significance of the change from initial to follow-up could have been done using factor scores. Since this was not the case, change from initial to follow-up was analyzed by means of multivariate analysis of variance using the vector of Bellak Ego Function Scales as the dependent variable. Since the sample was heterogeneous with respect to diagnostic category and initial level of health–sickness, we also introduced two blocking factors into the multivariate analyses of change. These two blocking factors were independent as indicated by a nonsignificant chi square test of association (see Table 8.9). In one analysis the blocking factor was diagnostic category and the levels chosen were Schizophrenic and Borderline, both represented by sizable numbers of cases in this sample; in this analysis differential change for Schizophrenics and Borderlines was tested for significance. In the other analysis the blocking factor was initial health–sickness with three levels, High, Middle, and Low; in this analysis differential change for groups starting out at different levels of severity was investigated.

The hypotheses stated earlier were tested by means of Pearson correlations between initial Bellak factor scores and follow-up outcome measures. Initial Bellak ego function ratings were also correlated with the follow-up rating of the same scales.

Initial and Follow-up Rating Comparisons Using the Bellak Scales

In correlating initial with follow-up Bellak scale ratings, those scales originally loaded on Factor I at admission were all highly correlated across time. The correlation was less true of those included under Factor II. Correlations of those loadings on Factor III were not statistically significant (see Table 8.4). The lack of correlation would suggest that not only were there changes in degree and kind on the Bellak scales at outcome, but the structure of relationships among Bellak scale ratings at outcome was changed as well.

Differences between initial and follow-up ratings on the Bellak scales

Table 8.4. *Correlation of Initial and Follow-up Ratings on the Bellak Scales (N = 78)*

Scales	r	p
Factor I: Freedom from Thought Disorder		
Reality Testing		
1. Distinction between inner and outer stimuli	.5366	<.001
2. Accuracy of perception	.5301	<.001
Thought Processes		
10. Ability to conceptualize	.5546	<.001
11. Primary-process thinking	.6173	<.001
Autonomous Functioning		
12. Freedom from impairment—primary	.4634	<.001
13. Freedom from impairment—secondary	.4006	<.001
Synthetic–Integrative Functioning		
14. Reconciliation of incongruities	.3965	<.001
15. Relating together of events	.4437	<.001
Mastery–Competence		
16. Competence	.4831	<.001
Factor II: Judgment and Impulse Control		
Judgment		
3. Anticipation of consequences	.3449	.002
4. Manifest behavior	.2510	.026
5. Appropriateness of behavior	.3302	.003
Regulation and Control of Drives, Affects, and Impulses		
6. Directness of impulse	.2645	.016
7. Effectiveness of delay and control mechanisms	.3766	<.001
Factor III: Superego Functioning		
Superego Scale		
17. Guilt	.1559	.170
18. Ego ideal	.1322	.245
Object Relations		
8. Degree and kind of relatedness	.5282	<.001
9. Object constancy	.3639	<.001

Table 8.5. Changes in Bellak Ratings—Initial and Follow-up

	Mean	
Scales	Initial	Follow-up
Reality Testing		
1. Distinction between inner and outer stimuli	3.61	4.55[a]
2. Accuracy of perception	3.52	4.46
Judgment		
3. Anticipation of consequences	3.00	4.17
4. Manifest behavior	2.90	4.17
5. Emotional appropriateness	3.18	4.27
Regulation and Control of Drives, Affects, and Impulses		
6. Directness of impulse expression	3.22	4.33
7. Effectiveness of delay mechanisms	2.97	4.26
Object Relations		
8. Degree and kind of relatedness	2.82	3.81
9. Object constancy	2.78	3.85
Thought Processes		
10. Ability to conceptualize	3.67	4.58
11. Primary–secondary process	3.83	4.80
Autonomous Functioning		
12. Freedom of primary autonomous apparatuses	3.78	4.63
13. Freedom of secondary autonomy	3.45	4.41
Synthetic Integrative Functioning		
14. Reconciliation of incongruities	3.21	4.06
15. Active relating of events	3.22	4.13
Mastery Competence		
16. Actual competence	3.06	3.97
Superego Scale		
17. Guilt	2.58	3.90
18. Ego ideal	2.54	3.98

[a] The vector of Initial–Follow-up mean differences was significant at $p < .001$. The largest contributors to the significant F for the multivariate analysis as indicated by the discriminant function coefficients were Regulation and Control of Drives: Effectiveness of Delay Mechanisms (1.327), Thought Processes: Primary–Secondary Process (1.092), and Superego: Ego Ideal (1.155).

were on the magnitude of about one point. Those scales defining Freedom from Thought Disorder (Factor I) had the smallest change while those defining Judgment and Regulation and Control of Drive, Impulses, and Affects (Factor II) produced slightly larger changes; and those defining Superego Functioning (Factor III) changed most of all (see Table 8.5). The vector of mean differences was significant at $p < .001$, which exceeded the level of confidence required by the PPS Core Group. The major contributions to the significant F for the multivariate analysis were made by Effectiveness of Delay Mechanisms, Primary–Secondary Process, and Ego Ideal.

When one compares the initial and follow-up ratings on *all* the Bellak scales, only 1 (1.3%) subject received a lower rating on all of the Bellak scales at follow-up; 55 (70.5%) subjects improved on 11 or more of the Bellak scales, whereas 14 members (17.9%) decreased on 10 or more Bellak scales (see Table 8.6). The two scales that showed the largest number of cases with improvement appeared to be Effectiveness of Delay Mechanisms and Ego Ideal. From these results one could surmise that patients felt better about themselves and were better able to control their behavior.

High–Middle–Low Initial Health–Sickness Groups

Results from the Psychotherapy Research Project (PRP) (Kernberg et al., 1972) and the Hospital-wide Follow-up Study (Harty et al., 1981) suggest that the ones who benefit most from treatment are probably the ones who need it the least. Their studies argue that high initial ego strength in patients implies a good prognosis for all modalities of treatment within a psychoanalytical frame of reference. The Multidimensional Scalogram Analysis of the PRP indicated that there exists an overriding relationship between overall outcome (change) and ego strength, especially regarding those aspects of ego strength related to the quality of interpersonal relationships. In the PRP study patients with low initial ratings on the Ego Strength Scale (particularly low initial ratings on the Quality of Interpersonal Relationships Scale) showed least improvement. This outcome remained true even when the researchers considered the skill of the therapist. The PRP study found that the skill of the therapist is of particular significance for the improvement of very ill patients while skill does not influence greatly the improvement of the "stronger" patients (Kernberg et al., 1972).

To test whether this phenomenon might also be true in the PPS study and whether a middle group might be obscuring changes made in the two extreme groups, the PPS sample was divided into three groups: High, Middle, and Low, based on their initial Health–Sickness ratings (see Table 8.7).

The multivariate test of differential change for the three different levels of initial health–sickness was borderline significant. Discriminant function coefficients indicated that the major contributions were made by Guilt and Blame, Reconciliations of Incongruities, and Anticipation of Consequences. In the case of Guilt and Blame and Anticipation of Consequences, the largest

Table 8.6.   Direction of Changes Between Initial and Follow-up Ratings on Bellak Ego Functions Scales for Individual Subjects (N = 78)

Scales	Number of Subjects		
	+	−	No Change
Reality Testing			
1. Distinction between inner and outer stimuli	54	18	6
2. Accuracy of perception	54	14	10
Judgment			
3. Anticipation of consequences	58	15	5
4. Manifest behavior	55	15	8
5. Emotional appropriateness	54	16	8
Regulation and Control of Drives, Affects, and Impulses			
6. Directness of impulse expression	57	13	8
7. Effectiveness of delay mechanisms	65	8	5
Object Relations			
8. Degree and kind of relatedness	54	13	11
9. Object constancy	56	17	5
Thought Processes			
10. Ability to conceptualize	58	14	6
11. Primary—secondary process	52	14	12
Autonomous Functioning			
12. Freedom of primary autonomous apparatuses	52	20	6
13. Freedom of secondary autonomy	56	16	6
Synthetic–Integrative Functioning			
14. Reconciliation of incongruities	59	17	2
15. Active relating of events	56	15	7
Mastery Competence			
16. Actual competence	54	18	6
Superego Scale			
17. Guilt	57	10	11
18. Ego ideal	61	11	6

change was for the Middle Health–Sickness group. For Reconciliation of Incongruities, both the Middle and Low Health–Sickness groups made the most change. The test of change for the total sample was significant at $p < .001$, with the largest contributors being Reconciliation of Incongruities and Effectiveness of Delay Mechanisms.

Although there was evidence of change when initial and follow-up ratings

Table 8.7. *High, Middle, and Low Initial Health–Sickness Group Mean Differences Between Initial and Follow-up Ratings on the Bellak Scales*

Scales	High Initial Health–Sickness Mean Difference	Rank	Middle Initial Health–Sickness Mean Difference	Rank	Low Initial Health–Sickness Mean Difference	Rank
Reality Testing						
1. Distinction between inner and outer stimuli	−.333	3	−.583	1	−.523[a]	2
2. Accuracy of perception	−.328	3	−.692	1	−.421	2
Judgment						
3. Anticipation of consequences	−.562	2	−.665	1	−.551	3
4. Manifest behavior	−.625	2	−.810	1	−.491	3
5. Appropriateness of behavior	−.531	2	−.675	1	.444	3
Regulation and Control of Drives, Affects, and Impulses						
6. Directness of impulse	−.594	2	−.595	1	−.519	3
7. Effectiveness of delay and control mechanisms	−.641	2	−.720	1	−.611	3
Object Relations						
8. Degree and kind of relatedness	−.630	1	−.490	2	−.403	3
9. Object constancy	−.656	1	−.565	2	−.394	3
Thought Processes						
10. Ability to conceptualize	−.312	3	−.535	2	−.542	1
11. Primary-process thinking	−.349	3	−.660	1	−.472	2
Autonomous Functioning						
12. Freedom from impairment— primary	−.271	3	−.515	2	−.523	1
13. Freedom from impairment— secondary	−.411	3	−.475	2	−.551	1

Table 8.7.   (Continued)

Scales	High Initial Health–Sickness Mean Difference	Rank	Middle Initial Health–Sickness Mean Difference	Rank	Low Initial Health–Sickness Mean Difference	Rank
Synthetic–Integrative Functioning						
14. Reconciliation of incongruities	−.453	2	−.455	1	−.380	3
15. Relating together of events	−.474	1	−.420	3	−.468	2
Mastery–Competence						
16. Competence	−.578	1	−.445	2	−.370	3
Superego Scale						
17. Guilt	−.610	3	−.710	1	−.671	2
18. Ego ideal	−.823	1	−.710	2	−.648	3

[a] The vector of Initial Follow-up mean differences for the total sample was significant at $p <$ .001. The largest contributors to the significant F for this multivariate analysis as indicated by the discriminant function coefficients were Reconciliation of Incongruities (−1.126) and Effectiveness of Delay Mechanisms (1.046).

The vector of Initial Follow-up mean differences for the three initial health–sickness groups was borderline significant ($p = .168$). The discriminant function coefficients indicated that the largest contributors of this differential change were Guilt and Blame (1.125), Reconciliation of Incongruities (−1.012), and Anticipation of Consequences (.941).

on the Bellak scales were compared for the High, Middle, and Low groups (see Table 8.7), the kind of change was different from that seen in the PRP (Kernberg et al., 1972), and the Hospital-wide Follow-up Study (Harty et al., 1981). According to the data, the "rich get richer" phenomenon does not seem to prevail in the PPS Follow-up Study. In this study the Middle HS group improved more than the High and/or Low groups, particularly on 10 of the 18 Bellak scales: the two Reality Testing scales; Distinction Between Inner and Outer Stimuli, Accuracy of Perception; the three Judgment scales: Anticipation of Consequences, Manifest in Behavior, and Emotional Appropriateness; the two Regulation and Control of Drives, Impulses, and Affects scales: Directness of Impulse Expression and Effectiveness of Delay Mechanisms; only one of the Thought Process Scales: Primary–Secondary Process; one of the Synthetic Functioning scales: Guilt. This group appears to have improved in its thinking and judgment and possesses a more reasonable superego.

The Low group improved the most on three scales: one of the Thought Process scales: Ability to Conceptualize; and on both Autonomous Functioning scales: Freedom from Impairment of Primary Autonomous Functioning and Freedom from Impairment of Secondary Functioning. This group's main improvement appears to be in the area of thought.

The Low group changed least on 10 of the scales*: those dealing with Judgment: Anticipation of Consequences, Manifest in Behavior, and Emotional Appropriateness; both Regulation and Control of Drives, Impulses, and Affects scales: Directness of Impulse Expression and Delay Mechanisms; both Object Relations scales: Degree of Relatedness and Object Constancy; one of the Synthetic Integrative Functioning scales: Reconciliation of Incongruities; Mastery–Competence scale: Actual Competence; and one of the Superego scales: Ego Ideal.

The High group improved the most on five of the 18 scales: both Object Relations scales: Degree of Relatedness and Object Constancy; one of the Synthetic–Integrative Functioning scales: Relating Together of Events; one of the Mastery–Competence scales: Actual Competence; and one of the Superego scales: Ego Ideal. These results suggest that these individuals were feeling better about themselves, had improved interpersonal relationships, and had higher aspirations for themselves. They were achieving more than previously, felt better about it, and had set higher goals.

Schizophrenia Versus Borderline Groups

To check further if a particular diagnostic group was accounting for most of the kinds of changes that were made within the total group, the patients with a similar diagnosis were grouped. Two groups emerged large enough to be considered: the Schizophrenias and the Borderlines. The remaining groups had too few members to be considered.

Inclusion in the Schizophrenia group was based on criteria as set forth in DSM-II (1968), which was in use at the time the patients were in treatment. Criteria for Borderline personality organization were based on those set forth by Kernberg (1975) regarding ego strength, the characteristic defensive operations of the ego, and the pathology of the internalized object relationships of these patients.

Using the criteria stated earlier, the group divided into 26 Schizophrenic patients and 39 Borderline patients (see Table 8.8).

The multivariate test of differential change for the Schizophrenic and Borderline diagnostic groups was significant at $p < .001$. Discriminant function coefficients indicated that the major contribution was made by Reconciliation of Incongruities. The largest change was for the Borderline group. The test of change for the total sample was also significant at $p < .001$, with the largest contributors being Reconciliation of Incongruities, Effectiveness of Delay Mechanisms, Ego Ideal, and Primary–Secondary Process.

---

* Thus regression toward the mean also did not seem to be a factor in the amount of change for a majority of the scales.

Table 8.8. Schizophrenia Group and Borderline Group Differences Between Initial and Follow-up Ratings on the Bellak Scales

	Mean Difference	
Scales	Schizophrenic	Borderline
Reality Testing		
1. Distinction between inner and outer stimuli	−.558	−.442[a]
2. Accuracy of perception	−.510	−.458
Judgment		
3. Anticipation of consequences	−.486	−.696
4. Manifest behavior	−.514	−.756
5. Appropriateness of behavior	−.399	−.673
Regulation and Control of Drives, Affects, and Impulses		
6. Directness of impulse	−.317	−.750
7. Effectiveness of delay and control mechanisms	−.389	−1.907
Object Relations		
8. Degree and kind of relatedness	−.197	−.708
9. Object constancy	−.159	−.804
Thought Processes		
10. Ability to conceptualize	−.471	−.500
11. Primary-process thinking	−.490	−.503
Autonomous Functioning		
12. Freedom of impairment—primary	−.428	−.462
13. Freedom of impairment—secondary	−.423	−.545
Synthetic-Integrative Functioning		
14. Reconciliation of incongruities	−.384	−.574
15. Relating together of events	−.337	−.590
Mastery Competence		
16. Actual competence	−.221	−1.625
Superego Scale		
17. Guilt	−.385	−.865
18. Ego ideal	−.457	−.933

[a] The vector of Initial-Follow-up mean differences for the total sample was significant at $p <$ .001. The largest contributors to the significant F for the multivariate analysis as indicated by the discriminant function coefficients were: Reconciliation of Incongruities (−1.515), Effectiveness of Delay Mechanisms (1.327), Ego Ideal (1.155), and Primary–Secondary Process (1.092).

The vector of Initial-Follow-up mean differences for the Schizophrenic and Borderline diagnostic groups was significant at $p <$ .001. The discriminant function coefficients indicated that the largest contributors to this differential change were Reconciliation of Incongruities (−.944) and, to a much smaller extent, Distinction between Inner and Outer (−.589), Emotional Appropriateness (−.562), Effectiveness of Delay Mechanisms (.561), and Object Constancy (.555).

Although both the Schizophrenia and Borderline groups indicated change, they changed differently, with Borderline patients improving considerably more than the Schizophrenic patients. The Schizophrenic group changed more only in the area of Reality Testing: in being able to detect the difference between Inner and Outer Stimuli, and in their Accuracy of Perception. The Borderline group changed more than the Schizophrenia group in regard to Object Relations, Regulation and Control of Drives, Actual Competence, and the Superego scales. Clinically, this finding has relevance in that it is in these areas that the Borderline patient is most incapacitated at the beginning of treatment; thus, if treatment has been successful, change would be most apparent in these areas.

One might question whether a halo effect may be at work in Schizophrenic patients receiving a lower rating at least at initial rating. To avoid such a situation as much as possible, the chart material used in making the original ratings had all identifying data removed, including all diagnoses before it was sent to the raters.

Schizophrenic–Borderline Groups Versus Initial High–Middle–Low Health–Sickness Groups

In examining the number of Borderline and Schizophrenic patients included in each initial Health–Sickness group, the two diagnostic groups did not differ significantly with respect to the proportions in each of the initial Health–Sickness groups. The Schizophrenic and Borderline patients were, on a percentage basis, closely represented within the Middle Health–Sickness group. As expected, Schizophrenic patients were more represented in the Low Health–Sickness Group than were the Borderline patients, and Borderline patients were more represented in the High Health–Sickness group than were the Schizophrenic patients (see Table 8.9).

Table 8.9. Comparison of Schizophrenic and Borderline Patients in Initial High, Middle, and Low Health–Sickness Groups

	Diagnoses			
Health–Sickness	Schizophrenia N	($N = 26$) %	Borderline N	($N = 39$) %
High	5	19.2	14	35.9
Middle	8	30.8	15	38.5
Low	13	50.0	10	25.6
Chi square =	4.3592	n.s.		

Factor Structures: Initial and Follow-up Using the Bellak Scales

Since initial factor structures were similar in both the 150-member group and the 78-member group (see Table 8.3), inferences made from this small group are assumed to be representative of the larger group. The validity of this assumption can only be tested when the follow-up interviews and statistical analysis of the 150-member sample have been completed.

At follow-up the three factors* obtained at the initial rating of the Bellak scales merged into one general factor for both the interviewer and the two raters.

Ratings on all follow-up scales were highly intercorrelated and merged into one general factor, a Follow-up Adjustment or Health–Sickness factor. Two separate analyses, one using the interviewer's ratings and another one using the two raters' ratings, produced the same results. How might we understand this finding?

Data Base. Although the Bellak scales were rated from clinical documents in both the initial treatment phases and the follow-up phase of the PPS study, the data source for these documents was different in each case. Initial ratings utilized clinical documents written by different individuals (hospital doctor, social worker, and nurse) whose source of information was the patient, the family, and the team observation of the patient over a period of time, usually the first four weeks prior to the diagnostic conference.

Follow-up ratings utilized discharge summaries from the hospital therapist, psychotherapist, social worker, and aftercare coordinator where applicable, to establish a baseline for evaluating the information contained in the follow-up interview. The follow-up interview, on the other hand, is the result of one or two contacts generally by telephone with the patient and/or his or her family and written by one individual. The data base for this document, therefore, is different from that of other documents used in the study.

Psychoanalytic Orientation. The raters in the PPS study did their analyses and rating from a psychoanalytic frame of reference, which inadvertently could have biased their ratings in the direction of a general factor. The psychoanalytic frame of reference suggests not only a theory of personality development but also a therapeutic technique, and by implication, a philosophical statement about the individual in regard to needs, desires, goals, and aspirations. Basic to this orientation is the concept of the unconscious. Although the definition of *unconscious* and its manner of influencing behavior may vary sharply, most behavioral scientists agree our day-to-day living is influenced by factors that are outside immediate awareness and reside in

---

* The first unrotated factor at this initial rating came close to being a general factor, however.

what might be termed the unconscious. The Unconscious influences one's thought, one's behavioral response to affect, instinct, and drive fueled by the presence or absence of unconscious guilt and one's self-perception. It is difficult to assess an individual within the psychoanalytic frame of reference without considering all these aspects of the individual. This bias could be reflected inadvertently in the manner of reporting and interpreting patient material.

Results of Treatment. A question might be raised in regard to treatment itself. Psychiatric treatment could be seen as a socialization process. We turn out individuals who can fit reasonably well into and not be disruptive of society. In most states individuals can be committed to a psychiatric hospital only if there is sufficient evidence that they are a serious danger to themselves and/or others (potential suicide or homicide). Our goals are much more ambitious than mere socialization but in reality may not be too frequently achieved, particularly with the growing emphasis on short-term treatment.

Bellak Scales. We could speculate that the Bellak scales are insensitive to the finer nuances of personality structuring that would be necessary to delineate subtle differences characteristic of patients at follow-up. Consequently, the specific ego functions of patients tend to be viewed in more global than specific terms. Because of this tendency additional scales were used in the PPS.

The issues discussed earlier present certain technical difficulties with the Follow-up study but do not invalidate its findings. What might be obscured in the findings due to the manner in which follow-up data are obtained and evaluated are the finer nuances of patient adjustment.

Predictions of Outcome at Follow-up

The initial Bellak scale factors were correlated with the Follow-up Adjustment Scale* to see how well they predicted outcome at follow-up. Both Freedom from Thought Disorder ($p < .001$) and Judgment and Impulse Control ($p < .036$) correlated significantly, but Superego Functioning did not correlate with anything (see Table 8.10). Thus, Factor I (Freedom from Thought Disorder) and Factor II (Judgment and Impulse Control) predict a certain amount of the outcome variance at follow-up. This condition is not true, however, for Factor III (Superego Functioning).

The two Object Relations scales—Degree and Kind of Relatedness and Object Constancy—that did not load on any of the Bellak factors at admission correlated significantly ($p < .001$) with Follow-up Adjustment. This

* Marker variable for the Follow-up Adjustment or Health–Sickness factor.

correlation was expected in accord with our Object Relations point of view. What was unexpected was their failure to attain status as an independent factor.

The fact that the follow-up outcome ratings factored into only one factor created a problem for testing the hypotheses, since these presupposed that follow-up ratings would be relatively independent. Thus, differentiation among the results for the follow-up outcome variables is less likely.

The hypotheses that ratings of General Adjustment (PPS) (Behavior, Symptoms, and Interpersonal Relationships) and the ratings from the Hospital-wide Follow-up Study Scales (Harty et al., 1981) (Extent of Separation from Family of Origin and Quality of Object Relations) would be related to Factor III were not confirmed. The PPS Core Group did somewhat better, with some of the other predictions, as indicated below (also see Table 8.10).

I. Ratings of General Adjustment
    A. Behavior appeared to relate to Factor II, but in fact related even more to Factor I.
    B. Symptoms, which the group had felt would be related to Factors I and III, related to Factor I and only slightly to Factor II.
    C. Drug and Alcohol Abuse was related to Factor II only.
    D. Sexual Interests related to Factor I.
    E. Interpersonal Relationships did not relate to Factor III but did relate to Factors I and II.
    F. Work Adjustment, which the group thought might relate to Factor II, related to Factor I.
    G. Dependence–Independence and Special Skills both related to Factor I.
II. Ratings from Hospital-wide Follow-up Scales (Harty et al., 1981)
    A. Health–Sickness (Luborsky, 1975), which the group thought would be related to both Factors I and II, was found to be related to Factor I only.
    B. Follow-up Adjustment was related to Factor II but was related much more to Factor I.
    C. Global Improvement was related to Factors I and II.
    D. Separation from Family of Origin was related to Factors I and II, not Factor III as predicted.
    E. Abstract and Conceptual Thinking was related to Factor I as predicted.
    F. Quality of Object Relations was related to Factors I and II.
    G. Acquisition of Skills and Interests, which the group thought would be related to Factor II, was more strongly related to Factor I.

The hypotheses made prior to follow-up were not totally confirmed, in part because they were made on the basis of the kind of differentiation in

Table 8.10. Correlations of Follow-up Scale Ratings Predicted to Relate to Bellak Factors from Initial Ratings

Scales	Factor I: Freedom from Thought Disorder (N = 78)		Factor II: Judgment and Impulse Control (N = 78)		Factor III: Superego Functioning (N = 78)	
	r	p	r	p	r	p
I. Ratings of general adjustment						
A. Behavior	−.3316	.003	−.2270	.046	−.0247	.830
B. Symptoms	−.4420	<.001	−.2297	.043	.0543	.637
C. Drugs and/or Alcohol Abuse	.0544	.636	−.2596	.022	−.0476	.679
D. Sexual Interests	−.4018	<.001	−.1854	.106	−.0235	.839
E. Interpersonal Relationships	−.4821	<.001	−.2230	.050	−.0349	.762
F. Work Adjustment	−.4747	<.001	−.2197	.053	−.0951	.408
G. Dependence–Independence	−.4789	<.001	−.2160	.058	−.0091	.937
H. Special skills	.4169	<.001	−.2146	.059	.1621	.156
II. Ratings from hospital-wide follow-up study scales						
A. Health–Sickness	.4356	<.001	.1420	.215	.0675	.557
B. Follow-up Adjustment	.4778	<.001	.2376	.036	.0940	.413
C. Global Improvement	.4485	<.001	.2080	.068	.1121	.228
D. Extent of Separation from Family of Origin	.4230	<.001	.3186	.004	−.0235	.838
E. Abstract and Conceptual Thinking	.6066	<.001	.1847	.105	−.0048	.966
F. Quality of Object Relations	.5329	<.001	.2865	.011	.0198	.863
G. Acquisition of Skills and Interests	.4589	<.001	.1889	.098	.0846	.461

Bellak Scales found at the initial ratings, which was no longer true at follow-up. Thirteen of the 15 follow-up scales correlated with Factor I at $p < .001$ and a 14th scale, "Behavior," at the $p < .003$ level. Only Drugs and/or Alcohol Abuse did not correlate with Factor I. This finding in part reflects the unexpectedly high correlation among outcome ratings.

Correlations with Factor I, "Freedom from Thought Disorder," were not a total surprise, since how a person thinks influences all that he does; his behavior is a response to his thinking. Those scales, however, describing special behavioral responses (Sexual Interests, Work Adjustment, Dependence–Independence, and Special Skills) would have been expected to relate to Factor II, "Judgment and Impulse Control." Although their correlation with Factor I is understandable, the small or zero correlation with Factor II was unexpected. Even more astonishing was Factor III's lack of correlation with any follow-up scale. One would have thought, since feelings of guilt and how one perceives his or her own ego ideal have such an influence on interpersonal relationships, that those scales that relate to object relationships especially (Interpersonal Relationships, Separation from Family of Origin, and Quality of Object Relations) would be related to Factor III.

Discussion of Results

The changes noted between initial and follow-up ratings were statistically significant ($p < .001$). This change was more apparent when the subsample was divided into Schizophrenia and Borderline groups. Clinically, these patients changed in areas and directions in which they would be expected to change. Schizophrenic individuals have significant difficulty with thought processes and object relations. A major goal of treatment is to help them learn to control their thinking even though difficulty remains. It is not uncommon to have individuals who carry the diagnosis of schizophrenia to report at the conclusion of treatment that they still have the same kinds of thoughts they had before. They just don't talk about them with others. Data from repeat psychological testing (Cerney, "Unraveling the Symbiotic Bond," manuscript in preparation) indicate that at a conclusion of treatment primary process material is still present but the patient maintains better control over its expression.

A rather disappointing finding to the clinicians in this study is the relative lack of change in Object Relations overall, particularly in regard to the schizophrenia sample. Object Relations was also expected to rank as one of the more important factors. Treatment emphasizes the importance of the development of object constancy and object relatedness to others. From these data it would appear either that we do not succeed in this area as much as we might wish or that the Bellak scales are not sensitive to the kinds of changes seen in the follow-up sample.

Preliminary analyses of individual subjects who improved markedly in the Schizophrenia study (Cerney et al., in process) seem to indicate that one facilitating aspect for their remarkable changes was the development of an enduring bond to one or more members of their treatment team. An in-depth examination of the Schizophrenia group members in the PPS who made marked change in the course of treatment may reveal the same finding.

The clinician's experience is that many schizophrenics remain rather isolated individuals who function marginally in society after treatment. Since the family in many cases has come to terms with what can be expected and has accepted the individual at his or her own level, the individual's behavior may be less disruptive to the family. Released of pressure to function at an impossible level of performance, many schizophrenic individuals chose occupations with minimal stress and low expectations. With permission to function at this lower level, some achieve marginal independence, become self-supporting, but do not circulate in the same social class as their parents.

Borderline personalities, on the other hand, initially have difficulty around judgment and impulse regulation. A major goal of their treatment is to help them learn to control their behavior and be more socially in tune with society. No longer at war with society, they get along better and experience major improvement in their object relations. Freed of psychological constraints, they are also better able to utilize their natural endowments.

That change should occur strikingly on the Superego scales is of interest. Patients often come to treatment with such severe superegos that their lives are a constant torture. Others arrive with what appears on the surface to be an utter lack of conscience. Both of these groups, according to the data, seem to benefit from treatment, with the severe superego becoming more benign and the lax superego becoming more responsible, as reflected in change on the Bellak scales.

No matter which way the data are examined, most improvement is evident in Judgment, Regulation of Drives, and Superego Functions. These are important areas if one is to function in a reasonable way in society without undue stress and with some measure of satisfaction.

CONCLUSION

The results of the analysis of these data are consistent with what is experienced clinically. We attempt to effect change in the thought structure of patients, but we know we only succeed in possibly socializing them. They learn to be more circumspect in how, when, and where they express their thoughts. It is, nevertheless, encouraging to see improvement in their reality testing, their control of their impulses, and how they apply their judgment to everyday situations. With a more reasonably balanced superego, neither too strict nor too lax, life is not the trial it once was.

One might question whether the outcome achieved in this study is the result of phone interviews and the possibility of halo effect or whether patients report themselves to be better than they are in actuality. In some instances it was possible to speak with parents and others who knew the patient. Where this contact occurred, there seemed to be general agreement in the patient's overall functioning, although the patients tended on the average to rate themselves somewhat lower than parents and others who knew them. However, these additional data were not available on the entire sample reported here.

It is notable that what turned out to be more differentiated criteria at the initial rating of the patients, did not turn out to be so at follow-up. According to the data, patients are more differentiated when they arrive for treatment, less so at follow-up. This finding may be attributable to the different data base used in each rating, clinical documents at the initial rating and self-report at follow-up. What appears to be the homogenizing effect of treatment may also be related to the data base, as well as the scales and/or the psychoanalytic bias of the raters inadvertently reflected in their rating.

At this point we have insufficient follow-up data to enable a meaningful comparison of the patient profile groupings at initial with follow-up outcome to test whether the patient profile is any more valid than any other diagnostic scheme as regards treatment response and outcome.

REFERENCES

American Psychiatric Association. *Diagnostic and statistical manual of mental disorders* (2d ed., DSM-II). Washington, D.C.: American Psychiatric Association, 1968.

American Psychiatric Association. *Diagnostic and statistical manual of mental disorders* (3d ed., DSM-III). Washington, D.C.: American Psychiatric Association, 1980.

Bellak, L., Hurvich, H., & Gediman, H. K. *Ego functions in schizophrenics, neurotics and normals: A systematic study of conceptual, diagnostic, and therapeutic aspects.* New York: Wiley, 1973.

Cerney, M. S. Unraveling the symbiotic bond: A comparison of repeat psychological testing on a schizophrenic patient, *Bulletin of the Menninger Clinic* (in press).

Cerney, M. S., Coyne, L., Poggi, R., Mittleman, F., & Zee, H. Outcome and follow-up study of 20 consecutive schizophrenic patient admissions, manuscript in preparation.

Frieswyk, S., Cerney, M., Coyne, L., Newsom, G., Novotny, P., & Schroeder, P. Quality of relations: An empirical measure, manuscript in preparation, 1981.

Frieswyk, S., Cerney, M., Coyne, L., Newsom, G., Novotny, P., and Schroder, P. Capacity for emotion: An empirical scale, manuscript in preparation, 1981.

Harty, M., Cerney, M., Colson, D., Coyne, L., Frieswyk, S., Johnson, S. B., and Mortimer, R.

Correlates of change and long-term outcome: An exploratory study of intensively treated hospital patients. *Bulletin of the Menninger Clinic,* 1981, *45,* 209–228.

Kernberg, O. F. *Borderline conditions and pathological narcissism.* New York: J. Aronson, 1975.

Kernberg, O. F., Bernstein, D., Coyne, L., Appelbaum, A., Horwitz, L., & Voth, H. Psychotherapy and psychoanalysis. *Bulletin of the Menninger Clinic,* 1972, *36*(1, 2), 3–195.

Comparison of Ego Function Scales and Symptom Ratings in Evaluating Long-Term Hospital Treatment

JON G. ALLEN, LOLAFAYE COYNE,
THOMAS M. MURPHY, GERALD TARNOFF,
JAMES BUSKIRK, AND N. WILLIAM KEARNS

We collected the data reported here in the initial phase of a treatment–evaluation project we are implementing in a long-term hospital setting. We wished to develop a set of scales to use on an ongoing basis to monitor patients' progress in treatment and assess the outcome at the point of discharge. We had two requirements for the set of variables to be selected: First, the variables should be comprehensive and encompass the major dimensions of psychopathology and psychological strengths in our patient population. Second, the set should contain a manageably small number of variables such that the process of rating them and interpreting their clinical significance would not be unduly time consuming.

We chose the Bellak Ego Functions Scales (Bellak, Hurvich, & Gediman, 1973) to be the cornerstone of our assessment procedure because our treatment aims at personality reconstruction and our goals include improvement in ego functioning. We added the Brief Psychiatric Rating Scale (Overall & Gorham, 1962) to complement the ego functions scales to enable us to compare symptomatic improvement with intrapsychic change. We also devised four scales to assess problem behaviors pertinent to our hospital population: Suicide Risk, Physical Self-destructiveness, Risk of Violence, and Substance Use. Finally, we included the Health–Sickness Rating Scale (Luborsky, 1975) to assess overall severity of psychopathology.

To pave the way for the prospective study, which involves ongoing assessments (Allen et al., 1983), we conducted a retrospective study of 52 patients consecutively discharged over a 2½-year period. We rated all of the scales mentioned above from clinical charts at admission and discharge. This paper compares the ego functions scales and the BPRS symptom ratings as initial assessment methods and contrasts the two approaches as they relate to changes observed at discharge.

METHOD

Setting and Patient Population

We conducted the research on a long-term unit in the C. F. Menninger Memorial Hospital, which emphasizes intensive treatment guided by psychoanalytic principles. The patients present a range of serious and chronic psychiatric disorders; most of them have had extensive previous treatment, often including many prior psychiatric hospitalizations. In our sample of 52 patients, the primary diagnoses were schizophrenic disorders (28 patients), personality disorders (18 patients), and major affective disorders (6 patients). Twenty-nine patients were female and 23 were male; the average age was 24.7 years; and the mean length of stay was 15.7 months. All of these patients were treated on our unit, which is comprised of two multidisciplinary teams who treat 10–11 patients each.

Instruments and Rating Methods

Ego Functions. We assessed the ego functions from the example-anchored component subscales that had been found previously to be reliably ratable from clinical charts in our setting (see Coyne et al., Chapter 6): Reality Testing (distinction between inner and outer stimuli; accuracy of perception), Judgment (anticipation of consequences, manifest behavior, appropriateness of behavior), Regulation and Control of Drives, Affects, and Impulses (directness of impulse expression, effectiveness of delay and control), Object Relations (degree and kind of relatedness, object constancy),

Thought Processes (ability to conceptualize, language and communication), Autonomous Functioning (apparatuses of primary autonomy; secondary autonomous functions), Synthetic–Integrative Functioning (degree of reconciliation, active relating), Mastery–Competence (competence), and Superego Adaptation (guilt and blame, ego ideal). We rated the patients' characteristic functioning around the time of admission (based on recent history prior to admission and functioning during the evaluation period) and characteristic functioning around the time of discharge.

Brief Psychiatric Rating Scale.   The Brief Psychiatric Rating Scale (BPRS) assessed 18 symptoms: somatic concern, anxiety, emotional withdrawal, conceptual disorganization, guilt feelings, tension, mannerisms and posturing, grandiosity, depressive mood, hostility, suspiciousness, hallucinatory behavior, motor retardation, uncooperativeness, unusual thought content, blunted affect, excitement, and disorientation. Each symptom is rated on a seven-point scale ranging from "not present" to "extremely severe." We departed from the customary use of this scale in making the ratings from clinical charts rather than psychiatric interviews. Nevertheless, the charts typically contained extensive documentation of the patients' mental status and behavior in interview situations such that the required material for the ratings was available.

Problem-Behavior Scales.   We devised four scales to assess the risk of potentially destructive behavior of central interest in our setting: Suicide Risk, Physical Self-destructiveness (not suicidal in intent), Risk of Physical Violence, and Substance Use. Each scale takes into account the potential dangerousness of the behavior, the patient's capacity to exercise control over the behavior, and the likelihood that such action will occur. These are 100-point example-anchored rating scales, modeled after the Health–Sickness Rating Scale (see below).

Health–Sickness Rating Scale.   The Health–Sickness Rating Scale (Luborsky, 1975) is an example-anchored rating scale assessing global severity of psychopathology. The scale ranges from zero ("any condition which, unattended, would quickly result in the patient's death") to 100 ("an ideal state of complete functioning, integration, of resiliency in the face of stress, of happiness and social effectiveness").

Global Improvement Ratings.   To measure staff perception of outcome, we included a 100-point example-anchored Global Improvement Scale that has been employed previously in our setting as a direct measure of change (Harty et al., 1981). These ratings were made independently and retrospectively by each member of the multidisciplinary team (i.e., hospital therapist, social worker, team nurse, and activity therapist). The Spearman–Brown corrected reliability for the average rating was .81.

Raters and Procedures

The raters were experienced clinicians working in the hospital unit on which the project is conducted. The majority of charts in the sample were rated by the unit psychologist (senior author); the remainder were rated by one of three unit psychiatrists (the unit leader and the two team leaders). Although the raters in many instances were familiar with the patients they were rating, to limit bias, cases were assigned to raters who had *not* been *directly* involved in the treatment (e.g., as team leader or hospital therapist). The raters used extensive material from the hospital charts (e.g., the diagnostic summary of the treating psychiatrist or psychologist, the nursing assessment, the social worker's family study, and results of psychological testing). Summaries from the multidisciplinary treatment staff were also used to make ratings at discharge.

Each patient was rated by only one rater; hence, we did not establish interrater reliability for our assessments. Nevertheless, the ego functions scales we employed had previously been shown to be reliably ratable by experienced clinicians in our setting for comparable, although somewhat less extensive, material (see Chapter 6). In addition, the reliabilities of the Brief Psychiatric Rating Scale and Health–Sickness Rating Scale have also been established previously (although the BPRS has been rated from interviews). Thus, the only untested scales in our assessment are the problem-behavior scales; nevertheless, the findings reported below support their construct validity.

RESULTS*

Overview

We shall present the following data analyses: (1) factor analyses of the ego functions scales and BPRS symptom ratings at admission;† (2) correlations between the ego functions scales and symptom ratings with the Health–Sickness Rating Scale and our problem-behavior scales at admission; (4) multivariate analyses of change (admission to discharge) for the ego func-

---

* A global description of our results is presented here; detailed tabulations of findings are available from the senior author upon request.

† We also factor analyzed the ego functions scales and BPRS symptom ratings at discharge. The factors were less differentiated and more difficult to interpret; hence, these are not discussed further.

tions scales and symptom ratings; and (5) correlations of the ego functions scales and symptom ratings with perceived improvement.

Factor Analyses

We conducted a separate factor analysis of the ego functions scales from that reported previously (Chapter 9) because we used different subjects and the data base for making our ratings was somewhat more extensive. Hence, the results and our factor labels are somewhat different. Four factors emerged from our analysis* of the ego functions assessed at admission. The first factor, best labeled Thought Organization, is a broad one, encompassing Thought Processes, Reality Testing, Autonomous Functions, and Synthetic Functioning. It is not surprising that this factor emerges as a central dimension in our population; a major differentiating factor among our patients is the presence (and degree) of psychosis. The second factor, best labeled Object Relations, encompasses the two Object Relations subscales, along with the Mastery–Competence and Ego Ideal subscales. This factor is also rather broad in scope; it appears to reflect the level of separation–individuation and capacity for functioning independently and autonomously. Again, this is a central dimension in our population, as our patients cover a wide range of the separation–individuation spectrum. The remaining factors are relatively narrow, the third being Judgment and the fourth being Drive Regulation. The Drive Regulation factor not only has high loadings on the Drive Regulation subscale but also has a high loading on Superego–Guilt, probably because many of our patients who have difficulty modulating drive are expressing this in suicidal and self-destructive behavior.

Five factors emerged from the factor analysis of the BPRS symptom ratings. Paralleling the ego functions scales, the first factor is best labeled Psychoticism, and it encompasses a relatively broad array of variables: unusual thought content, grandiosity, conceptual disorganization, suspiciousness, hallucinatory behavior, and disorientation. The remaining four factors are affective dimensions: Emotional Withdrawal (also including blunted affect, mannerisms, and posturing), Depression (also including guilt, somatic concern, motor retardation), Hostility (also including uncooperativeness), and Agitation (including tension, excitement, anxiety).

Comparison of Ego Functions and BPRS Symptom Ratings at Admission

To compare the ego functions and symptom rating assessment methods, the factor scores from each method were intercorrelated. These results are

---

* We employed a principal components factor analysis with normal varimax rotation of all factors with eigenvalues of 1 or greater.

Table 9.1. Correlations Between Ego Functions Factor Scores and BPRS Symptom Rating Factor Scores at Admission

Ego Function Factors	Symptom Rating Factors				
	Psychoticism (I)	Withdrawal (II)	Depression (III)	Hostility (IV)	Agitation (V)
Thought Organization (I)	−.61***	−.32*	.04	.24+	−.35**
Object Relations (II)	−.13	−.49***	−.14	−.30*	.07
Judgment (III)	−.33*	.15	.51***	−.29*	.03
Drive Regulation (IV)	−.01	−.10	−.01	−.05	−.21

Note: *** $p \leq .001$, ** $p \leq .01$, * $p \leq .05$, + $p \leq .10$.

displayed in Table 9.1. Note that the scales are keyed in opposite directions such that higher ego functions scores represent healthier functioning, whereas higher symptom rating scores represent more disturbance. Thought organization and psychoticism correlate most highly, reflecting a major area of overlap in the two methods. Thought organization is also associated negatively with emotional withdrawal and agitation, although it is associated positively with hostility (at a marginally significant level). As would be expected, higher-level object relations are associated negatively with emotional withdrawal and hostility. Interestingly, better judgment is negatively associated with psychoticism and hostility but *positively* correlated with depression. The likely explanation is that depressed patients internalize their conflicts whereas others are more likely to act them out in destructive behavior reflecting poor judgment. In contrast to judgment, drive regulation does not correlate with any symptom rating factors.

We also compared the ego functions and symptom ratings (factor scores) in relation to the Health–Sickness Rating Scale and our problem-behavior scales. These results are displayed in Table 9.2. Each ego function factor is positively correlated with Health–Sickness (higher scores on each represent greater health). Notably, the correlations are highest for Thought Organization and Object Relations, which suggests that these are two major, distinct dimensions of disturbance in our population. Appropriately, our problem-behavior scales are most negatively associated with Judgment and Regulation and Control of Drives, Affects, and Impulses (higher scores represent more disturbance). As we would expect, better judgment is associated with lower risk of self-destructiveness, violence, and substance use. Interestingly, better judgment (along with higher thought organization) is associated marginally with *higher* suicide risk. It is likely that depression (also associ-

Table 9.2. *Correlations of Ego Functions Factors and BPRS Symptom Rating Factors at Admission with Health–Sickness and Problem-Behavior Scales*

Factors	Health–Sickness	Problem-Behavior Scales			
		Suicide	Self-destructive	Violence	Substance Use
Ego Functions					
Thought Organization (I)	.56***	.30*	.09	.04	.17
Object Relations (II)	.54***	−.02	.11	.04	.05
Judgment (III)	.28*	.26⁺	−.43**	−.47***	−.36**
Drive Regulation (IV)	.36**	−.24⁺	−.41**	−.42**	−.09
Symptom Ratings					
Psychoticism (I)	−.57***	−.22	.14	.08	.16
Withdrawal (II)	−.37**	−.11	−.15	−.01	−.18
Depression (III)	.02	.51***	−.16	−.40**	−.31*
Hostility (IV)	−.13	.09	.18	.23⁺	.08
Agitation (V)	−.28*	.03	.18	−.02	−.05

Note: *** $p \leq .001$, ** $p \leq .01$, * $p \leq .05$, ⁺ $p \leq .10$.

ated with better judgment) is the mediating variable. Drive regulation correlates most strongly with self-destructive and violent behavior, although there is also a marginally negative correlation with suicide risk.

The relationships between symptom ratings (factor scores) and health–sickness parallel those for ego functions; psychoticism correlates most strongly, followed by emotional withdrawal (which corresponds partly to object relations). Depression is the only symptom-rating factor that relates strongly to problem-behavior scales; it is associated with higher suicide risk and lower risk of violence and substance abuse. This confirms the suggestion that depression lowers the risk of alloplastic destructive behavior.

Multivariate Analyses of Change

The multivariate profile analysis of variance revealed significant overall positive change in the ego functions scales from admission to discharge ($p <$ .001). Alternatively, the univariate F-tests revealed significant differences for each of the 18 scales ($p < .001$). Among the discriminant function coefficients, the strongest predictors are one of the Thought Processes scales (Ability to Conceptualize), Regulation and Control of Drives, Affects, and Impulses (Effectiveness of Delay and Control) and Mastery–Competence;

Superego Functioning (Guilt–Blame) and the other Thought Processes scale (Language and Communication) enter in prominently as suppressor variables (negative beta weights). The multivariate profile analysis of variance for symptom ratings also revealed significant overall positive change ($p <$ .001) and univariate F-tests revealed significant positive changes ($p < .05$) for all scales except Grandiosity, Hostility, and Uncooperativeness.

Relationship of Ego Functions Scales and BPRS Symptom Ratings to Perceived Improvement

The pattern of correlations of ego functions subscales with mean (multidisciplinary) global improvement ratings revealed modest relationships between assessments of ego functioning at admission and perceived improvement at discharge (i.e., higher levels of ego functioning at admission were associated with more improvement in treatment). The correlations for four subscales were statistically significant: Reality Testing (Accuracy of Perception), Judgment (Anticipation of Consequences), Synthetic Functioning (Reconciliation or Integration), and Mastery–Competence; the correlation for thought processes (language and communication) was marginally significant. Consistent with these generally low correlations, there was no significant relationship between admission ratings of health–sickness and perceived improvement ($r = .13$).

In contrast, all the ego functions assessed at discharge are significantly correlated with perceived improvement; similarly, change in each of the ego functions (residual change scores*) is significantly associated with perceived improvement. It is likely that this pervasive association between ego functions and perceived improvement at discharge in part reflects the relative lack of differentiation among the ego functions scales at that period (see second footnote, p. 153).

The correlation of BPRS symptom ratings at admission with mean global improvement revealed slightly stronger relationships than those observed for ego functions. Emotional withdrawal, grandiosity, suspiciousness, and, to a lesser extent, conceptual disorganization, hallucinatory behavior, and unusual thought content are negatively associated with global improvement. Interestingly, guilt and depression at admission are positively, although modestly, associated with improvement. This is consistent with the finding reported earlier that, in some respects, depression is a positive sign (i.e., associated with lowered potential for acting out). In addition, the relationships of symptom ratings at discharge to improvement are stronger (although not as uniformly positive as those found for ego functions). Further, the relationships of symptom-rating change to scores to improvement are quite consistently high.

* Residual change scores were obtained by partialing out initial level from the raw change scores (difference).

DISCUSSION

In many respects the results confirmed our expectation that the ego functions scales and symptom ratings would be complementary. The results of the factor analysis of the ego functions at admission were very compatible with our conceptualization of our patient population; Thought Organization, Object Relations, and Impulse Control (reflected in judgment and drive regulation) are dimensions of major import. The only area of redundancy between the ego functions and BPRS symptom ratings is in the overlap of the Thought Organization factor with several symptom scales reflecting "psychoticism." The other factors emerging from the symptom ratings, however, provide additional useful dimensions as they represent major areas of affective disturbance.

The pattern of correlations between the ego functions factors and symptom-rating factors supports the construct validity of each approach. The only surprising finding was the positive relationship of depression to judgment and its negative relationship to violence and substance use. Notwithstanding its positive correlation with suicide risk, depression was also a good prognostic sign. As mentioned earlier, this probably reflects the greater proclivity of depressed patients in our sample to internalize rather than act out conflicts, hence, to benefit from treatment.

Ego functions and symptom ratings assessed at admission were modestly predictive of perceived improvement at discharge. Both methods of assessment were highly sensitive to overall level of change, although neither was highly discriminating. That is, perceived improvement at discharge was associated with change in ego functions and symptoms almost across the board. Of course, our measure of improvement was a global one. Further, these global findings may partly reflect some limitations in our retrospective method. First, although the raters were not directly involved in the patients' treatment, they were identified with the work of the hospital unit and had general knowledge of the outcomes; hence, bias may have operated to produce a general halo effect. Perhaps more importantly, the discharge ratings were made from clinical charts and the material in the charts is usually less extensive at discharge than at admission (which includes a very thorough, multidisciplinary diagnostic evaluation). Thus, the information from which the ratings were made was less differentiated at discharge than it was at admission.

Despite the limitations of our retrospective method, the results provide a solid foundation for our prospective treatment-evaluation project (Allen et al., 1983). Guided by the factor analyses and comparisons of the two assessment approaches at admission, along with our conceptual preferences, we have selected key scales that capture the major dimensions of interest in our population. The ego functions scales are most useful to assess core aspects of structural personality change. For purposes of comprehensive treatment evaluation, however, our findings support the addition of supplementary scales to assess specific dimensions of affective disturbance (i.e., from the BPRS) and potentially destructive behavior (i.e., problem-behavior scales). We are using these selected scales to assess patients' functioning at admission, their progress during treatment (corresponding to regularly scheduled review conferences), and their condition at discharge. We graph the profiles that emerge from our numerical ratings on all of these scales. At admission, these graphs assist in the formulation of treatment goals; thereafter, the graphs contribute to the evaluation of change and the assessment of areas of continuing impairment that require further intervention.

REFERENCES

Allen, J., Tarnoff, G., Murphy, T., Buskirk, J., and Coyne, L. The benefits of integrating treatment evaluation and clinical practice in a long-term hospital setting. *Bulletin of the Menninger Clinic,* 1983, *47,* 225–241.

Bellak, L., Hurvich, M., & Gediman, H. K. *Ego functions in schizophrenics, neurotics, and normals: A systematic study of conceptual, diagnostic, and therapeutic aspects.* New York: Wiley, 1973.

Harty, M., Cerney, M., Colson, D., Coyne, L., Frieswyk, S., Johnson, S. B., & Mortimer, R. Correlates of change and long-term outcome: An exploratory study of intensively treated hospital patients. *Bulletin of the Menninger Clinic,* 1981, *45,* 209–228.

Luborsky, L. Clinicians' judgments of mental health: Specimen case descriptions and forms of the Health–Sickness Rating Scale. *Bulletin of the Menninger Clinic,* 1975, *39,* 448–480.

Overall, J. E., & Gorham, D. R. The Brief Psychiatric Rating Scale. *Psychological Reports,* 1962, *10,* 799–812.

CHAPTER TEN

A Study of Agreement Among Raters of Bellak's Ego Function Assessment Test

ALV A. DAHL

The present report is part of a larger investigation of the validity of the borderline class as a diagnostic category. As part of this project the Ego Function Assessment Test (Bellak et al., 1973) was applied to patients of several diagnostic groups with the aim of comparing borderline patients with patients in other diagnostic categories. With this goal in mind, it was first necessary to demonstrate that this measure could be reliably used with a Norwegian patient population. In constructing the Ego Function Assessment Test, scoring and administration procedures were standardized, and reliability studies demonstrating adequate interrater reliability were conducted (Bellak et al., 1973).

METHOD

Subjects

The data were collected from a sample of 231 inpatients, ranging in age from 18 to 40, who were consecutively admitted to two hospitals in Oslo.

Twenty-three patients (10% of the sample) was randomly selected from a sample of 156 patients, whose interviews were either videotaped or audiotaped.

The author divided the subjects into five diagnostic categories, according to operational criteria (RDC/DSM-III). Three subjects were assigned to the schizophrenic group, three to the affective disorder group, nine to the borderline group, two to the group of neurotics, and six to the "other disorders" category (other personality disorders and psychoses).

Data

The data considered for the current study consisted of a three-part interview: (1) an extended version of the Schedule for Affective Disorders and Schizophrenia (SADS) including the Schedule for Interviewing Borderlines (SIB), (2) a life and family history inventory, and (3) the Ego Function Assessment Interview.

Procedure

Independent evaluations were conducted by experienced psychiatrists and psychotherapists who had psychoanalytic training and substantial experience in differential diagnosis. Preparation and training for their task was fairly extensive. They read papers and met with the main investigator for discussions. In addition, two videotapes were shown and scored so that any obscurities in the scoring could be discussed and clarified. Finally, the group participated in a two-day seminar with Leopold Bellak on the Ego Function Assessment Scale. Each of the seven evaluators was given three audiotaped interviews to score for diagnosis on operational criteria (five categories), and in the categories of Mental Disorders in the Ninth Revision of the International Classification of Diseases (ICD-9), as well as to score on the Global Assessment and Ego Function Assessment Scale.

Two cases, which were videotaped and used for training purposes, were included in the diagnostic analysis, however, because the raters did not have prior experience with the other measures, only 21 cases were considered in the analyses for the other instruments.

RESULTS

On the diagnostic criteria there was a high degree of agreement among the independent raters in assigning subjects to diagnostic categories. Although the agreement expected by chance was calculated to be 20%, the raters agreed with the investigator on the diagnosis for 21 of the 23 cases, or on 91% of the subjects. (Two of these cases were the two training cases where all the raters agreed on the diagnosis although these were not independent assessments.)

For the ICD-9 system, 20 cases were scored and 18 of these were assigned to the same category by the rater and the investigator. Here the agreement expected by chance was calculated to be 20%, and the overall agreement achieved by the raters came to 91%.

On the Ego Function Assessment Test, the investigator's mean score was compared to that of the different evaluators. For raters 2, 4, 6, and 8, the differences were all within one scale point, and for raters 3, 5, and 7 the differences never surpassed a maximum of two scale points. Furthermore, only rater 4 assigned a lower mean score than the investigator.

For all other calculations the mean score for the seven raters was compared to the mean scores by the investigator. Table 10.1 shows the mean standard deviation and range of the investigator's scores, the raters' mean scores, the product moment correlation coefficient between the mean scores, and the percentage of cases with less than one scale point difference.

Table 10.1.   Comparison of Investigator's and Evaluators' Mean Scorings

	Investigator's Score			Evaluators' Score, Mean	Reliability Correlation	Percent Less than One Point Difference
	Mean	SD	Range			
Reality Testing	6.4	1.3	4–9	7.7	0.81	43
Judgment	5.8	1.8	3–9	7.1	0.45	43
Sense of Reality	6.4	1.2	5–9	7.1	0.65	52
Regulation and Control	5.2	1.6	3–8	5.9	0.45	67
Object Relations	5.7	1.0	4–8	6.6	0.50	67
Thought Processes	8.3	1.4	6–11	9.2	0.36	43
ARISE	6.2	1.6	4–10	6.6	0.25	43
Defensive Functioning	5.6	1.0	4–7	5.8	0.13	48
Stimulus Barrier	6.8	0.6	6–8	8.1	0.24	48
Autonomous Functioning	6.1	1.2	4–9	8.5	0.23	38
Synthetic Functioning	6.2	1.2	4–8	7.1	0.27	62
Mastery– Competence	5.7	1.2	4–8	6.4	0.30	52
Mean Score	6.2	1.0	4.3–8.2	7.2	0.47	50
Global Assess- ment Scale	36	4	29–43	42	0.61	71[a]

[a] Percent less than 10 points difference.

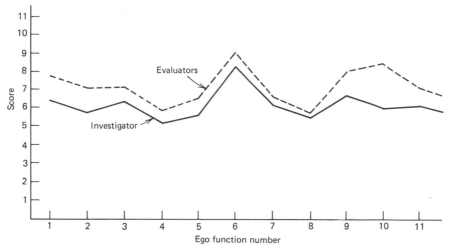

Figure 10.1.   Mean score on Ego Function Assessment by investigator and evaluators.

Figure 10.1 shows the investigator's and the raters' mean scores on the 12 ego functions. The profiles show a high degree of concordance, with the exception of ego function 10, Autonomous Functioning. The mean scores differ between 0.2 and 2.4 scale points, with a mean of 1.0 point. The investigator's mean scores are consistently lower than those of the raters. The raters' mean scores are quite similar to the investigator's scores, except for ego function 9, Stimulus Barrier, where the raters' mean is 0.1 point over the investigator's range.

Reliability estimates were obtained by the product moment correlation coefficient. Values higher than .50 indicated good reliability. This was achieved in the scorings of ego functions 1, 3, and 5. Values between .20 and .50 indicated some reliability. This is the level found for ego functions 2, 4, 6, 7, 9, 10, 11, 12 and for the mean ego function score. Poor reliability was indicated by a value below .20. This was found for only ego function 8, Defensive Functioning. (As a comparison, the value found for the Global Assessment Scale was .61.)

Reliability estimates were also calculated by computing the percentage of the investigator's and the raters' scores that differed by less than one scale point. That percentage varied from 43 to 67, with a mean of 50 on the 13-point scale used. On the Global Assessment Scale, 71% of the cases had a difference of less than 10 scale points on a 100-point scale. The extent of disagreement among the raters and the investigator on the various ego functions is shown in Table 10.2.

On the Ego Function Assessment Test, the investigator's mean range was 4.5 scale points, whereas that of the raters was 7.3 points. This reflects a greater variability in their scores.

Table 10.2.   Scale Points of Disagreement on Various Ego Functions

	Points of Disagreement						
	0	1	2	3	4	5	6
Reality Testing	2	7	8	2	1	1	
Cumulative	10	43	81	90	95	100%	
Judgment	3	6	7	2	2	1	
Cumulative	14	43	76	86	95	100%	
Sense of Reality	7	4	5	4	1		
Cumulative	33	52	76	95	100%		
Regulation and Control	3	11	5	1		1	
Cumulative	14	67	90	95		100%	
Object Relations	5	9	4	3			
Cumulative	24	67	86	100%			
Thought Processes	6	3	5	6	1		
Cumulative	29	43	67	95	100%		
ARISE	3	6	4	3	4	· 1	
Cumulative	14	43	62	76	95	100%	
Defensive Functioning	4	6	6	4	1		
Cumulative	19	48	76	95	100%		
Stimulus Barrier	5	5	8	2		1	
Cumulative	24	48	86	95		100%	
Autonomous Functioning	4	4	2	3	7	1	
Cumulative	19	38	48	62	95	100%	
Synthetic Functioning	4	9	3	2	3		
Cumulative	19	62	76	86	100%		
Mastery–Competence	3	8	4	4	1	0	1
Cumulative	14	52	71	90	95		100%
Mean	4.1	6.4	5.3	2.8	1.8	0.5	0.1
Cumulative	19	50	75	89	97	99.6	100%

DISCUSSION

Several factors may have influenced the results of this reliability study. First, the interviews by definition are clinical interviews and thus are not completely standardized. Additionally, the investigator, as opposed to the raters, had seen the patients and read their case records.

These sources of variance mean possible lower reliability, as compared to carefully preselected tapes, which also could have a diagnostic distribution matched to the investigator's diagnoses of the main material. On the other hand, the factors mentioned give an "everyday feeling" and contribute to reliability under normal circumstances, and not to the "artificial" high one found under optimal circumstances.

The agreement between the investigator and raters on diagnoses was astonishingly high for both diagnostic systems utilized. This may be attributed to the raters' extensive experience in diagnosis and to the breadth of the interviews.

Agreement on the scorings of the Global Assessment Scale regarding current psychopathology was greater than that for the Ego Function Assessment Test but less than that for diagnoses. Although the reliability coefficient for the Global Assessment Scale was good, it is lower than the coefficients typically found in other studies with joint assessment (Endicott et al., 1976). It is reasonable to expect comparable levels of agreement for diagnoses and for the Global Assessment Scale. The discrepancy found might be due to the raters being less familiar with the instrument than with diagnostic decision making. The lower reliability on the Ego Function Assessment Test can be explained by the greater complexity of that measure.

On the Ego Function Assessment some of the raters' scorings are consistent with the investigator's, whereas others display somewhat higher mean scores. This may be due to discrepancies between raters in their understanding of the manual. All kinds of hospitalized psychiatric patients were scored by the investigator so that he had scored all kinds of pathology with the instrument. This was not the case for the raters. However, an overall comparison of the mean ego function profiles derived by the investigator and the raters depicts a high degree of concordance, with the exception of Autonomous Functioning. Both the evaluators and the investigator made the lowest scores on the clinically sickest cases. This demonstrates that the scoring system of the Ego Function Assessment Test is relatively consistent when used by experienced psychiatrists.

Although reliability in the present study, as calculated by the product moment correlation coefficient, was generally good for the Ego Function Assessment Test, it was not as good as that reported by Bellak et al. (1973). Two possible explanations for this can be proposed. First, it is possible that Bellak et al.'s raters were better trained. Second, the larger sample size in Bellak's study may also have been a factor. In fact, the statistic of "percentage of cases with less than one point score difference" is probably a better indicator of reliability than the product moment correlation coefficient, as the latter tends to be unreliable when the number of cases is low. The "percentage index" does in fact indicate that the 12 ego functions have approximately the same reliability—with the possible exception of Autonomous Functioning.

Notably, whereas Bellak found that 60% of the cases were scored with less than one scale point difference, the finding was 57% in the present study. In light of the aforementioned differences between the two studies, it nevertheless can be concluded that the reliability scales, as determined by the percentage index, were comparable.

CONCLUSION

This study demonstrated that the Ego Function Assessment Test can be scored by experienced psychiatrists with good reliability. With the possible exception of Autonomous Functioning, the present study shows that the reliability was comparably good for all the other ego functions. Furthermore, the reliability scores approach those obtained with a fairly straightforward psychopathology scale (the Global Assessment Scale).

The guidelines for the interview provide adequate standardization for the test procedure and the scoring manual aided in the provision of scores that differentiated cases representing the most severe psychopathology from those with less severe disturbance. An adequate training procedure for the raters is crucial, and training was not optimal in the present study. That probably is the main explanation for the lower interrater reliability figures compared to those obtained by Bellak et al. (1973).

ACKNOWLEDGMENTS

The author wants to thank cand. real. Leiv Sandvik for doing the statistical analyses, and the following colleagues for being evaluators: Carl-Ivar Dahl, M.D.; Astrid Nøklebye Heiberg, M.D.; Ragnhild Husby, M.D., and Bjørn Østberg, M.D.

This study was supported by research grant no. C 38-65.020 from the Norwegian Council for Science and the Humanities, and with grants from Dr. med. Hans Evensen's Legacy, Oslo University, School of Medicine, and Karl Modalen's Legacy for Psychiatric Research at Gaustad Hospital.

REFERENCES

Bellak, L., Hurvich, M., & Gediman, H. *Ego function in schizophrenics, neurotics, and normals: A systematic study of conceptual, diagnostic, and therapeutic aspects.* New York: Wiley, 1973.

Endicott, J., Spitzer, R. L., Fleiss, J. L., and Cohen, J. The global assessment scale. *Archives of General Psychiatry*, 1976, *33*, 766–771.

Ego Function Assessment of Hospitalized Adult Psychiatric Patients with Special Reference to Borderline Patients

ALV A. DAHL

Following the recommendations of Robins and Guze (1970) and Perry and Klerman (1978), the aim of the present project is to compare the level of ego functioning in a group of borderline patients with the level in patients from other diagnostic categories.

The significance of this investigation derives from the observation that borderline patients characteristically show ego deficits. In seeking answers to two questions, (1) "What are the specific ego weaknesses in borderline patients?" and (2) "Do they differ from those of patients belonging to different diagnostic classes?" Bellak's Ego Function Assessment proved to be a useful instrument, and as suggested in the preceding paper, a reliable one.

SUBJECTS

The sample consisted of hospitalized patients, ranging in age from 18 to 40 years, who were consecutively admitted to two hospitals in Oslo. Patients with intelligence deficits, organic cerebral pathology, and serious physical defects were omitted from the sample. Chronic patients, defined by having spent more than 10% of their lives in mental health institutions, and foreigners living in Norway for under 5 years, were also omitted. Additionally, 8.3% of the patients admitted declined to participate in the study—this group was evenly distributed among diagnostic categories. The total sample then consisted of 252 hospitalized patients.

METHOD

As all patients were interviewed by the author during the second week of hospitalization, their most florid symptoms had dissipated or, in the case of

Table 11.1. Diagnostic Groups Compared in the Study

Group	N	RDC Diagnosis		DSM-III Diagnosis	
Borderline	62	—		Borderline personality disorder (p.d.)	$N = 22$
				Schizotypal p.d.	$N = 23$
				Mixed (bdl + scht)	$N = 17$
Schizophrenia	58	Schizophrenia		Schizophrenia	$N = 47$
				Schizophreniform	$N = 11$
Affective psychoses	25	Major depressive disorder		Major depressive	$N = 12$
		Bipolar I		Bipolar	$N = 10$
		Bipolar II		Atypical bipolar	$N = 3$
Neuroses	43	General anxiety disorder		General anxiety disorder	$N = 15$
		Phobic disorder		Agoraphobia	$N = 3$
		Briquet's disorder		Somatization disorder	$N = 2$
		Minor depressive disorder		Dysthymic disorder	$N = 19$
		$(N = 22)$		Adjustment depression	$N = 3$
		Intermittent depressive disorder		Cyclothymic disorder	$N = 1$
Personality disorders	27	Antisocial p.d.	$N = 14$	Antisocial p.d.	$N = 10$
		Labile p.d.	$N = 2$	Histrionic p.d.	$N = 5$
		Antisocial + labile	$N = 3$	Antisocial + Histrionic	$N = 5$
		Other psychiatric	$N = 8$	Other p.d.	$N = 7$

the drug abuse patients, their detoxification had been completed. They each had two 1-hour interviews, which were conducted on consecutive days. The interview consisted of three parts: (1) The Schedule for Affective Disorders and Schizophrenia (SADS) (Endicott & Spitzer, 1978) with the addition of the Schedule for Interviewing Borderline (SIB) (Baron, 1979); (2) life, family, and psychiatric history; and (3) Bellak's Ego Function Assessment interview.

On the basis of these data as well as a review of the case records from earlier and present hospitalization, diagnoses based on SADS and the diagnostic criteria of RDC and DSM-III were assigned; the life history form was completed, and the Global Assessment Scale (GAS) (Endicott et al., 1976) was scored, as were the 12 ego functions and the superego parameters of the Bellak test. The drug abuse patients received a primary personality diagnosis and a subclassification for the specific substance abuse problem. Five diagnostic categories were compared in this study: schizophrenia, affective psychoses, borderlines, neuroses, and personality disorders (other than borderlines). The various diagnoses in the five groups are shown in Table 11.1 with diagnoses in the RDC and DSM-III systems.

In the borderline group 20 patients (32.3%) got a RDC diagnosis of drug disorder, and 15 patients (24.2%) a diagnosis of alcoholism. In the personality disorder group 21 patients (77.8%) had a RDC diagnosis of drug use disorder and 7 patients (25.9%) a diagnosis of alcoholism. These disorders were rare in the other comparison groups.

INITIAL TESTING WITH THE INSTRUMENT

The interview guide and scoring manual for Bellak's Ego Function Assessment was translated into Norwegian by the author, since the instrument had never been used before in this country. Questions in the interview guide covered by the other two instruments were not repeated, which meant that the ego function interview could be done in 30–45 minutes. Nearly all patients found the questions meaningful and of relevance to their problems; very few had a feeling of being in a test situation.

Two additional and related scoring difficulties were found by the author. First, the separation by Bellak et al. (1973) of current, characteristic, highest, and lowest level of ego functioning requires that one differentiate current functioning in the interview situation from the more characteristic functioning based on the patient's past—a task that was found to be quite difficult in the setting. Second, because many of the hospitalized patients were functioning at their characteristic or lowest level, the assessment of highest level required high-order inferences. In summary, the investigator, finding the delineation of four separate levels of functioning to be arbitrary and difficult, chose to score only the current level of ego functions.

Table 11.2.   Summary of Background Variables of the Diagnostic Classes

	N	Sex Male	Female	Age Mean	Range	Mean social class, Hollingshead & Redlich	% N on medication
Schizo-phrenia	58	35	23	28	(18–38)	3.86	93*
Affective psychoses	25	8*	17	32*	(22–39)	3.19*	80*
Borderlines	62	31	31	27	(18–39)	4.11	56
Neuroses	43	11*	32	31*	(18–39)	3.27*	40
Personality disorders	27	23*	4	25	(18–35)	4.55*	44

Note: * $p < .05$, Student's t-test, borderlines compared to other categories.

RESULTS

The findings on background variables for the diagnostic classes are listed in Tables 11.2 and 11.3. The results of the ego function assessment scorings are shown in Figures 11.1 and 11.2.

The mean level of ego functions for schizophrenics is 4.4, with a standard deviation of .9 and a range of 3.0 (3.4–6.4); for affective psychoses, the mean is 5.8, with a standard deviation of 1.2 and a range of 2.7 (4.7–7.4); for borderlines, the mean is 5.5, with a standard deviation of .8 and a range of 3.3 (4.5–7.8); for neuroses, 7.3 with a standard deviation of .7 and a range of 3.2 (6.0–9.2); and for personality disorders, the mean is 6.2 with a standard deviation of .7 and a range of 4.2 (4.4–8.3).

Table 11.3.   Summary of Mean Scores on Measures

	GAS Score Mean	Range	Rehospitalization rate Mean	Range	Severity per episode Mean	Range
Schizophrenia	27*	(8–40)	0.7	(0–3)	77*	(0–343)
Affective psychoses	29*	(10–40)	0.7	(0–4)	28	(0–105)
Borderlines	33	(21–43)	0.5	(0–2.8)	32	(0–170)
Neuroses	39*	(31–52)	0.2	(0–2)	21	(0–300)
Personality disorders	36*	(30–45)	0.4	(0–2)	22	(0–91)

Note: * $p < .05$, Student's t-test, borderlines compared to other categories.

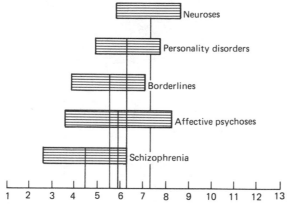

Figure 11.1.   Mean level of ego functions with two standard deviations for the various diagnostic categories in the study.

Three additional analyses were conducted. Among the subtypes of borderline including those with unstable, schizotypal, or mixed features, there were no differences of greater than 1 point observed on any of the ego functions. Borderline patients with drug use disorder did exhibit mean scores 1.0–1.4 lower on judgment, sense of reality, regulation and control, and thought processes than other patients diagnosed as borderline. Differences were minimal with regard to other ego functions.

The 21 patients with personality disorder and drug use disorder were compared to the 20 drug-using borderline patients. The drug-using borderlines had a mean ego function score of 5.4 with a standard deviation of .6

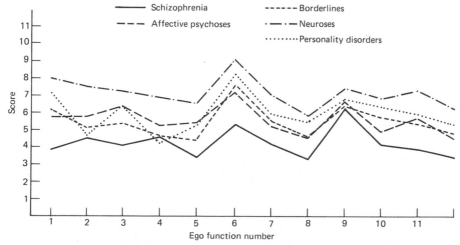

Figure 11.2.   Mean ego function levels of the various diagnostic categories.

Table 11.4. *Ego Function Assessment Scores of Various Diagnostic Categories*

	Schizophrenia N = 58		Affective psychoses N = 25		Borderlines N = 62		Neuroses N = 43		Personality Disorders N = 27	
	Mean	SD	Mean	SD	Mean	SD	Mean	SD	Mean	SD
Reality Testing	3.9*	1.1	5.8*	1.3	6.3	.9	8.1*	1.0	7.3*	.9
Judgment	4.6*	1.4	5.9	2.1	5.2	1.4	7.6*	1.6	4.9	1.3
Sense of Reality	4.2*	1.2	6.5*	1.3	5.5	.8	7.4*	1.4	6.9*	.7
Regulation and Control	4.7	1.1	5.4*	1.7	4.8	1.2	7.0*	1.1	4.4	1.0
Object Relations	3.5*	1.2	5.6*	1.6	4.5	.9	6.7*	1.1	5.5*	.8
Thought Processes	5.4*	1.4	7.4	1.8	7.8	1.2	9.2*	1.0	8.6*	1.1
ARISE	4.3*	1.2	5.4	1.9	5.7	1.1	7.1*	1.2	6.1	1.2
Defensive Functioning	3.4*	1.0	4.7	1.3	4.8	.9	6.0*	.8	5.6*	.8
Stimulus Barrier	6.4	1.0	6.8	.8	6.6	.8	7.6*	1.1	7.0	1.6
Autonomous Functioning	4.3*	1.0	5.1*	1.3	5.8	.7	7.0*	1.0	6.6*	1.0
Synthetic Functioning	4.0*	1.3	5.9	1.6	5.5	1.0	7.5*	1.0	6.1*	1.1
Mastery–Competence	3.5*	1.2	4.7	1.5	4.9	.9	6.4*	1.0	5.5*	.8
Mean	4.4	.9	5.8	1.2	5.5	.8	7.3*	.7	6.2*	.7

Note: * p < .05, Student's *t*-test, borderlines compared to other categories.

(range 4.4–6.5), whereas the patients with drug use and personality disorder attained a mean of 6.0 with a standard deviation of .6 on the ego function assessment (range 5.0–7.0). There were significant differences between these drug-using patients on most of the 12 ego functions.

DISCUSSION

The results must be interpreted cautiously. First, the ratings of the primary investigator were not blind as to diagnosis and thus may have affected the EFA ratings. However, because the seven other raters in the reliability study were blind to both diagnosis and ego functions, this bias appears to be of little significance.

A second limitation of the present investigation is that the influence of neuroleptic medication is not controlled. Simply on the basis of clinical experience, it is reasonable to suppose that neuroleptic medication may improve ego functions. It can be further speculated that reality testing, judgment, control and regulation of drives as well as thought processes are the ego functions most likely to be influenced by drugs. Most subjects in a sample of patients exhibiting serious psychopathology (e.g., schizophrenia and affective psychoses) are treated with medication and thus their ego function scores may be greater than those of a similar drug-free sample of patients.

Notwithstanding these limitations, the results give added empirical support to the view that some diagnostic groups demonstrate significant differences in their level of ego functioning. As expected, neurotic patients attained the highest ego function scores, whereas the schizophrenic subjects' scores were the lowest. Scores attained by borderline patients fell between the two classes, although closer to the schizophrenic group. This finding supports the view that borderline patients, as defined in the present study, occupy a position between neurotics and schizophrenics in terms of their level of ego functioning.

Patients with affective psychoses attained comparable scores on the ego function assessment to those of the borderline group, although this group showed greater variability as was evidenced by the standard deviation scores. This finding is consistent with the view that the level of ego functions in patients with affective psychoses is in rapid flux, although optimally it is quite high. These findings also lend support to the view that the level of ego functioning in borderline patients is closer to patients with affective psychoses than to patients with schizophrenia (Akiskal, 1981; Stone, 1980).

The personality disorder sample in this study consisted mainly of patients with histrionic and/or antisocial personality disorders. The personality disorder group has significantly higher ego function scores on 9 of the 12 variables. A study by Sheehy, Goldsmith, and Charles (1980) found that problems in object relationship, affect and impulse control, and a cohesive sense of self were more prominent among borderline patients than patients with nonborderline personality disorders. Those findings are partially confirmed in this study since the personality disorder patients score significantly higher on sense of reality of the world and the self and on object relations. The lack of significant differences on judgment and regulation and control of affects and impulse can be explained by the higher percentage of antisocial personality disorders in the present sample.

From the ego function scores of the borderline patients there are no specific ego weaknesses in these patients. They have a global ego weakness within a small range on the scale. This can also be explained by halo effect, or that the steps between the anchor points in the manual do vary among the various ego functions.

Spitzer et al. (1979) subdivided their borderline patients in the schizotypal and unstable type. The symptom picture of these two types are quite different. It is of interest that in the present study the subdivision into schizotypal, unstable, and mixed forms showed no significant differences in the various ego function scores. That finding supports a dimensional view of borderline patients, that although they have a variety of symptoms they have the same degree of ego weakness.

Additionally, when the subgroup of borderline patients with drug use disorder was compared as a group to the rest of the borderline group, no significant differences emerged.

Bellak et al. (1973) hoped to find differences in the pattern of performance on the different subscales for different patients, in addition to identifying patterns that might characterize diagnostic groups. Ego function assessment has been applied to schizophrenic patients in at least two other studies, including Bellak et al.'s (1973) original study and that of Docherty and Feister (see Chapter 5). By comparison with these other studies, the ego function scores derived in the present sample are significantly lower. The differences between Bellak's findings and the present ones might be attributed to differences in the sample. Twenty percent of Bellak's sample are questionable schizophrenics (10% borderline schizophrenics and 10% possible schizophrenics). Docherty's sample is similar to the present population, although his study used well-functioning, outpatient schizophrenics. This, his study concerns optimally functioning patients, whereas the present one concerns patients at their lowest level of functioning.

For the neurotic category the findings in Bellak's study were strikingly similar to those in the present study. His sample was drawn from a population seeking outpatient psychotherapy in New York City, whereas in the present study the sample was drawn from a group of hospitalized patients in Oslo. Despite the fact that in Bellak's study an outpatient group of neurotics was assessed, and in ours inpatients were evaluated, the similarity of the findings is quite noteworthy. One might speculate that treatment attitudes toward neurotics may differ in the two cities. In Oslo psychotherapists in private practice are few, and one can presume that they would take care of the neurotic patients in New York.

There are no other studies in which the ego function assessment was applied to patients with affective psychosis, so no comparisons could be made. In another study (Dahl, 1983) it was found that patients with schizoaffective disorder (RDC) had ego function scores close to those in patients with schizophrenia (RDC) and schizophreniform disorder (DSM-III). However, the schizoaffective sample had significantly higher scores on seven ego functions than the sample of patients with schizophrenia (DSM-III). Also the schizoaffectives had lower scores on six ego functions as compared to the affective psychoses group.

A comparison of the borderlines and other personality disorder patients with drug use disorder showed that the latter group had significantly higher ego function scores. These results were consonant with those of Frosch & Milkman (1977) in hospitalized drug abusers. Taken together these results suggest that hospitalized drug addicts display general ego weakness, which is more severe for the borderline group.

In conclusion, the ego function assessment test was found to be a practical tool for use with hospitalized patients. The significance of these results as well as the reliability data reported in the previous paper, do point to the cross-cultural potentialities of the use of ego function assessment in clarifying the diagnostic and clinical questions that all psychiatric practitioners face. Still it remains essential that future research aim at further validation of the subscales and their standardization on different patient groups.

ACKNOWLEDGMENTS

This study was supported by research grant no. C. 38–65.020 from The Norwegian Research Council for Science and the Humanities, a grant from Dr. med. Hans Evensen's Legacy, University of Oslo, School of Medicine, and from Karl Modalen's Legacy for Psychiatric Research at Gaustad Hospital.

REFERENCES

Akiskal, H. S. Subaffective disorders: Dysthymic, cyclothymic and bipolar II disorders in the "borderline" realm. *Psychiatric Clinics of North America*, 1981, *4*(1), 25–46.

Baron, M. *Schedule for interviewing borderlines*. New York: New York State Psychiatric Institute, 1979.

Bellak, L., Hurvich, M., & Gediman, H. *Ego functions in schizophrenics, neurotics, and normals*. New York: Wiley, 1973.

Dahl, A. A. Ego function assessment of schizo-affective patients as compared to schizophrenic and affective psychotic patients. *Psychiatria clin.* (in press).

Endicott, J., Spitzer, R. L., Fleiss, J. L., & Cohen, J. The Global Assessment Scale: A procedure for measuring overall severity of psychiatric disturbance. *Archives of General Psychiatry,* 1976, *33,* 766–771.

Endicott, J., & Spitzer, R. L. A diagnostic interview: The schedule for affective disorders and schizophrenia. *Archives of General Psychiatry,* 1978, *35,* 837–844.

Frosch, W. A., & Milkman, H. Ego functions in drug users. In *Psychodynamics of drug dependence,* NIDA Research Monograph 12. Washington D.C., 1977.

Perry, J. C., & Klerman, G. L. The borderline patient. A comparative analysis of four sets of diagnostic criteria. *Archives of General Psychiatry,* 1978, *35,* 141–150.

Robins, E., & Guze, S. B. Establishment of diagnostic validity in psychiatric illness: Its application to schizophrenia. *American Journal of Psychiatry,* 1970, *126,* 983–987.

Sheehy, M., Goldsmith, L. A., & Charles, E. A comparative study of borderline patients in a psychiatric outpatient clinic. *American Journal of Psychiatry,* 1980, *137,* 1374–1379.

Spitzer, R. L., Endicott, J., & Gibbon, M. Crossing the border into borderline personality and borderline schizophrenia. *Archives of General Psychiatry,* 1979, *36,* 17–24.

Stone, M. H. *The borderline syndromes: Constitution, personality and adaption.* New York: McGraw-Hill, 1980.

CHAPTER TWELVE

The Use of Ego Function Assessment in the Long-Term Treatment of Depression with Lithium Carbonate

LIESELOTTE SCHWINDL, E. OPGENOORTH, AND P. SCHUSTER

Disorders of personality structure that persist after depressive phases have been a central topic of research. In the present paper special attention is focused on endogenous depressive patients who are exposed to long-term treatment with lithium carbonate. The treatment may be carried out over years, and perhaps a lifetime. This research concentrates on the personality structure of these patients at the end of a depressive phase; on the psychodynamic change in personality under lithium treatment; and on the personality of the social partner of these patients.

Two personality tests (Gieben, FPI) and a psychoanalytic interview (Ego

---

Translated from the German by Peter Stastny.

Function Assessment, Bellak et al., 1973) were used to obtain information on the personality structure of the sample patients. The personality structure on the social partner was assessed through the Giebentest. Empirical testing showed that patients after an acute endogenous depressive episode, and shortly before leaving the clinic, continued to exhibit an unstable personality structure with considerable weakness in ego strength. This population, when treated with lithium, displayed a stable personality structure, evidenced sufficient adaptation in the area of ego functions, and psychic conflict along neurotic lines. Albeit, there were manifestations of exaggerated perfectionistic strivings and marked signs of anxiety and aggressiveness. The personality structure of the social partner proved to be stable over time but nevertheless also displayed exaggerated superego demands.

POPULATION

Patient group I (PG I) consisted of nine male and six female patients with a mean age of 36 years. All had a diagnosis of endogenomorphic depression and were treated a few days prior to discharge from the hospital. All testing occurred while the patients were on a lithium regimen and adjudged to be in a "decline of the depressive phase." Partner group I consisted of a marital or common-law partner of each of the 15 patients.

Patient group II (PG II) also consisted of nine male and six female patients with a mean age of 39 years. All had a diagnosis of endogenomorphic depression and had been on a successful lithium prophylaxis from 2 to up to 10 years, requiring no hospitalization since the start of lithium treatment. Although in some cases subclinical depression or "hypomanic phases" were observed, no additional medication had been required in our sample group. (Those patients who very quickly relapsed or required antidepressant medication were excluded from further study.) Partner group II also consisted of a marital or common-law partner of each patient.

EGO FUNCTION ASSESSMENT

The data, examined statistically, were derived from an in-depth ego function assessment interview as outlined in Bellak et al. (1973). Interviews were audiotaped and rated "blindly" according to the Bellak et al. (1973) rating manual. Each of the 12 ego functions was rated according to three levels of ego functioning—the characteristic, current, and lowest level. The rating of each function and components thereof is based on a scale of 13 points.

The Bellak scales were chosen because of their derivation from psychoanalytic concepts. Their clinical use was evidenced by their capacity to differentiate between schizophrenic, neurotic, and normal subjects. Additionally, Bellak's interrater reliability was quite high (a Spearman–Brown correlation coefficient of .77) and has been replicated in a research project by Ciompi (Chapter 13, present volume). The scale is being used for the first time in a German-speaking country and approximates a small-scale effort at validation of the instrument. We felt that an examination of the patients' personality structure using an in-depth psychological approach was essential; particularly so in light of the fact that "premorbid" levels of adaptation could be included in the evaluation.

It might be useful to keep in mind the manner in which Bellak et al. (1973) grouped the scale values on a continuum of psychopathology: from the psychotic range of 1–6, to the borderline range of 4–8, to the neurotic range of 6–10, and finally, the normal range, 8–13.

RESULTS

Patient Group I

Since the data obtained were based on a scale with ordinal rankings, we first computed the median Z for each ego function.

The level of functioning for all 12 ego functions in PGI fell between scale points 6 and 9, with scale IV (Regulation and Control of Drive, Impulse, and Affect) showing the lowest value ($Z = 6.86$) and scales I (Reality Testing) and II (Judgment) achieving the highest values ($Z = 8.80$). Thus, in using Bellak's categories, 6 of the 12 ego functions showed values below 8, namely, outside the normal range. The other six ego functions fell between 8.08 and 8.80 and were at the lower margin of the normal range.

In terms of current level of functioning the median values computed for

Table 12.1. *Median Z Ego Function Ratings for Patient Groups I and II*

Function	Characteristic		Current		Lowest	
	PG I	PG II	PG I	PG II	PG I	PG II
I	8.80	9.67	9.00	10.08	5.00	6.88
II	8.80	9.00	8.44	9.43	6.83	7.20
III	8.00	9.92	8.21	9.80	3.43	4.88
IV	6.86	7.92	6.63	8.95	3.92	4.88
V	7.00	8.00	7.58	8.94	3.06	4.63
VI	8.06	9.80	8.50	10.30	5.90	7.20
VII	7.00	7.67	6.62	8.38	5.33	6.88
VIII	7.56	7.60	6.38	8.88	3.60	3.42
IX	7.75	9.06	7.20	8.63	5.33	7.40
X	8.08	8.75	7.33	9.80	4.92	5.29
XI	8.20	8.78	8.38	9.00	6.57	7.00
XII	8.08	8.75	7.67	9.63	4.00	5.17

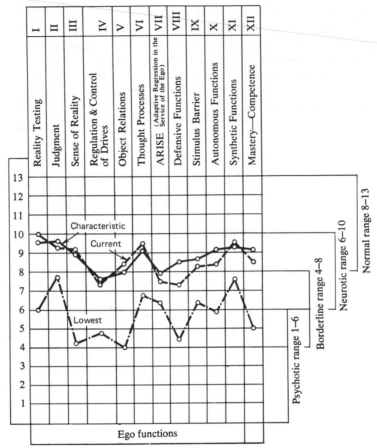

Figure 12.1.   Characteristic, current, and lowest levels of ego functioning in Patient Group I.

the performance on the 12 ego functions fell between 6.38 and 9.0 on the scale. The lowest ($Z = 6.38$) median was observed on scale VII (Adaptive Regression in the Service of the Ego—ARISE), and scale IV (Regulation and Control of Drive, Impulse, and Affect), $Z = 6.63$. The highest levels of performance were evidenced on scale I (Reality Testing), with a median score of 9.0.

The median for the lowest level of functioning fell between the scale points 3 and 7. The lowest value was measured for scale V (Object Relations), with $Z = 3.06$; a score clearly within the psychotic range. The highest value was found on scale II (Judgment).

Patient Group II

In terms of the level of functioning, the median for this patient group fell between 7 and 10 points on the scale. The lowest value was 7.60 for function

VIII (ARISE) and the highest 9.92 for function III (Sense of Reality of the World and the Self). Here too we measured values below 8 points in four of the scales, which according to Bellak constitutes a deviation from the normal range and must be interpreted at least as neurotic.

As for current level of functioning, the 12 ego functions in this group of long-term lithium-treated patients was higher than those ratings for PG I. The values for each ego function ranged between 8 and 11 points on the scales and are thus within the normal range. The lowest values were found for function VII (ARISE) at 8.38 and the highest for function VI (Thought Processes) at 11.0.

For lowest level of functioning the median scores fell between 3 and 8 on the scales. The lowest values computed were for function VIII (Defensive Functioning), $Z = 3.42$. The highest value was for ego function IX (Stimulus Barrier), $Z = 7.40$. Given Bellak et al.'s (1973) groupings, these values fall within the psychotic or borderline range for 6 out of 12 functions.

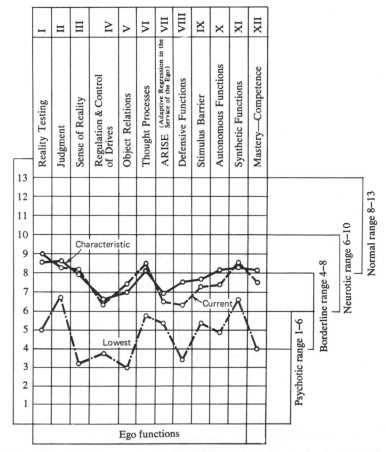

Figure 12.2.   Characteristic, current, and lowest levels of ego functioning in Patient Group II.

Comparison of PG I and PG II

We used the Mann–Whitney U-test for ordinally ranked data for all comparisons between groups. For function VI (Thought Processes) we could not produce precise results for all subjects, thus reducing the *N* in some cases to below 15. This was taken into consideration when computing the U-tests and is annotated separately in the charts.

Comparison of the Characteristic Level of Functioning in the Two Patient Groups. The characteristic level of functioning was considered to tap the level of adaptive ego functioning that prevailed before the onset of the acute phase of the illness. Thus, we might regard such measures as approximations of the premorbid level of functioning. It is necessary to consider the lapses and distortions of memory that may occur. We hypothesized that the

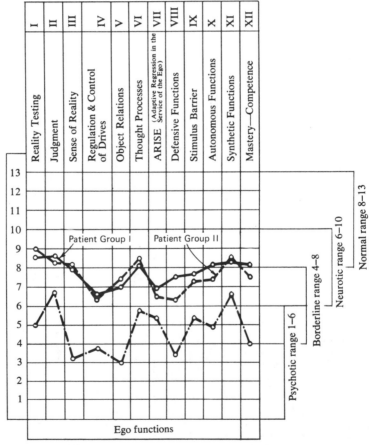

Figure 12.3.   Median values for characteristic levels of ego functioning for both groups.

two groups would not appear significantly different regarding their characteristic level of functioning.

The comparison of the two groups in terms of characteristic level of functioning revealed only two significant differences; the PG II received significantly higher scores on function III (Sense of Reality) and function IX (Stimulus Barrier) than did PG I. One might hypothesize that as the PG II subjects had not experienced a psychotic decompensation for many years, there may have been some retrospective distortion as to past illness, possibly as a result of repressive processes. However, we would be more certain in our statements if we could undertake a longitudinal analysis of the same patient population, starting after the onset of the illness and extending for years on lithium maintenance therapy. Nevertheless, we have confirmed the hypothesis for 10 of the 12 functions and in these areas the groups did not differ significantly in regard to their characteristic level of functioning.

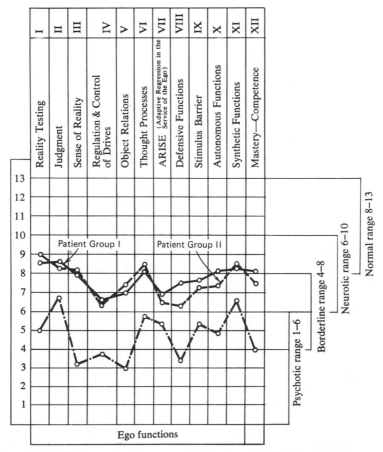

Figure 12.4. Median values for current levels of ego functioning for both groups.

The graphical arrangement of the median values in Figure 12.3 illustrates this concordance of levels of functioning in the two groups rather nicely. The graphs for each group run almost exactly parallel to each other and reach their lowest values for function IV (Drive Regulation) while both groups score highest on function I (Reality Testing).

Comparison of Current Levels of Functioning in PG I and PG II. The current level of functioning represents the performance on the 12 ego functions at the time of the interview. We hypothesized that the two groups would show significant differences when assessed at this level, as lithium prophylaxis should lead to a stabilization of personality functioning (Rüger, 1976).

PG II did in fact score higher on 11 out of 12 functions with the exception of function XI (Synthetic–Integrative Functioning). On this function, the

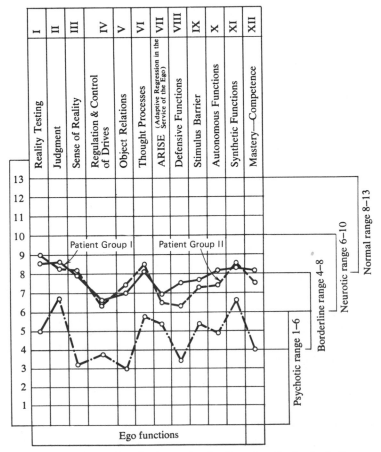

Figure 12.5.   Median values for lowest levels of ego functioning for both groups.

PG I group barely scored within the normal range (8.38) even though it appeared to be one of their better-adapted functions.

Comparison of the Lowest Level of Functioning for PG I and PG II.   As patients of both groups showed at least two psychotic episodes in their life history in the form of endogenomorphically depressive episodes, we can assume that they would not differ significantly at this level. In fact, in 9 out of 12 ego functions PG I and II showed no significant differences. Both groups showed a pervasively low performance, well below the normal range, and mostly within the psychotic or borderline ranges. Only three ego functions revealed differences between the two groups: function IV (Thought Processes), function IX (Stimulus Barrier), and function XII (Mastery–Competence).

It has already been mentioned that the comparison of patient groups on the characteristic level of functioning yielded a difference in function IX (Stimulus Barrier). PG II seemed to exhibit some amnesia or repression of past deficiencies, as was suggested by the following comments: "I am certainly not fond of remembering these times," "I already forgot the way it was." Other explanations might also be posited. It could be that the group that responded favorably to a lithium prophylaxis already started out with a less severe deficit in the aforementioned areas of functioning. It would require a longitudinal or prospective study to supply hard data for any of these assumptions.

In general, we can say that our hypothesis was confirmed as the groups did not differ significantly with regard to their lowest level of functioning except for the exceptions cited.

DISCUSSION

Lauter (1969) and Glatzel and Lungershausen (1970) point out that disorders of personality structure often persist after affective psychotic phases and over the course of months or years may contribute to the repeated emergence of endogenous depressive episodes. Lauter posits that after the acute phases of the illness recede, certain chronic depressive attitudes persist and can be observed in the ways patients enact their "social role."

The treatment with antidepressants proves useful mainly during the acute phase but shows little reliable prophylactic effect (Angst, 1970). By contrast, a prophylactic effect is provided by a long-term treatment with lithium carbonate. Schou (1969) states that with most patients no relapses occurred at all. This report seems a bit too optimistic when compared with reports of Angst (1969) and Mueller-Oerlinghausen (1976). Nevertheless, the prophylactic effect of lithium treatment today is no longer called into question. The treatment has to be continued for years, and perhaps a lifetime, if a repeated psychotic decompensation is to be prevented. Unfortunately, little is known of the psychodynamic changes of personality that occur with long-term lithium treatment. The reports are primarily case studies. On the basis of an analytic interview Rüger (1976) reports that a patient on lithium treatment for over 7 years exhibited a picture of a stable, neurotic adaptation without an upsurge of symptomatology.

In sum, in the present study the effects of lithium on two groups of endogenously depressed patients were compared by means of the EFA of Bellak et al. (1973). One group (PG I) was evaluated at the end of a depressive phase, and shortly before the beginning of the lithium treatment. All of these patients were on antidepressants at the time of the investigation. Our comparison group (PG II) was evaluated after lengthy treatment with lithium carbonate (mean duration of treatment 5 years). These patients did not require any additional antidepressant medication.

The characteristic, lowest, and current level of ego functions were assessed in both groups. Although no differences were expected in the adaptive level of ego functions on the characteristic and lowest level, it was expected that the current level of functioning in the lithium group would be higher than in the other group of patients. This hypothesis follows the assumption of Rüger (1976) that by means of long-term treatment with lithium, a stabilization in functioning can be achieved.

The data gained by means of the ego function assessment revealed the following results: There were no differences between the two groups with regard to their characteristic level of functioning. The same held for the "lowest level of functioning"; only 3 of the 12 ego functions showed a significant difference. By contrast, a significant difference between groups was found on the "current level of functioning." The ratings of the ego functions for PG II ranged from above 8 to 10.3, and thus were in the "normal range." Hence, Rüger's assumption that long-term therapy with lithium leads to a stabilization of personality functioning is supported.

REFERENCES

Angst, J. Ruckschläge und Erfolge einer revolutionären Therapie. *Weltwoche,* Nr. 39, 1978.

Angst, J., et al. Verlaufsgesetzlichkeiten depressiver Syndrome. In H. Hippius & E. Sellbach (Eds.), *Das depressive Syndrom.* Vienna: Urban and Schwarzenberg, 1969.

Bellak, L., Hurvich, M., & Gediman, H. *Ego functions in schizophrenics, neurotics, and normals.* New York: Wiley, 1973.

Glatzel, J., & Lungershausen, N. *Arch. Psychiat. Nervenkrankheiten,* 1970, *213,* 388–395.

Lauter, H. Phasenüberdauernder Persönlichkeitswandel und persistierende Symptome bei der endogenen Depression. In H. Hippius & E. Selbach (Eds.), *Das depressive Syndrom.* Vienna: Urban and Schwarzenberg, 1969.

Mueller-Oerlinghausen, B., et al. Untersuchung uber die Bedeutung neurosenpsychologischer Faktoren bei der Lithium-Dauerbehandlung. *Arzneimittelforschung,* 1976, *26,* 1160–1180.

Rüger, U. Tiefenpsychologische Aspekte des Verlaufs phasischer Depressionen unter Lithium-Prophylaxe, *Nervenarzt,* 1976, *47,* 538–543.

Schou, M. Lithium als Psychopharmakon. *Fortschr. Neurol. Psychiat., 36,* 1969, 349.

Objectifying Psychodynamic Changes in Psychotherapy with a Simplified Version of the Ego Function Scales

LUC CIOMPI, CLAUDIO AGUE, AND JEAN-PIERRE DAUWALDER

In the last analysis one can say that all psychotherapy rests on a reinforcement of the ego, despite the fact that the term often designates a poorly defined and equivocal entity. An objective measure of the effects of psychotherapy often involves the need to measure changes in certain dimensions of ego functioning. Such dimensions relate to adaptation to external reality, degree of impulse control, and others, which, in their totality, can be called ego strength. As a result, all tentative evaluations of ego strength deserve our interest (Ciompi, 1974).

In the framework of a research project that was not specifically focused on psychotherapeutic questions, but studied ego strength as one of several possibly favorable and unfavorable factors in socio-vocational rehabilitation of the mentally ill, we have examined and surveyed over 30 procedures for the evaluation of ego strength proposed in the literature—notably the rating scales of Barron (1953), Luborsky (1962), Prelinger and Zimet (1964), Jacobs et al. (1968), Semrad et al. (1973), the Camarillo Dynamic Assessment Scales of May and Dixon (1969), and the methods used in the famous study on the effects of different psychotherapies at the Menninger Clinic (Kernberg et al., 1972). Although it is clearly not possible to elaborate here the specific details of each procedure and despite the undeniable quality of some of them (especially the four most recent ones), a common omission, in our opinion, is in the area of construct validity. The procedures do not appear to be grounded in a concept of the ego that is clearly defined and delimited. Consequently, the proposed scales often have a somewhat arbitrary character.

There is, however, one procedure that does seem to avoid certain methodological pitfalls, namely, the work of Bellak et al. (1973). These researchers, over several years, carefully studied the psychoanalytic literature, and notably that of modern ego psychology (Hartmann, 1939; Hartmann et al., 1964; Rapaport, 1955; Jacobson, 1964, and others). They elucidated a concept of the ego in terms of a specification and definition of the principal functions of the ego. They then converted each function into a scale of 13 steps for the purposes of evaluation, ranging from the least to the most adaptive level of functioning. The 12 following functions were considered to be necessary and sufficient for the determination of ego strength.

1. Reality Testing
2. Judgment
3. Sense of Reality of the Self
4. Impulse Control
5. Object Relations
6. Thought Processes
7. Adaptive Repression in the Service of the Ego
8. Defensive Functioning
9. Stimulus Barrier
10. Autonomous Functions
11. Synthetic–Integrative Functions
12. Mastery–Competence

Bellak based his evaluation procedures on a semistructured interview that was analytic in orientation and in each case lasted approximately 2 hours. He also utilized clinical records and other clinical measures as well as a battery of psychological and perceptual tests. The reliability coefficient between the evaluations of several expert raters was around .77, with a range from .61 to .88. The construct validity seemed impressive to us as the methodology was firmly rooted in psychoanalytic theory and, in turn, the clinical validity was demonstrated by the instrument's ability to discriminate between patterns of ego functions among normals, neurotics, and schizophrenics (Bellak et al., 1973).

For our purposes the instrument, which we translated into French, seemed quite long and proved difficult for those without advanced psychoanalytic training. We were also initially unable to replicate the same degree of reliability as that of Bellak's group. Despite such difficulties, and in light of the potentialities and advantages of the technique, we developed a shortened and simplified version based as much as possible on those aspects from the original version that were clearly observable (see Appendixes 1 and 2; further information available on request from the author). In doing so, we hoped to add to the clear definition and standardization of the evaluation process. On the basis of a good previous knowledge of each patient, acquired through extended daily contacts in a clinical setting and through additional information from relatives, clinical files a.s.o., our final version allows us to evaluate each patient in 15–20 minutes. After more than a year of experimentation with over a hundred cases, the clinical and conceptual validity of the procedure now seems quite good. The reliability data between two independent observers proved satisfactory and in our last study with 39 cases, the reliability coefficient reached, as in Bellak's work, .77 for the average score of the 12 functions that constituted our primary interest; concerning the particular functions, our reliability ratings, while always statistically significant, were slightly less satisfactory (between .43 and .75, see Table 13.1.)

In evaluating the results it is necessary to mention certain sampling features (e.g., a preponderance of midscale ratings) that reflected the nature of

Table 13.1. Reliability Coefficients[a] of the Simplified Version of Bellak et al.'s Rating Scale (N = 39)

1.	Reality Testing	0.72***
2.	Judgment	0.75***
3.	Sense of Reality of the Self and the World	0.64***
4.	Impulse Control	0.56***
5.	Object Relations	0.55***
6.	Thought Processes	0.43**
7.	Adaptive Regression in the Service of the Ego	0.51***
8.	Defensive Functions	0.44**
9.	Stimulus Barrier	0.59***
10.	Autonomous Functions	0.56***
11.	Synthetic–Integrative Functions	0.61***
12.	Mastery–Competence	0.53***
	Global rating score	0.77***

Note: ** = $p < .01$, *** = $p < .001$.
[a] Reliability coefficients were derived from two independent observers.

the examined sample population. The degree of reliability of the ratings is therefore perhaps better expressed in another way: Among 468 (39 × 12) judgments made by the two observers on each 13-point scale, disagreement was about .57 points on average (as opposed to Bellak's 1.5 points), which seems to us adequate in assessing the relatively subtle changes that can occur over the course of psychotherapy. As is demonstrated in Figure 13.1, on the basis of a profile of ego functions of a patient in psychoanalysis who was evaluated initially and then after a year of treatment, it becomes possible to localize particular areas of ego weakness and consequently to develop priorities for therapeutic work.

In conclusion, the ego function scales of Bellak et al. (1973), especially in their modified form, seem to us to be useful in evaluating dynamic changes in treatment. The methodology has begun to approach a degree of validity, reliability, practicability, and applicability sufficient for its use in clinical

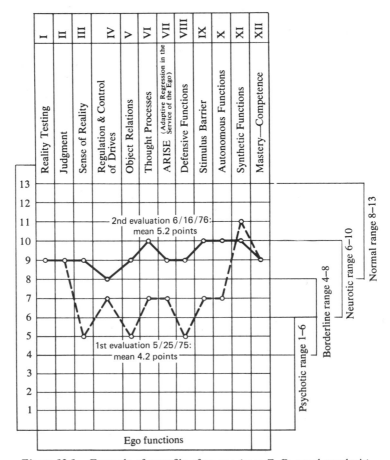

Figure 13.1.   Example of a profile of an ego (case Z. B. psychoanalysis).

practice. We therefore feel that the technique can readily be recommended for the clinical practitioner, as well as for the psychodynamic researcher.

SUMMARY

A simplified version is presented here of the Ego Strength Rating Scales of Bellak et al. (1973), which are based on ratings of 12 ego functions defined according to psychoanalytic concepts. Reliability, validity, and practicability of the instrument were satisfactorily demonstrated in its modified version. It was found to be useful and sufficiently sensitive in measuring psychodynamic changes for large numbers of patients in intensive psychotherapy.

REFERENCES

Barron, M. An Ego Strength Scale which predicts response to psychotherapy. *Journal of Consulting Psychology*, 1953, *17*, 327–333.

Bellak, L., Hurvich, M., Gediman, H. *Ego functions in schizophrenics, neurotics, and normals*. New York: Wiley, 1973.

Ciompi, L. Paut-on évaluer l'efficacité da la psychothérapie? *Rev. méd. de la Suisse romande*, 1974, *94*, 533–544.

Hartmann, H. *Ego psychology and the problem of adaptation*. 1939; repr. New York: International Universities Press, 1958.

Hartmann, H., Kris, E., & Loewenstein, R. Comments on the formation of psychic structure. *Psychological Issues*, 1964, *4*(14), 27–55.

Jacobs, M. A., Pugateh, D., & Spilken, A. Ego Strength Scale (EES): Ego strength and ego weakness. *Journal of Nervous and Mental Disease*, 1968, *147*, 297–307.

Jacobson, E. The self and the object world. New York: International Universities Press, 1954.

Kernberg, O. F., Burstein, E. D., Coyne, L., Appelbaum, A., Horwitz, L., & Voth, H. Psychotherapy and psychoanalysis. Final report of the Menninger Foundation psychotherapy research project. *Bulletin of the Menninger Clinic*, 1972, *36*, 1–275.

Luborsky, L. Clinical judgments of mental health: A proposed scale. *Archives of General Psychiatry*, 1962, *7*, 407–417.

May, P. R. A., & Dixon, W. J. The Camarillo Dynamic Assessment Scales. I. Measurement of psychodynamic factors. *Bulletin of the Menninger Clinic*, 1969, *33*, 1–35.

Prelinger, E., & Zimet, C. *An ego psychological approach to character assessment*. New York: Free Press, 1964.

Rapaport, D. The development and the concepts of psychoanalytic ego psychology. Twelve seminars given at the Western New England Institute for Psychoanalysis. S. Miller (Ed.), mimeographed, 1955.

Semrad, E. V., Grinspoon, L., & Fienberg, S. E. Development of an Ego Profile Scale. *Archives of General Psychiatry*, 1973, *28*, 70–77.

APPENDIX 1: SIMPLIFIED DEFINITIONS OF THE 12 EGO FUNCTIONS

1. *Reality Testing.* The capacity to perceive and to distinguish correctly external and internal reality.

2. *Judgment.* The capacity to anticipate the consequences of one's acts, to behave adequately, to comprehend the reactions of the environment, and to profit from previous errors.

3. *The Sense of Reality of the World and of the Self.* The capacity to feel oneself part of the real world, with a real identity and self-boundaries.

4. *Impulse Control.* The capacity to express and to control adequately impulses (especially sexual and aggressive ones, including intra-aggressive-depressive ones) and to be able to bear frustrations and delay.

5. *Object Relations.* The richness and the quality of interpersonal relations. The capacity to comprehend the sentiments and the autonomous needs of others. The capacity to tolerate loneliness, separation, loss.

6. *Thought Processes.* The capacity to utilize the memory; the ability to concentrate, conceptualize, engage in abstract thinking, to utilize the language, to be able to communicate.

7. *Adaptive Regression in the Service of the Ego* (*ARISE*). The capacity to let go, to suspend controls with pleasure and to permit ideas and fantasies to emerge in a regressed state thus furthering imagination, play, humor, inventiveness, and creativity.

8. *Defensive Functions.* The quality and efficacy of the mechanisms of defense against anger, fear, depression, dysphoria, compulsions, and disquieting fantasies.

9. *Stimulus Barrier.* Sensitivity, excitability, and tolerance for sensory stimuli, noise, light, temperature, odors, tastes, pain, and so on.

10. *Autonomous Functions.* Capacity to utilize psychomotor abilities cognitively and intellectually (coordination, walk, language, perception memory, attention, concentration, capacity to understand, etc.).

11. *Capacity to Synthesize and Integrate.* Capacity to organize, to plan, and to work in a coherent fashion, to be able to integrate a number of circumstances, concepts, points of view, and so on, concurrent ones and contradictory ones.

12. *Mastery–Competence.* The capacity and the competence to master life actively on the basis of realistic appraisals of one's abilities and capacities.

APPENDIX 2: EXAMPLES OF ONE SCALE OF EVALUATION

1. *Reality Testing*

   Capacity to perceive and to distinguish correctly external reality from internal reality.

   1 = Maximal distortions of reality that are constant and that preoccupy and, in effect, disturb total functioning and self-critique

   (hallucinations, delirium, confusional states, dreamlike states, disorientation, spatial-temporal disorientation)

   2 = Severe disturbance of reality testing, almost constant, but limited in certain aspects/without any self-critique.

   (hallucinations, delirium, confusional states, dreamlike states, spatial-temporal disorientation)

   3 = Important disturbances of reality but limited to certain aspects or circumstances (e.g., under stress, fatigue, the effect of alcohol, self-critique is partially present but inconstant.)

   (many illusions and a partial confusion and partial disorientation)

   4 = Moderate disturbance of reality, but more frequent in certain circumstances, (e.g., intense needs, stress, fatigue, alcohol) self-critique possible but insufficient.

   (projections, distortions, imprecise perceptions, difficulties of orientation but not hallucinations, delirium or disorientation)

   5 = Minor disturbances of reality testing, occasional under certain circumstances (e.g., stress, fatigue, half-sleep) that are easily corrected and self-critique is quite good.

   (perceptual errors, selective perception, imprecise perceptions, sporadic difficulties with orientation)

   6 = Normal functioning on the average: none of the disturbances of reality except minor difficulties, occasionally under exceptional stress, easy correction and good self-critique, realistic attitude.

   7 = Optimal functioning, well above the average, flexible and automatic without disturbances of reality itself, even under exceptional stress, self-critique is optimal, realistic.

— *CHAPTER FOURTEEN* —————————————

Ego Function Assessment of Analytic Psychotherapy Combined with Drug Therapy

LEOPOLD BELLAK, JACK CHASSAN,
HELEN K. GEDIMAN, AND MARVIN HURVICH

In some forms of psychotherapy, and even in some forms of modified psychoanalysis, the psychotropic drugs often play the role that anesthetics play for surgery: they often constitute the conditions that enable the intervention to be carried on. For, just as somatic pain may make survival unbearable, or extensive or subtle surgery impossible, so psychic pain may make the verbal operations of psychotherapy extremely difficult. Just as good anesthesia provides the right tonus and generally the optimal field for surgery, so properly used psychotropic drugs may provide for the patient the

We are grateful to the *Journal of Nervous and Mental Disease* for permission to use material for this chapter. This material was previously published as Ego Function Assessment of Analytic Psychotherapy Combined with Drug Therapy by Leopold Bellak, Jack B. Chassan, Helen K. Gediman, and Marvin Hurvich, *The Journal of Nervous and Mental Disease*, 1973, *157*(6), 465–469.

optimal mixture of enough freedom from anxiety or its dread without interfering with ego functions (including the anxiety signal) so much as to interfere with motivation or learning in the therapeutic sense. At times a single drug may be enough; at other times antagonists, such as tranquilizers and energizers, or antidepressants, may have to be used in varying proportions to maintain the best therapeutic climate.

This present study is focused on an assessment of the effects of diazepam (Valium), a well-known antianxiety agent, on ego functioning in psychotherapy. The method employed is the intensive design. The main hypothesis, that Valium can affect ego functioning, is based on the assumption that Valium reduces anxiety, and that lowering a high level of anxiety can result in more adaptive ego functioning. Psychoanalytic theory holds that anxiety impairs ego functions. A similar conclusion may be reached from other theoretical frameworks. Mednick, for example, writing from a behaviorist viewpoint, has suggested that anxiety as an operant conditioner leads some persons to avoid anxiety-arousing thoughts, which can eventuate in overinclusive thinking and other disorders of thought (1969).

The intensive design is a methodological approach for assessing changes within a subject over time and has been most fully developed by J. B. Chassan (1967). The focus is on variation of variables within the person over a given time span and in relation to whatever experimental treatments are being evaluated. Bellak and Chassan (1964) have employed this methodology in a study of the effects of chlordiazepoxide (Librium) on a psychotherapy patient. Other discussions of the intensive method used in psychotropic drug research can be found in Bellak (1965) and Bellak and Chassan (1964).

Procedures for rating ego functions from interview and other material have been developed by Bellak, Hurvich, and Gediman as part of a study on ego functions in schizophrenics, neurotics, and normals (1969, 1973). Indices of rater reliability and construct validity have been established in the context of that study. The utilization of an ego function assessment approach for the evaluation of psychotropic drug effects has been discussed in an earlier paper (1968).

Case Report

Patient A, a woman of about 40 with a diagnosis of severe psychoneurosis, was seen in the study twice weekly in psychoanalytically oriented psychotherapy sessions over a period of about $5\frac{1}{2}$ months (with three missed sessions). During this course of treatment the patient was alternated, on a double blind basis, between diazepam, 10 mg, t.i.d. and matching placebo. The alternations between the two medications took place after 1 or after 2 weeks, with each such length determined on a random basis. The patient was rated on each ego function scale each time she was seen, that is, at each psychotherapy session. Out of a total of 44 sessions she was rated with respect to Valium on 23, and in relation to placebo in the other 21 sessions.

Table 14.1. Sequence of Treatment Observation Periods

Observation Period	Average Ego Function Score on:		Observation Period	Average Ego Function Score on:	
	Valium	Placebo		Valium	Placebo
1	4.5		23	5.5	
2	3.8		24		5.2
3		3.4	25		4.7
4		3.3	26		4.9
5		3.4	27		5.6
6	4.5		28	5.7	
7	4.7		29	5.6	
8	4.2		30	4.9	
9	4.2		31	5.0	
10		3.9	32		4.7
11		3.8	33		5.0
12		4.6	34		5.5
13		3.9	35	5.9	
14	5.4		36	5.7	
15	5.0		37	5.4	
16		4.4	38	5.5	
17	4.6		39		4.8
18	4.9		40		5.1
19		4.4	41	5.5	
20		4.5	42	5.8	
21	5.3		43		4.9
22	5.5		44		5.5

Table 14.1 shows the sequence of treatment of observation periods, the medication patient A was on during each period, and the corresponding average of the 11 ego function scores.

Table 14.2 contrasts patient A's average results over the course of the study with respect to each ego function on Valium, with the corresponding averages on placebo. As can be seen from the table, statistically significant differences favoring Valium were obtained in all but two of the scales: Object Relations and Adaptive Regression in the Service of the Ego (ARISE). The two ego functions showing the greatest differences between diazepam and placebo were (1) Regulation and Control and (2) Defensive Functioning. The last column of Table 14.2 presents the averages, on diazepam and placebo, respectively, of the individual ego function averages. The global ego function averages thus obtained show a clear significant difference between diazepam and placebo (as would be expected on the basis of the component averages). It is noted that in the statistical analysis that has been presented, no attempt was made to eliminate the variance due to trend. In all likelihood

Table 14.2. *Average Ego Function Scores on Seven-Point Scale*

	Reality Testing	Reality Testing Judgment	Sense of Reality	Regulation and Control	Object Relations	Thought Processes	Adaptive Regression in the Service of the Ego	Defensive Functioning	Stimulus Barrier	Autonomous Functioning	Synthetic Functioning	Global, or Average Ego Function Score
Valium	5.52	5.41	5.26	5.00	4.93	5.35	5.57	4.87	4.02	5.09	4.89	5.09
Placebo	4.86	4.83	4.81	4.31	4.60	4.70	5.53	4.24	3.55	4.48	4.36	4.55
Difference	.66	.58	.45	.69	.33	.65	.04	.63	.47	.61	.53	.54
t	2.88	2.79	1.85	3.41	1.42	2.79	0.23	3.00	2.51	2.70	2.13	2.78
p<	.002	.003	.04[a]	.001	N.S.[b]	.003	N.S.	.003	.01	.005	.02	.003

[a] Single-tailed.
[b] N.S., not significant.

significant levels would have been strengthened *a fortiori* had this been done.

Ego function ratings obtained by one rater on the basis of a therapeutic session and the ratings by another rater obtained on the basis of a two-hour standard interview (designed specifically for a larger research project on schizophrenia) at the beginning of treatment correlated .72 (Spearman–Brown formula). This correlation provides some validity for the clinical rating of ego functions, as the reliability and validity of the standard interview had been extensively established in the schizophrenia research project on neurotics as well as schizophrenics and normals (Bellak et al., 1973).

In Figure 14.1 the ratings at the end of treatment are superimposed upon the ratings at the beginning of the treatment. As these figures and accompanying tables show, the patient shows overall improvement as well as specific improvement in relation to diazepam.

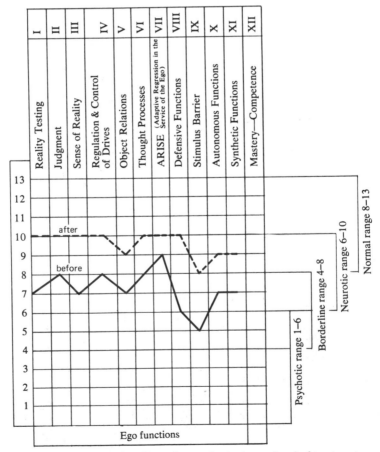

Figure 14.1.   Ego function ratings at beginning and end of treatment.

SUMMARY

A double blind assessment, using the intensive design method, was made of ego functions in a single patient in psychoanalytic psychotherapy who was receiving diazepam and placebo as well. Overall improvement as well as specific improvement in relation to diazepam are demonstrated.

REFERENCES

Bellak, L. Intensive design drug therapy and the psychotherapeutic process. *Psychosomatics,* 1965, *6,* 287–289.

Bellak, L., & Chassan, J. An approach to the evaluation of drug effect during psychotherapy: A double blind study of a single case. *Journal of Nervous and Mental Disease,* 1964, *139,* 20–30.

Bellak, L., & Chassan, J. An approach to the evaluation of drug effect during psychotherapy: A double blind study of a single case. In P. Davidson & C. Costello (Eds.) N-1, *Experimental studies of single cases.* New York: Van Nostrand Reinhold, 1969.

Bellak, L., & Hurvich, M. A. A systematic study of ego functions. *Journal of Nervous and Mental Disease,* 1969, *148,* 569–585.

Bellak, L., Hurvich, M., & Gediman, H. *Ego functions in schizophrenics, neurotics, and normals.* New York: Wiley, 1973.

Bellak, L., Hurvich, M., Gediman, H., & Crawford, P. The systematic diagnosis of the schizophrenic syndrome. *Dynamic Psychiatry,* October, 1969, 148–157.

Bellak, L., Hurvich, M., Silvan, M., & Jacobs, D. Towards an egopsychological appraisal of drug effects. *American Journal of Psychiatry,* 1968, *125,* 593–604.

Chassan, J. *Research design in clinical psychology and psychiatry.* New York: Appleton-Century-Crofts, 1967.

Mednick, S. A learning theory approach to research in schizophrenia. In A. Buss & E. Buss (Eds.), *Theories of schizophrenia.* New York: Atherton Press, 1969.

CHAPTER FIFTEEN

Ego Function Assessment and Analyzability

LEOPOLD BELLAK AND BARNETT MEYERS

For psychoanalysis as a system of therapy, analyzability is probably the single most important concept and factor: It is but a synonym for curability, at least by that particular technique. Curability in general, and analyzability in particular, is neither easy to determine nor an all-or-none proposition. With the possible exception of some acute infectious disorders, there is a quantitative spectrum of curability for most illnesses if the criteria are strict.

For an analyst, then, it is important to be able to determine as soon as possible if a patient is analyzable, to what extent, and what vicissitudes are likely to be encountered in the process. Even within the confines of the most classical model of analysis there must be allowance for individual differences, let alone allowing such in the broadened scope of psychoanalysis. Therefore, technical variations must also be contemplated as a function of the individual aspects of analyzability.

Assessment of analyzability intrinsically involves a prediction, namely,

We are grateful to *The International Review of Psycho-Analysis* for permission to use material for this chapter. This material was previously published as Ego Function Assessment and Analysability by Leopold Bellak, M.D., and Barnett Meyers, M.D., *The International Review of Psycho-Analysis,* Vol. 2, Part 4, 413–427, 1975.

that the patient is likely to respond to psychoanalytic treatment. Analysts have been somewhat reluctant to make explicit this particular implicit prediction, as well as the many other predictions involved in each of the conceptual and methodological propositions basic to the field (Bellak, 1961b).

Ego function assessment offers a systematic basis for prediction based on past and present functioning. The more clear-cut the conceptualization and the planning of treatment, the more success one can expect, the less stalemate (Glover, 1955), the fewer broken-off analyses and undesirable results.

The literature on analyzability is replete with statements regarding the "fragmentary and contradictory knowledge" (Namnun, 1968) and the "lack of well-defined criteria" (Limentani, 1972) regarding the indications and contraindications for psychoanalysis. Waldorn's (1960) review of the subject speaks to the "need for some better-organized and precise approach."

The specific role of the ego in the analytic process could be neither appreciated nor studied prior to the development of the structural theory. Before 1923 Freud conceptualized the goal of analysis as the lifting of repression and making the unconscious conscious. With the development of the structural theory these goals became the building of ego at the expense of id. This allowed Freud to consider the "obstacles that stand in the way of such a cure" (Freud, 1937). He spoke of an unfavorable alteration in the ego acquired in its defensive struggle as "prejudicial to the effectiveness of analysis." Freud was still primarily speaking of the ego as a structural entity. Nevertheless, a number of authors were concurrently defining this entity in terms of its functions (A. Freud, 1936; Hartmann, 1939).

We have since had a continuation of the description and definition of the ego functions. Parallel developments have included a concern about the "widening scope of psychoanalysis" (Stone, 1954) and a consequent increasing focus on the problem of analyzability. The relationship between these areas of investigation has become more apparent. Nunberg (1955) has spoken of the significance of overall ego strength and particularly of the synthetic function in determining a favorable outcome. Waldhorn (1960) considered it logical above all to evaluate ego functions in assessing analyzability. Aarons (1962), as Nunberg and Hartmann had done previously, emphasizes the importance of the synthetic function in determining motivation for analysis. Namnun (1968) elaborates on this theme with the term "the will to be analysed," which he sees as a manifestation of ego autonomy and capacity for mastery. He sees this autonomy as critical to the working through of the transference.

Shuren (1967), in his paper on the preanalytic patient, describes how disturbances in separation and individuation lead to deficits in ego functions that can prevent a successful analysis.

A number of other authors have discussed the role ego functions play in the analytic process without specifying them as such (Stone, 1954; Levin, 1960). Knapp et al. (1960) found evidence suggesting that a team of "experienced clinicians are able to assess suitability for analysis in advance." Although ego strength was "recognized as important" in the study, assessment of it "was left to the interviewer's intuitive clinical judgment." More recently, Lower et al. (1972) reported the high frequency with which "good ego strength" was described as a reason for acceptance for analysis and the higher frequency with which "poor ego strength" was cited as the reason for rejection.

We will address ourselves to the evaluation of specific ego functions as they relate to analyzability and possible parameters to be introduced into an analysis for specific problems.

SYSTEMATIC EGO FUNCTION ASSESSMENT

The systematic technique for the evaluation of ego functions, as developed by Bellak et al. (1973a), was utilized in the present study.

THE EGO FUNCTIONS AND THE ANALYTIC PROCESS

Reality Testing

Reality testing is considered here as a function that is distinct from sense of reality and judgment. Other authors have discussed reality testing as a component of a larger function, the "relation to reality" (Beres, 1956; Frosch, 1964). Nevertheless, the systematic study of the ego mentioned earlier substantiates consideration of reality testing as a separate function on phenomenologic grounds. We feel that such a distinction is warranted on genetic and metapsychological grounds as well.

One principal component of reality testing concerns the perceptual and cognitive capacity to distinguish internal from external stimuli. The loss of the capacity is most clearly demonstrated by one of its most extreme forms, as in the formation of a hallucination. It is more subtly seen in illusions or other phenomena where the perception of external reality is significantly altered by an internal affective state.

A more common yet more subtle form of confusion between internal and external stimuli occurs when contemporary external reality is perceived in terms of the internalized past, as when infantile fantasies or object representations determine the response to a here-and-now situation. Freud (1924) has discussed this loss of reality as a foundation of neurosis. It is a goal of analysis to repair such distortions and thus enable the individual to distinguish internal from external and past from present.

Other important components of reality testing include the intrapersonal and interpersonal validation of perceptions. This is largely a cognitive testing process. Intrapersonal validation refers to the check of data perceived from one sense against that perceived by others, as is lacking in hallucinations. Interpersonal validation involves the comparison of one's own perceptions with those of others, as is lacking in delusions. Any idiosyncratic beliefs that become evident in the consultation must be thoroughly examined with regard to the patient's capacity to test and validate them.

Another principal component is inner reality testing: The analytic process works through an increasing focus on understanding internal reality. It requires a shift of attention from external to internal without losing the capacity to separate the two. The patient is expected to become increasingly aware of how external perceptions are influenced by internal states. The depth and accuracy of internal perceptiveness are related to what we call "psychological-mindedness." Impaired defensive functioning, as manifested by excessive use of denial or projected-introjective mechanisms, limits this perceptiveness and thereby limits the analytic result. Here as elsewhere, we have to keep in mind the interrelationships of different ego functions and how strengths or weaknesses of one influence others.

Reality testing is integral to other aspects of the analytic process. Bellak's (1961a) conception of the "oscillating function of the ego" can be considered as a "macrofunction," contributed to by both adaptive regression and reality testing. The adaptive regression allows for the suspension of secondary process, ensuing free association and the emergence of previously unconscious material, while the observing reality testing function is required for the recognition and understanding of external and internal reality based on the data of the association.

Reality testing is also critical to the understanding and working through of the transference. At appropriate times the analysand must be able to distinguish internally from externally derived perceptions of the analyst. The regression that produces transference distortions must also be largely reversible at the end of the analysis so that functioning can resume in the patient's daily reality. Borderline and psychotic patients often continue to respond to the internal stimulation of the transference to the point where excessive and unmanageable acting out ensues. It is thus apparent that a parameter to be used in analyzing patients with deficient reality testing is the modulation of the developing transference by the analyst. Rapid clarification and interpretation of severely distorted transference phenomena become indicated.

JUDGMENT

The function of judgment refers to the ability to be aware of the likely consequences of intended or actual behavior and is reflected by the extent to which manifest behavior reveals such awareness. In this sense, judgment is a "social" and "conscious" function involving the ego's capacity to appreciate its interaction with external reality. Impaired judgment results in what is referred to as inappropriate behavior, relative to a specific cultural setting.

Logic, which involves the awareness and understanding of cause and effect relationships, is integrally related to judgment. Although logic is generally an aspect of "autonomous functioning" and "thought processes," its relevance to judgment has to do with the individual's capacity to appreciate the external effects of behavior.

The analyst must appraise the patient's judgment regarding the analysis itself. How realistic are the patient's expectations of goals? Does the patient appreciate the type of financial, geographic, and temporal commitments that are being made? To what extent does the patient undergo the voluntary "suspension of disbelief" that relates to the acceptance and awareness of the "as if" (Tarachow, 1963) nature of the transferential relationship? It is this faculty that permits, for example, the appreciation of and identification with theatrical drama without involvement to the point of running on to the stage to join the performance. Despite the regressive forces inherent in the analysis, the function of judgment must be maintained in order for the patient to synchronize the inner and outer realities of the analytic situation and thereby to respond accordingly.

Another significant aspect of judgment is its role in acting out. Patients with impaired judgment can be expected to act out in a socially inappropriate and perhaps harmful way. The consultation should evaluate the patient's judgment in regard to the resolution of past conflictual situations. Similar behavior can be expected to be acted out during the analysis. In such cases the analyst may have to supplement the patient's deficiencies in judgment with the analyst's own awareness of the consequences of intended behavior. This awareness can then become internalized as a signal that the patient can rely on when, for example, self-destructive behavior might otherwise be imminent. (See also Regulation and Control of Drives.)

Sense of Reality

The ego function referred to as sense of reality will be discussed both in terms of its phenomenology and its dynamics. Phenomenologically it is manifested by the extent to which external events are experienced as real and embedded in a familiar context as well as the extent to which one's body and its functioning are experienced as familiar and belonging to the self. Depersonalization, derealization, déjà vu, and dissociative experiences are all examples of a defective sense of reality. Another aspect is faulty self-esteem regulation because of the lack of a constant, cohesive concept of self. The result here is that the patient's self-esteem is quite mutable because of its dependency on daily experiences and the opinion of others. We see these clinical phenomena most clearly in narcissistic personality disorders.

The Sense of Reality is dynamically and structurally determined by the degree to which an individual has mastered separation and individuation, thus allowing for the distinction between self and object representations. Insofar as this developmental task has been mastered, both self and object representations can remain "constant" and relatively independent of changes in reality.

A question arises as to the distinction between sense of reality and reality testing. We have called both of these "ego functions" and both deal with the ego's ability to distinguish internal from external and its "awareness" of body boundaries. It is clear that the two functions are interrelated. There is, in fact, preliminary evidence from factor analysis that reality testing, judgment, sense of reality, and regulation and control of impulses form a "group" of functions whose strengths and weaknesses correlate closely in a particular patient (Bellak et al., 1973a). And yet one function relates to the way the ego senses and experiences reality, whereas the other involves the ego's ability to "test" these experiences against fixed internal percepts and ideas of what is real.

The significance of disturbances in the sense of reality in assessing analyzability has yet to be clearly ascertained. Nevertheless, defects in this area also suggest an overall problem with what Beres (1956) and Frosch (1964) have described as the "relationship to reality." Patients who give a history of responding to stress by regressively losing ego boundaries with resultant perceptual distortions will presumably have this difficulty in the analysis. A particular difficulty could ensue in the transference wherein severe transference distortions occurring under the influence of a regressive refusion with the analyst could result in an unmanageable transference psychosis. It is probable that parameters have to be introduced into the analysis of patients with severe defects in this function as a means of maintaining the observing ego, the working alliance, and the patient's ability to test his or her reality. One such parameter is the analyst's "lending" his or her ego to help the analysand perceive reality at times when it seems irretrievable.

Another parameter is the substitution of face-to-face sessions for the use of the couch. This becomes necessary for patients in whom disturbances in the sense of reality readily produce depersonalized or derealized states associated with such severe anxiety that analysis of the state becomes impossible.

The use of the couch need not be an all-or-none proposition. The patient may be able to use the couch most of the time, but may need to sit up when feelings of depersonalization or derealization emerge to a disturbing degree. When the relevant problems are analyzed, the patient is usually able to return to the couch.

Regulation and Control of Drives, Affects, and Impulses

Regulation and control of drives, affects, and impulses comprise the ego's capacity to cope with impulses impinging on it. It takes into account the directness of drive expression, the degree of frustration tolerance, and the extent to which drive derivatives are channeled through ideation, affective expression, and manifest behavior. The latter closely relates to, and can overlap with, defensive functioning.

Impaired regulation of drives is directly related to a tendency toward acting out. Acting out becomes a too easily used means of remembering and, as such, an alternative to analyzing and understanding conflicts within the analysis. Thus, in order for the analysis to progress, the frustration of not acting out transference wishes must be tolerated. The interpretation of the wishes within the analysis then results in a second loss and resultant frustration. As Tarachow (1963) points out, all transference interpretations result in a loss vis-à-vis transference wishes as the patient must accept the "as if" transference quality of the relationship. It is a difficult set of steps for the analysand to (1) first feel the impulses, (2) then renounce the gratification offered by acting them out, (3) bring the wishes into the analysis, (4) accept the loss that results from interpretation, and (5) use the interpretation to synthesize a new understanding and relinquish old object wishes.

Bellak (1963), in describing the psychology of acting out, suggests a number of points in its treatment, some of which are directly relevant here: Even at the beginning of the analysis it can be important to predict for patients who appear to have a tendency to act out that this is likely to arise, and can in fact include a desire to interrupt the analysis. This desire may emerge for seemingly external reasons or as a result of hostile feelings toward the analyst. It may be appropriate in the initial interviews, or early in the analysis, to point out to the patients the situations in which they are especially likely to act out and thus to increase their signal awareness. In this way an important therapeutic alliance can be established that may make the difference between a successful and an unsuccessful analysis.

Patients who give historical evidence of requiring immediate relief from anxiety or depression have difficulties in analysis. These are often the same patients who have histories of overstimulation and have constitutional or experiential deficiencies in stimulus barrier.

Patients who evidence deficient drive regulation combined with overtly gratifying symptomatology present specific problems. This relates to some of the difficulties encountered in the treatment of drug abuse and the perversions.

A parameter to be considered in dealing with weaknesses in this function is the addition of medication at times when excessive anxiety combined with deficient affect modulation has a particularly disorganizing effect. The amount and duration of such psychopharmacologic interventions must be carefully monitored so as to allow for an optimal effect while preserving cognitive functioning that would permit analytic work to continue.

Object Relations

Object relations is a complicated ego function that comprises both the degree and kind of relatedness to others. Specifically, it involves the extent to which others are perceived as separate entities rather than extensions of the self and the extent to which present relationships are influenced and patterned by past infantile ones. The unifying principle is the degree to which the patient has mastered separation and individuation and achieved object constancy.

Failures in the development of these spheres and object relations have particular effects on an analysis. Failure to differentiate self from object is the distinguishing characteristic of the psychosis, but is a more subtle manifestation of narcissistic personality disorders. In these narcissistic nonpsychotic disturbances, the separation of internal self and object representations has occurred, and consequently the individual can distinguish internal from external reality (reality test). However, because of both incomplete mastery of separation and unresolved wishes for refusion, the narcissistic patient is liable to transiently *feel* external objects to be extensions of the self. The result, in both psychosis and narcissistic disturbance, is that within the analysis, losses resulting from absence, silence, vacation, and transference interpretations lead to a severe anxiety that recapitulates infantile separation anxiety.

Disturbances in object relations can lead to transference resistance or resistance to transference. In the former, the analyst is perceived and maintained as the projection of an all good idealized "real" object. Analysis of this fusion would lead to a profound narcissistic loss. In the latter, the analyst is perceived as a powerful threatening figure via projective identification and such a transference makes a working alliance impossible. The severe forms of disturbance are classically seen in narcissistic and borderline conditions.

Kohut (1971) has specifically described the vicissitudes in object relations of the patient with a narcissistic character disorder and the analytic modifications and technical measures that follow from these considerations. Kernberg (1968) has discussed parameters that may become necessary during the analysis of both narcissistic and borderline disturbances. Jacobson (1971), in turn, has described the psychodynamics of the transference relationship of the severely depressed patient. In patients described by these authors, it is important to be fully aware of all the factors that are likely to appear as problems of analyzability so they can be identified at the earliest possible opportunity. In many cases the analyst must make decisions as to the feasibility of focusing on the vicissitudes of object representations, as opposed to a less classical approach that would aim at internalizing a new object by identification with the analyst. Naturally, this is never an all-or-none phenomenon.

Less severely distorted object relations are seen in neurotic disorders and, prototypically, in the transference neurosis. It is through the transference that we have most direct access to an examination of how internalized mental representations from childhood influence current perceptions and object relations. This can be contrasted to the hypothetic optimal level of object relatedness in which the perception of external objects remains constant regardless of affective or instinctual changes. It is noteworthy that for an analysis to take place there must be a regression in just this area. The patient must regress from his or her own optimal level of object relatedness in order to develop the transference distortions essential for an analysis. The limiting factor must be the level of individuation already achieved so that the transference distortions do not become symbiotic refusions or do not require the use of intransigent splitting, denial, idealization, or other primitive defenses that make the transference unanalyzable.

Classical theory of analyzability has been somewhat divergent from actual practice. According to the most classical, and undoubtedly most gratifying model of an analysis, interpretation of the defenses leads to the establishment of a transference neurosis. This transference neurosis is not only a renaissance of the childhood neurosis, but also the somewhat varying model of the patient's conflicts and problems in general, reproduced like a laboratory preparation in the analytic setting. In this ideal situation the interpretation of the transference neurosis leads by automatic generalization to a corrective therapeutic restructuring of the personality of the patient via this model. It is as if a calibrator were directly to transfer the learning from the small transference analysis model to the large, life-sized scale of all relationships. The fact is, however, that a majority of the patients currently seen in Western cultures rarely produce a classical transference neurosis unless they suffer from a hysterical disorder, possibly close to a borderline condition. Although most patients do not produce a full-blown transference neurosis, they do so to a small extent from time to time throughout the analysis. It would be a mistake to consider a limited ability to produce any kind of transference neurosis as a preclusion to analysis.

Thought Processes

The thought processes function concerns the ability to think clearly and is most plainly manifested by the capacity to communicate one's thoughts in an intelligible way. The adequacy of processes that guide and sustain thought, such as attention, concentration, concept formation, language, and memory as well as the relative primary–secondary process ratio in thinking are components of this process.

Many aspects of this function interrelate with other functions. Memory and language, usually considered under the heading of "autonomous functions," are considered here insofar as they have lost their autonomy and impair thinking. The ability to concentrate is also usually autonomous, but disturbances in concentration have a deleterious effect on thinking. This is irrespective of whether the disturbed concentration is secondary to marked anxiety, organic defect, or clouding of the sensorium, or excessive pressure of thoughts. Defensive functioning affects thinking as well, for example, by the mechanisms of displacement, condensation, and projection.

Denial, as particularly described by Lewin (1953), produces centrifugal thinking, while elliptical thinking occurs to an extreme degree in schizophrenics but may occur in minor degrees in all kinds of disorders of lesser pathology. Disturbances in thinking have traditionally been associated with the schizophrenic. There is evidence that some schizophrenics do not have a thought disorder and some nonschizophrenics do (Bellak et al., 1973a).

Especially noteworthy is an increasing awareness that mild neurological conditions, which in childhood probably manifested themselves as dyslexia or other learning disabilities with some soft neurological signs (minimal brain dysfunction), may also result in thought disorders under the impact of flooding by emotions. Patients with such conditions not only need to be specifically diagnosed with regard to their analyzability, but they also need to understand the origin of their disorder. Such patients may at times sound psychotic to themselves and others. A decreased tendency to be flooded by neurotic emotions will decrease their tendency toward confused thinking. At the same time, awareness and understanding of this tendency is essential. In this case a neurological deficit contributes to poor control of drives and affects, with a consequent disturbance in thinking.

Defects in the thinking process have clear-cut effects on the analytic process. Free association requires controlled regression of thought processes. The ego must be capable of an oscillating process whereby secondary process thought can take over for the purpose of perceiving and understanding primary process material that has emerged. The analysand must be able to use attention, concentration, memory, and concept formation in order to be aware of his or her associations, be capable of recalling them, and, finally, be able to decipher themes and form concepts regarding his or her internal reality. *The capacity to think syllogistically is relevant here.* The analyst's use of, and the patient's understanding of, syllogisms is critical to interpretation and insight.

Adaptive Regression in the Service of the Ego

The function of adaptive regression in the service of the ego involves the two phases of the oscillating process described by Kris (1952) and Bellak (1961a) and alluded to in the discussions of reality testing and thought processes. As Kris (1952) and others since have pointed out, adaptive regression is an essential aspect of the creative act and thus has a critical role in the analytic process. While this function allows for the relaxation of cognitive acuity and secondary process modes of thought, thus permitting the emergence of more mobile preconscious and unconscious ideation, it also involves the ego's capacity to interrupt and reverse the regression and return to secondary process thought. The third aspect of this function is the ego's capacity to utilize the regression adaptively by inducing new configurations and creative integrations.

Defects in any of these aspects of adaptive regression result in specific difficulties in the analysis.

The obsessive-compulsive personality will have great difficulty suspending secondary process thought because of the anxiety produced by affects, instincts, and the fluidity of cathexes. His or her thinking will remain concrete. This same anxiety about the unknown (unconscious) will impair such a patient's ability to form creative and new integrations adaptively. Schizophrenic and borderline patients can readily regress to primary process modes of thought but have difficulties reversing the process. The anxiety resulting from the loss of control of the thinking process in such patients impedes the adaptive utilization of the regression as well.

The initial interview is an invaluable tool here. Can the patient fantasize? Is he aware of his dreams and how does he respond to them? Is the patient capable of the regressions called for in the appreciation of art, sex, or humor, or are they felt as threatening and ego-alien? Alternatively, does the patient regress "too readily" and not in the service of the ego? Does the patient evidence primary process thought in a structured interview? Is there a history of fantasies interrupting intended concentration in a disabling fashion or of a preoccupation with and "being carried away by" fantasies?

Regarding the second phase of the oscillating process, the interviewer can investigate whether the patient has been able to use discoveries from dreams, fantasies, or other regressed states for planned or creative actions. How does he go about problem solving? Does he discover imaginative solutions via ego regression or can he only approach solutions by rote learning?

Finally, the question arises as to how smoothly the patient can make the transition from regression to control. Can the ego use regression and its controls in a complementary fashion that can lead to adaptation? A microcosm of this occurs in the consultation itself, where the patient relinquishes usual inhibitions to speak of emotionally charged anxiety-producing material. The interviewer must attend to how the patient responds to this regression and to the thoughts it evokes. A patient who is able to regress in a limited fashion, who finds this pleasurable, and, most importantly, who can use the consultation to form limited yet new understandings about the self creatively, is demonstrating evidence for a positive prognosis—at least in regard to how the patient's functioning in this area contributes to the outcome of the analysis.

In many cases the analyst can help the patient modulate the degree of regression during an hour so as to achieve an optimal regressive level for adaptive utilization. In some patients medication can be considered that might decrease the effect of anxiety on the oscillating function. Excessive and maladaptive regression can be interrupted by the analyst's increased activity or by the temporary substitution of face-to-face sessions for the couch.

Defensive Functioning

We consider defensive functioning a binary function that includes the extent to which defenses are successful in reducing dysphoric affects such as anxiety and depression and the degree to which in turn the defenses themselves adaptively or maladaptively influence ideation and behavior. The formation of a hierarchy of defensive functioning, based on either the chronological development of defenses or particular levels of psychopathology, is an unresolved issue for psychoanalytic theory. We are concerned here with an empirical operational assessment of defensive functioning. We are concerned with the effectiveness with which the defenses cope with drives and affects and the adaptability of the responses. Finally, we are concerned with the extent to which vicissitudes in this function facilitate or impede the analytic process. We must consider how deficits here can be identified during the initial consultations and what parameters are available for dealing with such deficits during the course of the analysis.

Incapacitating dysphoria will have a disruptive effect. Severe depression will result in retardation of thought and associations, as well as a general impairment of cognition. Excessive anxiety has an obvious disorganizing effect. Patients presenting such severe affective symptoms are often suffering from a failure of repression and necessitate, at least initially, a more "supportive" psychotherapeutic approach. The use of psychoanalysis can be reconsidered later, but even then the introduction of parameters that would help to bind dysphoria might be required.

Patients who bind their dysphoria but at the cost of maladaptation present the converse problem. The lack of anxiety and depression decreases the motivation toward analysis. The alloplastic tendency lends itself to acting out. In the obsessive-compulsive the defenses of isolation and intellectualization, by preventing the emergence of affects, mitigate against the development, awareness, and understanding of transference feelings. Patients suffering from pervasions or psychosomatic illnesses, because of the rapid discharge of affect inherent to their conditions, can be expected to present similar difficulties.

The more primitive defenses produce the greatest reality distortions and are therefore the most difficult to analyze. A patient whose presentation reveals an extensive use of denial can be expected to be quite resistant to perceiving, much less analyzing, the disturbing internal reality. The tendency to perceive problems as externally caused is associated with denial and projection and presents similar difficulties. This not only applies to overtly manic or paranoid patients but is also seen in what are often referred to as "acting-out" forms of character disorders. Finally, the borderline patient's tendency to split will be revealed in the consultation by a history of defensive overidealization or denigration of significant objects. The transference distortions resulting from splitting are often intransigent to analysis (Kernberg, 1967, 1968).

Stimulus Barrier

The ego function referred to as stimulus barrier also has two basic components: a receptive and an expressive one. The receptive is the individual's threshold for sensitivity to and awareness of sensory stimulation. The expressive component relates to how the individual responds to different degrees of stimulation with particular emphasis on whether coping mechanisms are adaptive or maladaptive. In the latter case deficient coping plus overstimulation leads to disorganization and withdrawal.

The receptive component includes sensitivity to internal and external stimulation with the common final pathway being impingement of the sensory nerves. Examples of internal stimulation include changes in body temperature, and visceral and muscular pain, whereas external stimulation includes light, sound, drugs, and other forms of inanimate stimuli.

Drives and impulses can also be conceptualized as stimuli, albeit internal ones; however, sensitivity to and regulation of them is considered a separate ego function. Stimulus barrier is more closely related to the sensory motor nervous system than the psychological realm. It is only when we see failures in sensory threshold or in motor responsiveness to the stimuli that we get "sensory overload." It is at this point that drive and affect changes occur and the function of their regulation becomes operative.

As mentioned above, the expressive component concerns the individual's capacity to cope with different levels of stimulation. A critical aspect of this is the individual's ability to regulate the stimulus threshold, which entails the modulation of and selective attention to stimulation. This screening mechanism allows for adaptive changes in sensitivity to stimulation, thus facilitating periods of heightened acuity, focused concentration, and the general filtering out of stimulation necessary for sleep. Other aspects of the expressive component include the degree of cognitive and motoric adaptation to high levels of stimulation versus motoric and cognitive disruption. Persons with a low stimulus threshold plus poor coping mechanisms are easily "overstimulated." This may lead to impaired sleep habits, concentration, mood and drive regulation, synthetic functioning, and so on. It is thus clear that overflow from defects in this function can influence the other ego functions as well.

The ego's capacity to regulate stimulus input plays a critical role in the analytic process. The analytic setting is designed to reduce external stimulation and thereby promote regression and an increased attention to internal phenomena. Patients with impairments in this area are easily distracted and such distractions can become a major obstacle to the analysis. The emphasis here is not on the psychic meaning of such distractions, but that some patients lack the ego capacity adequately to screen out adventitious stimulation.

Patients with such impairments often give histories of daily experiences in which sensory overstimulation has led to disorganization. Not being able to cope with the impact of small children or of having to orient oneself while driving in a new environment are commonplace examples of this.

In this context we want to refer to the previously mentioned and too rarely recognized problem of adults who, as children, suffered from a minimal brain dysfunction and may still have, on the one hand, a low stimulus barrier and, on the other hand, some problems in orientation. For example, there are cases when because of problems in spatial orientation a spouse may tend to get lost when driving to a destination; marital discord may ensue.

Another aspect of this is sensitivity to the effects of internal changes. How disorganizing does the consultee find the experience of pain or discomfort, or, in the case of women, premenstrual tension? The analysand must, rather than being overwhelmed by internal stimulation, have the capacity to perceive and utilize such stimulation in the service of self-understanding. Patients with strengths here can more readily understand the relationship between sensations that are perceived and their psychological meaning.

Conversely, the concept of a required minimal stimulation relates to this function. The classical example of deficient stimulation disrupting psychic functioning is in the sensory deprivation syndrome, and persons vary in regard to their sensitivity to this. Patients requiring moderate amounts of stimulation to preserve psychic integration can be expected to manifest symptoms of derealization or have transient psychotic experiences in the face of the sensory deprivation inherent in the analytic situation. Such patients may require a well-lit room or increased verbal activity by the analyst to prevent such experiences.

A paradigm for the evaluation of stimulus barrier can be how the consultee deals with the task of falling asleep. Is sleep too readily prevented by minimal external stimulation? Conversely, has the lack of stimulation inherent to falling asleep required the use of hypnotic agents or the auxiliary stimulation of the television or radio? The dynamic significances of sleep disturbances are myriad. Nevertheless, a critical element is how well the patient can regulate the stimulus barrier to achieve the level of stimulation necessary for sleep and how this regulatory capacity will facilitate or impede the analysis.

Autonomous Functioning

We are concerned here with the relative lack of impairment of what have been described as primary and secondary autonomous ego functions. Primary autonomous functions include perception, attention, intelligence, intentionality, memory, language, sensation, and motoric expression. Secondary autonomy refers to habits, skills, and behavior patterns that are either combinations of primary autonomous functions or have become secondarily autonomous by sublimation (Hartmann, 1939, 1955). Autonomy refers to the freedom from impairment of these operations by the intrusion of conflict, ideation, affect, and/or impulses. It takes into account a degree of resistance to regression and reinstinctualization that would result in such intrusions.

One can conceptualize the autonomous ego functions as the tools the patient brings to the therapeutic alliance to accomplish the analytic work. Deficits in these tools can severely limit the amount of work done. This is clearly true when we consider impairments in intelligence, language, memory, and attentiveness and their influence on the analytic process. The same is true for the complex patterns, subsumed under the heading of secondary autonomous functions. What acquired intellectual and perceptual skills (which include communication, the ability to symbolize and understand symbols, etc.) does the patient bring to the analysis? To what extent are other major ego functions, such as reality testing, judgment, and thought processes, operating free from conflict? How likely are these functions to regress and in what conflictual areas? A patient who develops severe anxiety with loosened associations when discussing overtly sexual material may have episodic impairments in reality testing, thinking, object relations, and his or her primary functions such that the capacity to perceive or understand his or her difficulties is lost.

We can always anticipate a degree of regressive instinctualization of what had previously been autonomous functions during the course of an analysis. What we must consider are the autonomous starting points and the autonomous reserves the patient will maintain. This will help decide the kind and degree of effort and equipment the patient has available for the analysis. Persons who already suffer from inability to perform simple work or intellectual tasks, for whom such tasks now seem a burden, and who have lost the ability to concentrate or communicate clearly, are usually not ready to start an analysis. In such cases a preparatory course of therapy is often indicated, followed by a reassessment to determine whether a patient's autonomous functioning would enable him or her to withstand the rigors of an analysis.

Synthetic–Integrative Function

The synthetic–integrative function will also be described in terms of two principal components. The first is the capacity to integrate potentially discrepant or contradictory experiences. Such experiences can be behavioral, psychological, or both, and can involve thoughts, feelings, actions, and perceptions. Psychological aspects include the ability to integrate: (1) apparently divergent self-representations, (2) distortions between internally perceived object representations and externally perceived objects, and (3) affects with incongruent ideation or internal perceptions. The resolution of such distortions plays a large role in reality testing, sense of reality, and object relations as well as other ego functions. It is also crucial to the resolving of ambivalence.

The second major component of this function is the ability to interrelate and integrate psychic or behavioral experiences that need not be contradictory. This aspect of the function facilitates the experiences of connections and continuity, in addition to allowing for planning and organizing operations. Psychologically, it enables the perception of the relationship of past to present, mood to idea, and percept to experiences.

As Beres (1956) has pointed out, synthetic operations are ubiquitous in human thought and action. This function works so closely with other functions that its examination in isolation is nearly impossible. This has been alluded to earlier. Nevertheless, the critical nature of this function's contribution to the analytic process makes such a dissection and investigation imperative. Without adequate synthetic–integrative functioning, the reductive dissective aspects of the psychoanalytic process would lead to dissolution and psychosis rather than resynthesis and ego growth.

The associative process by which connections occur also depends heavily on this function. Without it, the second phase of the oscillating function does not occur and free association becomes the loosened autistic associative process of the schizophrenic. The synthetic function allows for the linkage of initially causal associative data in order to arrive at causal and dynamic themes and understanding.

The psychoanalytic process is itself a dissociative experience: the patient is asked to observe himself and report on himself (Bellak, 1961). This involves both phases of the oscillating function, that is, adaptive regression followed by synthesis. In some people with poor synthetic functioning, the analytic process actually increases a tendency toward pathological dissociation. Having previously been self-observing in an unskilled way, they now substitute analytic self-observation. In the absence of a sufficient ego synthetic function, they are unable to utilize interpretations in a constructive way. They are primarily the people who do well intellectually, but are unable to integrate and synthesize the experience emotionally into the necessary gestalt that, indeed, is ultimately responsible for a restructuring of the personality. For that reason, when the capacity to synthesize is insufficient, it impairs the ability to use insight and is thus a contraindication to analysis and calls for psychotherapy with limited associating, limited self-observing, and other forms of intervention. Very often people who have been unsuccessfully analyzed, with a specific complaint of constant self-analysis and no symptom resolution, need postanalytic psychotherapy, specifically to undo the dissociative aspects of analysis.

Appraisal of this function during initial interviews should include evaluation of the frequency and severity of dissociative states. How well does the patient integrate affects with thoughts? How well has the patient been able to sort out excessive stimulation by specifically synthesizing the various stimuli to arrive at an understanding of the specific situation? Patients with neurological defects, particularly involving minimal brain dysfunction, may present difficulties here.

One parameter that can be introduced into the analysis of some patients would be the analyst's lending his or her own synthesizing function to the patient. The analyst could thus concretely review and synthesize significant elements of the session. The analyst would have to help the patient integrate the affective state and the thought content. The hoped-for result would be a strengthening of the patient's own integrative function so that the patient could then carry out such processes independently.

Mastery–Competence

The function of mastery–competence relates to the individual's capacity to master his environment relative to his resources (White, 1967). The resources are largely subsumed under the other ego functions, and by mastery–competence we are referring to how well an individual's ego assets are utilized in interaction with the environment. This function has three components: (1) objective performance relative to assets, (2) subjective sense of competency or expectation of success, and (3) the degree of concordance between actual performance and expectation.

The mastery we are considering here is of the analytic task. In essence, we are considering how well an individual utilizes the analytic insights to work through and resolve conflicts. Difficulties with this late step in the analytic course account for the difference between patients who understand the infantile origins of their conflicts while continuing neurotic patterns, and patients who, by working through conflicts, become free to achieve behavioral and characterological changes.

The preanalysis evaluation must assess this function and consider the potential analysand's sense of competency and its relation to actual achievement. Is the patient unrealistically grandiose or unduly pessimistic? Does he or she "underachieve" and why?

Patients with character traits marked by strong passive and/or masochistic wishes have problems in this area. The literature has considered these issues and the related topic of the negative therapeutic reaction (Freud, 1937). The resistances that develop in such patients are usually considered in terms of their psychodynamic origins or manifestations in the transference. We are not minimizing such issues but are rather focusing on another perspective through which to view them. That is, masochistic and passive-dependent character pathology may lead to impairments in a patient's functioning, specifically in the capacity to achieve mastery and competence. We would predict that without a minimal level of functioning in this area, regardless of the strengths of the other functions, a weakness in the so-called analytic utilization factor would result with a consequent limitation on potential analytic achievement. A corollary to this is that some relatively more disturbed patients who bring a particularly strong utilization factor to the analysis, as evidenced by a history of past environmental masteries, may be surprisingly good candidates for analysis.

SUMMARY AND CONCLUSIONS

Systematic evaluation of ego functions for the assessment of analyzability has been discussed. In concentrating on these aspects of the personality, evaluation of superego factors, and, to some extent, drive factors have not been considered. Similarly, reality factors, specific maturational phase or general life situation, intelligence, various handicaps such as speech difficulties, hearing difficulties, and congruence or incongruence of a given patient with a given psychoanalyst were also not discussed. It is in the nature of this paper that its scope is limited. In no way should this selected focus be construed as a willingness or suggestion that factors other than ego function assessment should be ignored or considered unimportant, or even less important.

On the other hand, we suggest that systematic ego function assessment is a valuable tool for all analysts. Though it is a very formal rating scheme with detailed definitions, it includes suggestions for inquiry and criteria for rating. Thus, it is possible and may be sufficient for any analyst to engage in some clinical rating without much more effort than listing these 12 functions and clarifying their definitions and criteria for evaluation, that is, using the list and criteria as a frame of reference in a clinical interview.

Of the ego functions discussed, stimulus barrier, mastery–competence, and ARISE are the only ones that may not routinely be kept in mind by analysts. With regard to stimulus barrier, certain neurological or generally physiological factors and their effect on organizing ability—and its absence—were especially stressed. Minimal brain dysfunction was given special attention particularly with regard to its impact on thought processes, impulse control, and some specific symptoms.

Mastery and competence so conceptualized may be a new consideration for many analysts because, among other things, the concept does not come from strictly psychoanalytic sources. Nevertheless, we feel that it is an important aspect of analyzability. Mastery–competence seems to be sufficiently autonomous to require its own assessment and not to be viewed simply in the light of dimensions of pathology.

ARISE (adaptive regression in the service of the ego), as originally formulated by E. Kris, needs only to be brought more fully to the attention of the analyst as a factor in considering analyzability.

In sum, we have suggested that the systematic and careful use of ego function assessment has specific applicability in assessing analyzability. Furthermore, ego function assessment may be as good a way as any for the systematic comparison of the status of many patients at the beginning, the middle, and the end of an analysis.

REFERENCES

Aarons, A. Indications for analysis and problems of analysability. *Psychoanalytic Quarterly,* 1962, *31,* 514–531.

Bellak, L. Free association: Conceptual and clinical aspects. *International Journal of Psychoanalysis,* 1961a, *42,* 9–20.

Bellak, L. Research in psychoanalysis. *Psychoanalytic Quarterly,* 1961b, *30,* 519–548.

Bellak, L. Acting out: Some conceptual and therapeutic considerations. *American Journal of Psychotherapy,* 1963, *17,* 375–389.

Bellak, K., & Hurvich, M. A systematic study of ego functions. *Journal of Nervous Mental Disease,* 1969, *148,* 569–585.

Bellak, L., Hurvich, M., & Gediman, H. *Ego functions in schizophrenics, neurotics, and normals.* New York: Wiley, 1973a.

Bellak, L., Chassan, J. B., Gediman, H., and Hurvich, M. Ego function assessment of analytic psychotherapy combined with drug therapy. *Journal of Nervous Mental Disease,* 1973b, *157,* 465–469.

Beres, D. Ego deviation and the concept of schizophrenia. *Psychoanalytic Study of the Child,* 1956, *2,* 164–235.

Freud, A. *The ego and the mechanisms of defence.* New York: International Universities Press, 1936; 1946.

Freud, S. Loss of reality in neurosis and psychosis (standard ed., Vol. 19). *The complete psychological works of Sigmund Freud* (J. Strachey, trans.). London: Hogarth Press, 1924.

Freud, S. Analysis terminable and interminable. (standard ed., Vol. 23). *The complete psychological works of Sigmund Freud* (J. Strachey, trans.). London: Hogarth Press, 1937.

Frosch, J. The psychotic character: Clinical psychiatric considerations. *Psychiatric Quarterly,* 1964, *38,* 81–96.

Glover, E. *The technique of psychoanalysis.* New York: International Universities Press, 1955.

Hartmann, H. *Ego psychology and the problem of adaptation.* New York: International Universities Press, 1958.

Hartmann, H. Notes on the theory of sublimation. *Essays on ego psychology.* New York: International Universities Press, 1955; 1964.

Jacobson, E. *Depression: Comparative studies of normal, neurotic, and psychotic conditions.* New York: International Universities Press, 1971.

Kernberg, O. Borderline personality organization. *Journal of the American Psychoanalytic Association,* 1967, *15,* 641–685.

Kernberg, O. The treatment of patients with borderline personality organization. *International Journal of Psychoanalysis,* 1968, *49,* 600–619.

Knapp, P. H., Levin, S., McCarter, R. H., Werner, H., Zetzel, E. Suitability for psychoanalysis: A review of one hundred supervised analytic cases. *Psychoanalytic Quarterly,* 1960, *29,* 459–477.

Kohut, H. *The analysis of the self.* New York: International Universities Press, 1971.

Kris, E. *Psychoanalytic explorations in art.* New York: International Universities Press, 1952.

Levin, S. Problems in the evaluation of patients for psychoanalysis. *Bulletin of the Philadelphia Psychoanalytic Association,* 1960, *10,* 86–95.

Lewin, B. *The psychoanalysis of elation.* New York: Norton, 1953.

Limentani, A. The assessment of analysability: A major hazard in selection for psychoanalysis. *International Journal of Psychoanalysis,* 1972, *53,* 351–361.

Lower, R., Escoll, P., & Huyster, H. Bases for judgement of analysability. *Journal of the American Psychoanalytic Association,* 1972, *20,* 610–621.

Namnun, A. The problem of analysability and the autonomous ego. *International Journal of Psychoanalysis,* 1968, *49,* 271–275.

Nunberg, H. *Principles of psychoanalysis.* New York: International Universities Press, 1955.

Shuren, I. A contribution to the metapsychology of the preanalytic patient. *Psychoanalytic Study of the Child,* 1967, *22,* 103–136.

Stone, L. The widening scope of indications for psychoanalysis. *Journal of the American Psychoanalytic Association,* 1954. *2,* 567–594.

Tarachow, S. *An introduction to psychotherapy.* New York: International Universities Press, 1963.

Waldhorn, H. F. Assessment of analysability: Technical and theoretical observations. *Psychoanalytic Quarterly,* 1960, *29,* 478–506.

White, R. W. Competence and the growth of personality. In J. II. Masserman (Ed.), *Science and psychoanalysis,* Vol. II, New York: Grune & Stratton, 1967.

CHAPTER SIXTEEN

Ego Function Assessment of the Psychoanalytic Process

VERNON SHARP AND LEOPOLD BELLAK

In the current climate of social, medical, and psychiatric change, objective and rapid clinical assessment of the ongoing psychoanalytic process has become increasingly vital for a variety of pressing reasons. These include analytic education, supervision, research, third-party inquiries, and peer review.

At least two factors make psychoanalytic clinical assessment unique. First, more than anyone else in the healing professions, analysts are reluctant to invade the privacy of the patient–doctor relationship, since it is fundamental and crucial to the treatment process. Second, the psychoanalytic appraisal of the patient's progress in treatment involves great difficulties because of the complex variables involved, far beyond manifest symptomatology.

The need for systematic assessment of psychoanalytic patients has been noted and responded to by others. Notably, Greenspan and Cullander described an excellent systematic metapsychological scheme for the assess-

We are grateful to *The Psychoanalytic Quarterly* for permission to use material for this chapter. This material was previously published as Ego function assessment of the psychoanalytic process by Vernon Sharp and Leopold Bellak, *The Psychoanalytic Quarterly*, 1978, *XLVII*, 52–72.

ment of analyzability (1973) and another for the assessment of the course of an analysis (1975). Regrettably, their scheme is not presented in a form that permits quantification readily enough to provide a basis for interrater reliability and validity. Some of their verbal statements could easily be translated into numerical ones in the future, but whether their scheme can attain statistically desirable characteristics has yet to be determined.

A method described by Endicott et al. (1976) as the Global Assessment Scale attempts to measure overall severity of psychiatric disturbance. They based their ratings, in essence, on a list of symptoms. In their study three groups were inpatients and the subjects in the fourth group were seen at an aftercare clinic—that is, they had been inpatients. The reliability of the GAS for this sample appears quite satisfactory. The authors discuss some reasons for technical doubts about the validity of their data. Be that as it may, the nature of their sample involved more severe symptomatology in a group of inpatients than psychoanalysts are likely to find in their patients. The more subtle the symptomatology, the more difficult it is to make discriminatory judgments. Even more critical for psychoanalytic assessment is the fact that a scale using only *symptoms* as criterion measures lacks meaning in a psychoanalytic, psychodynamic way.

The strength of the method suggested in this paper, ego function assessment (EFA), lies precisely in the fact that it constitutes a bridge between descriptive psychiatry and the dynamic propositions of psychoanalysis (cf. Strauss, 1975). It not only lends itself to operational definition and statistical study but can in fact now be related to an existing body of data with demonstrable reliability and validity. Independent observers have been shown to achieve high agreement on the status of the ego functions of a patient (Bellak et al., 1973; Ciompi et al., 1976; Milkman & Frosch, 1977). Ego functions have been carefully defined in previous research by Bellak, Hurvich, and Gediman (1973). From this work, an interview guide and scoring manual have been developed covering basic concepts readily familiar to all psychoanalysts. For experienced clinicians these materials need only serve as a systematic frame of reference.

In reporting ego functions to a committee or any third party, virtually nothing of personal significance or intimate meaning in the life of the patient is revealed. Scores on ego functions are highly impersonal matters, and yet to the expert they relate precisely to the complexities of psychoanalytic theory and practice and to the functioning of a person in treatment. The method is therefore suggested as a rapid, reliable, and global approach to the clinical assessment of the analytic process.

ASSESSMENT OF THE PSYCHOANALYTIC PROCESS

In collaborative work the authors have used the EFA method to continuously monitor the progress of two patients seen simultaneously in supervised analyses. The determination of EFA patterns at regular intervals has not only introduced a desirable element of precision into the ongoing analytic work, but has also provided a broad overview of specific trends in treatment and a focus for predicting future trends. In addition, this process has made possible the planning of future treatment goals in a flexible and methodical way.

In the following two case histories each patient entered treatment during a developmental crisis: late adolescence in the first and a midlife crisis in the second (cf. Jaques, 1965). Both were seen four times weekly, using the couch.

Case Histories

Patient A, a 22-year-old, bright, active, single female college graduate, entered analysis complaining of mild depression, problems with interpersonal relationships, and a generalized feeling of loss of purpose in her life. She had done well in college but had maintained a symbiotic tie to her mother through daily phone calls from her college in the mid-West to her parents' home on the East Coast. In her interpersonal relationships she was passive, compliant, and emotionally distant.

Following the death of her mother during her third year of college, the patient took a college-sponsored trip to France where she began to use a variety of drugs and engaged in a series of sexual affairs, all new activities for her. During this time, she experienced no conscious grief over the death of her mother. Following her return to college for her senior year, she experienced a number of troublesome but not disabling symptoms, for which she sought and received group and once-weekly individual therapy. After graduation, although she had planned to be a guidance counselor, she took a job as a trainee in a large advertising agency. At this point she sought analysis, in part because other members of her family had been in analytic treatment.

Patient B is a 39-year-old successful attorney. He has been married 14 years and has two daughters. He sought analysis on the advice of his internist when he complained of moderate depression, generalized feelings of dissatisfaction, and superficiality in his interpersonal relationships, especially with his children and his wife. He had not had sexual relations with his wife for months and was considering divorce. He said that although he had attained all the hallmarks of social and professional success, he felt he was "only going through the motions." A trial period of analysis was begun. It soon emerged that the patient was constantly preoccupied with the details of an incident that had occurred in the course of a long-standing love affair with his secretary, a casual sexual contact the secretary had had with a stranger at a time when the patient had been out of town, after which the relationship had deteriorated. During the analysis, it became clear that the patient's painful preoccupations, feelings of rage, deep distrust, and periodic punitive retaliation toward this woman were highly overdetermined and related specifically to childhood abandonments.

The patient had been abandoned by his natural father before his birth, and he had seen this man on only three occasions in early childhood. For the first 4 years of life, he was reared by his mother and another woman, a warm, interested person whom the mother had taken into the apartment as a boarder. When the patient was 4, however, the mother suddenly remarried, and at the insistence of the new husband, the patient was sent to a distant city to be raised by his maternal grandparents. He saw little of his natural mother thereafter. As with the first patient, there was little evidence of overt grief following parental abandonment.

Both patients were evaluated at the beginning of analysis using the EFA

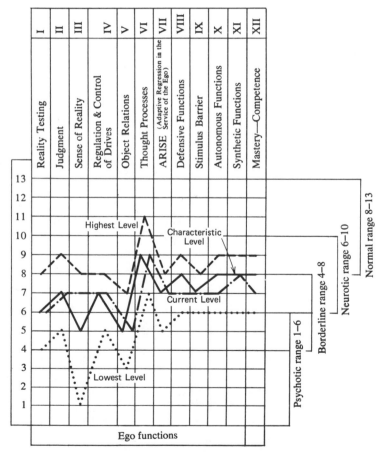

Figure 16.1.   Patient A. Onset of analysis.

method. (See Figures 16.1 and 16.2 for the ego function rating forms for each patient along with the approximate ranges of normality, neuroses, borderline conditions, and psychoses.)

Both patients have undergone periods of crisis, depending on vicissitudes in environmental stress and the analytic work. For example, patient A went through a suicidal period shortly after the third anniversary of her mother's death. During this time, conflicts over dependent needs were in the forefront of the analysis and her self-esteem was at a profoundly low ebb. On one occasion she became suicidal following an hour in which her anger over the analyst's fees began to emerge but was not sufficiently worked through because of an intervening weekend. At the same time, her confused relationships with several young men had taken a turn for the worse, and she had recently been promoted to a position of increased responsibility at her job, a change about which she was ambivalent. The regressive movement of her

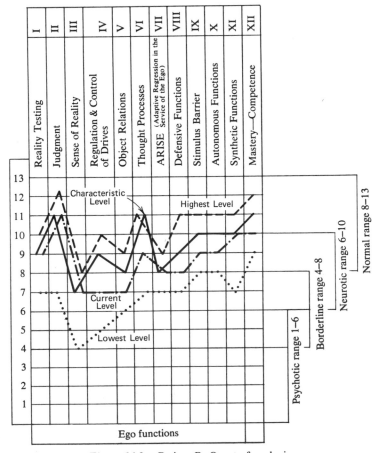

Figure 16.2.   Patient B. Onset of analysis.

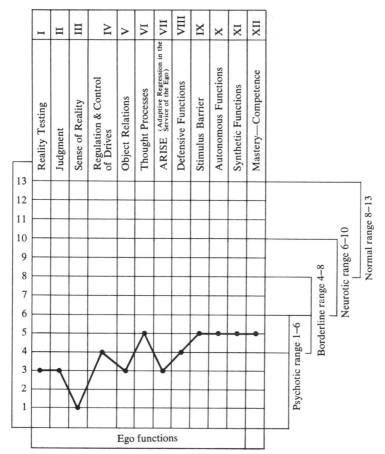

Figure 16.3.   Patient A. Rating during a suicide crisis.

ego functions under the combined pressures of internal conflict and external stress can be seen in Figure 16.3.

Having the scheme of ego functions clearly in mind was helpful to the supervised therapist in assessing his countertransference responses during such stormy periods in the course of treatment. In this instance the trainee was able to correlate the precise changes in the patient's manifest anxiety and altered ego functions with his own perceived anxiety, altered perceptiveness, and therapeutic effectiveness, a process that was quite valuable in the supervision. The systematic use of EFAs in the training of analysts and other therapists has yet to be explored.

Figure 16.4 illustrates an increase in the ego functioning capacity of patient B during an episode of especially strong positive transference. This event occurred 6 months after the analysis had begun. The patient had received a substantial raise in salary and for the first time in his life felt

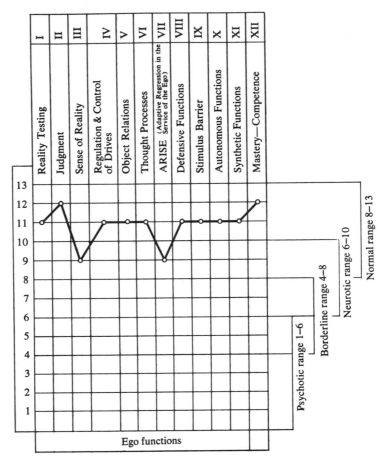

Figure 16.4. Patient B. Rating during a positive transference episode.

financially secure. However, he was experiencing great pressure to terminate the analysis. He was profoundly doubtful about his work and about his relationships with women and with his male superiors; he wished to withdraw from them all because he felt dangerously overinvolved. Underlying these currents of feeling was an increased sense of comfort and closeness with the therapist, which was being vigorously denied. In spite of his previous accomplishments in the analytic work and his improved financial status, he professed an inability to pay for further treatment, claiming it was an unbearable financial burden. In addition, he felt frustrated in the analysis and was deeply resistant to free associating.

Nevertheless, as work continued over several sessions, he began to perceive his pervasive distancing in all previous relationships, his fears of emotional closeness and terror of abandonment, and finally his sense of never having experienced secure parenting, only a succession of "guardians," from which he felt no direction or depth of commitment. During a particular hour the following dialogue occurred:

Patient: While my grandparents were bringing me up, I ran away from their apartment several times. I didn't really want to leave; just wanted to get my way, which I always did. They couldn't handle me. I always did what I wanted to do. They were older and I could always persuade or manipulate them. (pause) . . . And yet I guess I really wanted them not to give in so easily. I needed some kind of direction, a commitment from them, like a stamp of approval.

Therapist: Do you want me to tell you not to stop the analysis?

Patient: Yes, I think I do. Yes, I'm sure of it.

Therapist: If I'm really interested in you and care about your well-being, I won't let you run away?

Patient: Yes, that's it. I'd already decided to continue therapy, but I wanted you to affirm my decision, give it a stamp of approval.

Therapist: You wanted me to be a stronger parent and give you directions . . . not let you do self-defeating things.

Patient: Yes, I wanted you to sense that, without my having to tell you. I couldn't say it outright, but I guess I was testing for some kind of commitment from you. I've been constantly looking for okays all my life.

Therapist: At the same time that you're terrified of getting attached to somebody.

Patient: Yes, I've had just as much trouble with that in here with you as I have with people outside.

Therapist: In quitting the analysis you'd be reliving the same scenario as when you were a little kid . . . by running away.

Patient: Sure.

Therapist: Well, I don't think you should stop now and I strongly recommend that you don't. As you've already said there still remains a lot to do in our work here.

In the next hours he began to say that he had hit on something vitally important to him. He had begun to feel quite good and self-confident. He had started to feel a new level of being close to people. At the same time he felt himself losing the need to be superficially close to too many people at once. He was feeling more in charge of his life at work, at home, and in his other relationships. In relations with his superiors he felt his frustration and anger subsiding and the pressure to withdraw from them diminishing. He experienced an increase of concern and caring for his wife and a renewed closeness to his children. In another area he reported that for the first time he was not embarrassed by the emotionality of the Italian singing waiters at a nightclub where he had taken a client.

Although many ambivalent feelings regarding the continuing love affair with his secretary remained, he experienced a reduced sense of urgency to either fire her or obtain a divorce from his wife—a prominent feature in his original complaints. Finally, there occurred a renewed commitment to the analysis and a marked reduction in his resistance to free association. These changes are charted in Figure 16.4.

At the outset of analysis (Figure 16.1), patient B was highly dependent on praise and complements from clients, employees, and the community. He worked in many ways to obtain this feedback and was quite successful at it. Yet he often felt out of place, undeserving, and "phony." He was overly sensitive to criticism from superiors and often felt demeaned by them. During the episode of positive transference, patient B was rated at stop 9: "More . . . stable identity, self-image, and self-esteem noted here. There are signs of an independent sense of self with a moderately good sense of inner identity continuity, and internalized self-representation."

By contrast there was patient A, who had ingested 200 milligrams of secobarbital during her suicidal crisis on the anniversary of her mother's death. Her father and stepmother were out of town, and she was alone in her apartment. She felt strangely empty inside herself and began to experience a global floating feeling of being inside her mother's body. At the same time, important living people seemed very distant, like small statues or dwarfs. Previously, she had gone to her old home searching for a picture of her mother, but had been unable to find one because her stepmother had disposed of them all. She felt everything had been changed in a bizarre way. She returned to her apartment feeling totally alone and enraged at her father and stepmother. As the medication took effect she had a dreamy fantasy that by taking the whole bottle of secobarbital capsules she could blend and merge with her mother, each being inside the other's body. She thought of a male friend who had committed suicide with sleeping pills and envied the clever way he had done it. She repeatedly looked in her mirror and saw her mother's face.

She wanted to die, yet restrained herself by thinking how embarrassed she would be if she failed to kill herself. All of this was related in the next hour in a calm and accepting manner.

This transient episode was rated at stop 1 under Sense of Reality of the Self and the World:

> Surrounding people and things feel unreal, changed in appearance, as though they weren't there. . . . Very slight environmental changes may produce strange sensations. There may be oceanic feelings of nothingness, feeling dead, inanimate, selfless. Parts of the body feel unreal. . . . Feeling literally or physically empty inside. . . . May experience states of extreme fusion or

merging with others, suggesting near-total loss of boundaries between the self and the outside world. At this stop, body boundaries may be extremely fluid and vulnerable.

The patient's report of seeing her mother's face in her mirror had a nightmare-like quality about it, yet the experience was quite ego-syntonic.

DISCUSSION

The evaluation of the psychoanalytic process would greatly benefit from the use of EFAs. In practice, a patient in treatment with one analyst could be interviewed at any time by another analyst and both analysts could make their independent ego function ratings. If there were two peers evaluating a third one's patient, they could "conference" their findings and report agreed-on ratings as a basis for comparison with those of the treating analyst. Conferencing of findings is an accepted method among researchers. Utilizing this method of objective evaluation would further protect the treating analyst from arbitrary or poor rating.

In turn, it would be quite feasible, after independent ratings, for the treating analyst and the evaluating analysts to conference their separate assessments. This procedure would bring to the analytic situation the often-missed richness of shared observations that play so constructive a role in other forms of medical practice and progress.

In addition, the EFA approach to clinical assessment would make it possible to report behavioral operational concepts to interested nonanalytic audiences, such as general psychiatrists, county medical societies, insurance companies, and so on. Reporting findings to such nonanalytic third parties would have the advantage of protecting the privacy of the patient: quantitative statements about a patient's ego functions do not have the emotional charge of intimate life history data. Furthermore, concepts such as reality testing, judgment, and impulse control, as well as the majority of the other functions, are more readily intelligible to nonpsychoanalysts than other subtleties of psychoanalytic conceptualization.

Another advantage consists of the global inclusiveness of EFAs as opposed to the exclusiveness of diagnostic labels, which could be avoided entirely.

The recent establishment of the Research Foundation of the American Psychoanalytic Association strongly relates to the thrust of new interest in clinical analytic research, an area in which EFA holds great promise. Although these assessment procedures might create temporary distracting effects in the treatment, these are likely to be outweighed by the benefits of periodic consultation and the sharing of observations.

There are additional unique problems inherent in assessing the analytic process. Informed allowances must be made for the downward fluctation in ego functions as normal variables in treatment (see preceding patient A). Indeed, the proper assessment of the normal regression (e.g., of autonomous and synthetic ego functions in the course of any successful analysis) poses particular problems in the assessment of all clinical data.

SUMMARY

The current climate of social and medical change has brought about the need for clinical validity, accuracy, and speed in the assessment of psychoanalytic treatment and patient response. Peer review, insurance and other third-party inquiries, analytic education and research, all require objective evaluation of the analytic process.

Ego function assessment is presented as a reliable and easily applied quantitative method of psychoanalytic evaluation. EFA procedures are directly derived from psychoanalytic theory and clinically grounded in psychoanalytic practice. These procedures are described and their uses with patients in analysis are detailed. Two case histories are presented and examples are given of specific changes in ego functions during clinical crises in the treatment.

EFA is a dynamically sophisticated, easily applied approach to psychoanalytic assessment. Its applicability to a variety of current analytic problem areas is discussed.

REFERENCES

Bellak, L., Gediman, H., & Hurvich, M. Ego function assessment of analytic psychotherapy combined with drug therapy. *Journal of Nervous and Mental Disease*, 1973, *157*, 465–469.

Bellak, L., Hurvich, M., & Gediman, H. *Ego functions in schizophrenics, neurotics, and normals: A systematic study of conceptual, diagnostic, and therapeutic aspects.* New York: Wiley, 1973.

Bellak, L., & Meyers, B. Ego function assessment and analysability. *International Review of Psychiatry*, 1975, *2*, 413–427, and this volume.

Bellak, L., and Sheehy, M. The broad role of ego functions assessment. *American Journal of Psychiatry*, 1976, *133*, 1259–1264.

Ciompi, L., Ague, C., & Dauwalder, J. L'objectivation de changements psychodynamiques: Expériences avec une version simplifée des "Ego Strength Rating Scales" de Bellak et al. Paper read at the Tenth International Congress of Psychotherapy, Paris, October 7, 1976.

Endicott, J., Spitzer, R. L., and Cohen, J. The global assessment scale: A procedure for measuring overall severity of psychiatric disturbance. *Archives of General Psychiatry*, 1976, *33*, 766–771.

Greenspan, S., & Cullander, C. A systematic metapsychological assessment of the personality—its application to the problem of analyzability. *Journal of the American Psychoanalytic Association*, 1973, *21*, 303–327.

Greenspan, S., & Cullander, C. A systematic metapsychological assessment of the course of an analysis. *Journal of the American Psychoanalytic Association,* 1975, *23,* 107–138.

Jaques, E. Death and the mid-life crisis. *International Journal of Psychiatry,* 1965, *46,* 502–514.

Milkman, H., & Frosch, W. A. The drug of choice. *Journal of Psychedelic Drugs,* 1977, *9,* 11–24, and this volume.

Strauss, J. Review of ego functions in schizophrenics, neurotics, and normals. *Journal of Nervous and Mental Disease,* 1975, *159,* 216–218.

CHAPTER SEVENTEEN

Assessment of Object Relations in Selection for Brief Dynamic Psychotherapy: A Validation Study

MARGARET S. WOOL

Short-term anxiety provoking psychotherapy (STAPP) is a specific method of brief dynamic psychotherapy developed by Dr. Peter E. Sifneos (1979). Although it employs principles of psychoanalytic theory, it involves increased activity on the part of the therapist as compared with the traditional psychoanalytic stance. In this modality, anxiety is generated with the goal of rapid resolution of clearly circumscribed emotional conflict.

STAPP is one of a number of forms of brief psychotherapy, some of which share little more in common than time limitation. These therapies range from supportive to dynamic, with STAPP and the work of some others, including David Malan and Habib Davanloo, at the dynamic end of the spectrum.

Historically, there has been controversy regarding the application and claims of short-term psychotherapy. The arguments can be grouped into "conservative" and "radical" camps, in which beliefs about parameters of the treatable population as well as views of anticipated outcome span a wide spectrum. According to the conservative view, patients with mild emotional disturbance could be offered symptomatic relief but not conflict resolution. The radical view suggests that a wider population can be treated with a dynamic approach in a brief course of treatment and achieve lasting change. David Malan (1976) conducted empirical studies of treatment outcome. While he found that milder illnesses were treated successfully, he also observed that chronic dysfunctional patterns could be altered and improved as well.

One theme that cuts through the opposing views of brief therapy is the issue of selection. This study explored how certain criteria are measured by the selection instrument for STAPP. STAPP was chosen in particular because of the availability of a selection questionnaire that can be used as an instrument for comparison. This selection questionnaire, Criteria for Selection of Patients, was developed by Dr. Sifneos (1979) as part of the research he is conducting to document the effectiveness of STAPP both at the point of outcome and in later follow up. The selection criterion receiving the most attention was the capacity for object relations. This was based, in part, on its recognized significance in the selection of suitable patients for brief dynamic psychotherapy. The role of object relations has been dealt with in terms of clinical judgment but not empirically (Malan, 1976).

The hypothesis of the present study was that a significant positive relationship exists between mutuality in object relations as measured by the Bellak Ego Function Assessment Scale (Bellak, Hurvich, and Gediman, 1973) and suitability for STAPP as assessed by the Sifneos selection instrument. Specifically, the aim of the project was to examine the part that an individual's capacity for object relations, as measured by Sifneos's scale, plays in determining whether a patient is recommended for STAPP. This focus involved looking at criteria for selection outlined by Sifneos, which include focality—defined as a circumscribed issue for the therapy, motivation, capacity for object relations, and psychological-mindedness; and assessing their relative importance in the selection process.

In practice, STAPP involves an effort early in the treatment to develop a positive transference and therapeutic alliance to facilitate the working relationship.

> Time is the essence in STAPP. The therapeutic work must be done quickly before the transference neurosis makes its appearance. The best way to avoid such an occurrence is to use the patient's transference feelings early. This helps to make the crucial parent–therapist links which create what Alexander and French (1946) call a "corrective emotional experience" and facilitate the resolution of the patient's psychological problem. [Sifneos, 1979]

In light of these considerations, the patient's capacity for mutual object relationships is quite a significant factor in his or her suitability for therapy.

For Malan (1963), a history of "real and good relationships" is necessary, and the "willingness to become involved and bear the tension that ensues" is essential. The ability to achieve the necessary transference relationship and working alliance as well as to make use of interpretations would be facilitated or impeded, depending on the patient's capacity to relate in a mutual, give-and-take fashion.

Assessment of the capacity for mutuality in object relationships is clearly a critical factor in the selection of good STAPP candidates. Clarifying the selection process for short-term dynamic psychotherapy involves: (1) clarifying the parameters of the population most suited for STAPP, (2) refining evaluative techniques for reaching treatment decisions, and (3) matching patients to the most appropriate treatment modalities.

General criteria to be met by candidates for short-term dynamic psychotherapy are fairly consistent in the literature. The criteria for selection of STAPP candidates, listed in Sifneos's most recent book, include:

1. The ability of the patient to have a circumscribed chief complaint.
2. Evidence of a give and take, or "meaningful relationship" with another person during early childhood.
3. Capacity to relate flexibly to the evaluator during the interview and to experience and express feelings freely.
4. Above-average intelligence and psychological application.
5. Motivation for change and not for symptom relief. [1979, p. 24]

Davanloo supports the "radical" view, namely, "that it is possible to achieve not only symptomatic change but even characterological change by less intensive, short-term techniques, at least with selected patients" (1978, p. 2). In matching a patient to the therapy of choice, Davanloo cites diagnosis as significant but not a sufficient criterion. "Dynamic structural understanding" is the necessary additional component. He seeks to determine the degree of regression in the patient's presenting symptomatology, the patient's ability to relate to and interact with the interviewer, the ability to tolerate anxiety, in addition to factors relating to motivation, response to interpretation, and the flexible use of defenses.

In assessing the capacity for object relations, Davanloo depends primarily on the patient's ability for involved interaction with the therapist. He found that the capacity to relate during the interview correlated with positive outcome, while the patient's report of relationships in his or her life proved to be a less reliable indicator.

Small (1971) selects patients for brief therapy when the presented material is understandable and the therapist can negotiate a treatment plan with the patient. High motivation and the ability to tolerate involvement, and the tension it brings, are positive prognostic indicators for brief therapy. Small looks for the ability to use interpretative interventions in his patients and an early development of transference that is not overly dependent.

Research in the area of selection for short-term dynamic psychotherapy is not abundant. Most empirical work has focused on outcome, seeking correlative relationships between selection, therapeutic techniques, and the success or failure of treatment. In these studies, as cited earlier, the selection process is based on clinical judgment and has not been validated against other more standard or objective measures. In this respect there may be variation in selection decisions based on differing clinical assessments of the fulfillment of various criteria.

Bellak and Small (1965) organized follow-up studies of brief therapy that were carried out by social workers. The findings revealed lasting results for various disturbances, including some severe emotional problems. Bellak and Small suggested that longer therapy be recommended for character-disordered patients; the motivation in these patients is likely to be insufficient for brief therapy because of the "subtle" nature of the patients' discomfort.

Malan (1976) has conducted outcome studies that have attended to selection criteria. These were reported in 1963 as "a study of brief psychotherapy." He used the following criteria for selection: "Static" criteria include (1) mild pathology, (2) recent onset, (3) propitious moment, (4) good outside relationships, (5) absence of deprivation, and (6) heterosexual experience. "Dynamic" criteria include (1) motivation for insight, (2) cooperation, (3) contact, (4) response to interpretation, and (5) ability to focus.

Malan found that one factor that correlated highly with positive outcome in brief dynamic psychotherapy was motivation for insight. Neither the degree of psychopathology nor length of illness showed any significant correlation with failure of treatment, and it appeared that motivation could supercede the effects of these factors. Recent onset, assumed to be a favorable factor, showed a small inverse correlation with successful treatment.

It could be asserted that motivation for insight requires the patient's recognition that his or her symptoms or problems are psychological in nature along with a willingness to take some responsibility in the therapeutic process. This attitude implies emotional maturity in that the patient has chosen to develop a mutual interaction and not exclusively a passive-dependent one. One would suspect that an individual manifesting high motivation for insight might also manifest certain qualities, as, for example, those measured by Bellak's scale that are indicative of mature object relations.

These findings might have significant implications regarding the boundaries of the treatable population. The work reviewed suggests that short-term dynamic psychotherapy can be an effective treatment for individuals with severe psychopathology providing they fulfill specific criteria, and particularly so in the area of object relations. It is further suggested that patients capable of benefiting from a brief course of dynamic therapy may comprise a larger group than previously thought.

METHOD

In the interests of developing an increased standardization of the selection process for brief psychotherapy, the study examined, through a comparison of Sifneos's selection questionnaire for STAPP (see Appendix 1) and Bellak et al.'s 1973 object relations scale, how the assessment of object relations was associated with the recommendations for STAPP. The research model was directed toward a validation of Sifneos's selection instrument, particularly in regard to those items designed to assess the capacity for object relations. In general, this study hoped to clarify the degree to which the evaluator's assessment of the patient's capacity to form meaningful relationships agreed with the patient's score on the Bellak Object Relations scale. It was also expected that by looking at item scores on the Sifneos scale in relation to the overall rating for STAPP, one would assess the degree of importance the evaluator placed on capacity for object relations in making decisions about the suitability for STAPP.

The instrument to be validated, the Criteria for Selection of Patients designed by Sifneos, is a questionnaire filled out by the clinical evaluator at the conclusion of every psychotherapy patient's evaluation. The evaluators rank their impression of the patient's candidacy for STAPP. A ranking of 70–100% would constitute an indication for referral to Dr. Sifneos or a colleague for further evaluation. Ten evaluators referred patients to the study and submitted questionnaires.

The Criteria for Selection of Patients questionnaire contains items designed to assess each of the criteria considered significant and/or essential to candidacy for STAPP. It constitutes a standardized summary of the evaluator's subjective clinical assessment. The items included are:

1. A circumscribed chief complaint
2. At least one meaningful relationship
3. Ability to interact flexibly with interviewer
4. Psychological-mindedness
5. Motivation—assessed by seven different measures
6. An oedipal problem or other focus (e.g., loss)

It is noteworthy that item 6, "an oedipal problem or other focus," is included to ascertain homogeneity in the STAPP population when outcome research is being conducted, and that it is not itself a criterion of selection for the therapy: Individuals who are "preoedipal" may be STAPP candidates on the basis of meeting other criteria. This is a point that has been misunderstood by some clinicians.

According to Sifneos,* the following configuration on the questionnaire

* Personal communication.

indicates a rating of 80–100% for the patient's candidacy for STAPP: affirmative assessments for focality (item 1 above), capacity for good object relations (items 2 and 3), and at least six of the seven measures of motivation (item 5). As was previously suggested, the capacity for object relations was selected as the focus for validation because it was cited by many practitioners of short-term dynamic psychotherapy as an essential factor in assessing suitability for this therapeutic modality. Use of positive transference, the primary therapeutic tool, would by definition develop within the context of an interpersonal relationship, and, therefore, give additional support to the relevance of object relations as a focus for study.

The Bellak scale was chosen to serve as the "standard measure" of capacity for object relations largely because it has been validated against other more objective measures (Bellak et al., 1973). In the present study the Object Relations scale was compared with the following psychological tests in the interests of assessing validity: Tomkins Faces-Recognition and Response to Affect, Embedded Faces, Cattell Friends and Acquaintances Test. In Bellak et al.'s work the interrater reliability factor for the Object Relations scale, with 100 subjects and two judges, was .83 (product-moment correlation coefficient) with a mean correlation of .77.

The Object Relations scale is a structured interview comprising 22 open-ended questions. The questions address present and past significant relationships in the subject's life, as well as the subject's experience of being alone and general preferences for interpersonal distance. Sensitivity, the experience of rejection, and the wish or expectation that other people should change for the benefit of the subject are also tapped.

Data from the interview are organized and scored according to four "stops" or dimensions. The dimensions are (1) Symbiosis to Separation–Individuation; (2) Primary Narcissism to Need Gratification to Object Constancy; (3) Stability, Quality, and Differentiation of Self-representations from Object Representations; and (4) Degree of Separation or Fusion of Good and Bad Object Representations. These dimensions are viewed as continua and are divided into seven intervals each, from low to high object relations.

POPULATION

The study was conducted at the outpatient psychiatry clinic of Beth Israel Hospital in Boston. The research sample of 14 subjects was 66% female, with ages ranging from 18 to 58 years. All subjects were Caucasian, except one, who was of Asian descent. Hollingshead and Redlich socioeconomic categories I through IV were represented, with 50% in category II and 32% in category III.

FINDINGS

The following is a brief description of the pairs of variables that were submitted to statistical analysis:

1. Selection for STAPP by scores on Bellak's Object Relations instrument. STAPP selection was defined as a rating of 70–100% on the Sifneos instrument. All others were "not recommended." The distribution of scores on the Bellak scale was bimodal with peak frequencies at scores of 3 and 4.5. Scores of 3.5 and below were rated "immature" and 3.6 and above were "mature."

2. Selection for STAPP by object relations items from the STAPP selection instrument. In the STAPP selection instrument, items 2 and 3 refer to capacity for object relations.

3. Bellak object relations score by object relations from the STAPP selection instrument.

4. Selection for STAPP by presence of an oedipal-level problem. The question involving an oedipal problem is item 6 on the selection instrument for STAPP.

5. Bellak object relations score by presence of an oedipal level problem.

The Fisher's Exact Test was performed on the paired variables.

Regarding the major question, that is, whether the capacity for object relations is significantly related to the selection for STAPP, the hypothesis was supported with marginal significance ($p < .07$), indicating that the capacity to relate was associated in the expected direction with the assessment of a patient's capacity to use brief dynamic psychotherapy. Yet the object relations items in the Sifneos Criteria for Selection of Patients questionnaire did not show a significant role in the selection for STAPP ($p < 0.4$).

These findings on these two comparisons raise the question as to whether Sifneos and Bellak approach the measurement of object relations in the same way.

A Fisher's Exact Test comparison of the two measures of object relations yielded a nonsignificant finding ($p < .7$), suggesting that Sifneos and Bellak are tapping independent qualities with their respective instruments. The findings do indicate that Bellak's measurement of object relations has a stronger relationship to selection for STAPP than does the Sifneos questionnaire items designed to assess the same quality.

The variable correlating most strongly with selection for STAPP was the presence of an oedipal problem ($p < .005$). This is interesting in light of the fact that the presence of an oedipal problem is not a selection criterion per se, but is included in Sifneos's selection questionnaire to aid empirical studies of outcome by clarifying homogeneity in the population for that research.

Presence of an oedipal problem was significantly correlated with scores on the Bellak scale as well ($p < .01$), indicating a strong positive relationship between the ability to relate in a mutual, reciprocal fashion and the attainment of an oedipal level of development.

DISCUSSION

The results of the study supported the hypothesis that a positive relationship exists between mutuality in object relations as measured by the Bellak (1973) scale and suitability for STAPP as assessed by the overall rating score on Sifneos's selection instrument. However, the two particular items in the STAPP instrument that are designed to assess object relations, that is, quality of relationships and interaction with the interviewer, were independent of the Bellak Object Relations scale and the overall selection rating for STAPP. Thus, it appears that although the ability to form a give-and-take relationship was found to be relevant to patients' suitability for STAPP, this capacity was not being assessed by items 2 and 3 in the STAPP instrument.

Considering its positive association with selection for STAPP, the Bellak instrument may be used to give the object relations items a more salient role in the selection process. A more detailed analysis of the relationship between rating for STAPP and particular items on the Bellak scale would probably be necessary to accomplish this task. As it stands now, the two object relations items in the STAPP instrument are not being adequately used in the selection process. This finding merits further empirical exploration. Replication on a larger sample could indeed suggest an indication for possible modifications in certain items of the STAPP instrument. It is possible that evaluators are including an assessment of object relations in their overall clinical impression, but evaluation of this criterion is not apparent from the selection questionnaires.

In terms of the relative importance of the items on the Criteria for Selection of Patients questionnaire, presence of an oedipal problem bore a highly significant relationship to selection for STAPP, exceeding the role of the other criteria. Scores on the Bellak scales were highly related to the question of an oedipal problem as well, underlining the association between developmental level and capacity for relationships.

It is possible that the item regarding oedipal development may have been given too great a weight by the evaluators in making their recommendations and particularly so relative to other criteria. There is some indication, for example, that patients suitable for STAPP on the basis of their motivation, capacity to form relationships, and ability to choose a focus, are not referred when the evaluator notes the absence of an oedipal-level problem. This suggests that the number of patients suitable for STAPP may exceed the number actually referred for further evaluation. Clearly, the evaluators valued the oedipal problem item over others. One way to explore this might be to offer STAPP treatment to an experimental group that meets basic theoretical criteria but does not evidence a clear-cut oedipal problem.

In summary, it is apparent from the study that there was a discrepancy between generally accepted criteria for selection for brief dynamic psychotherapy and the practical application of these criteria in the selection process. The method employed in the study revealed the discriminatory power of the individual criteria and offers some clarification of the degree to which theory can be integrated with practice. The validity of the measurement of object relations on the basis of the STAPP questionnaire was brought into question, in contradistinction to the Bellak scale.

The significant findings observed do point to areas for further empirical work. Increasing the validity of object relations items on the STAPP selection instrument and gaining further clarity as to the effectiveness of particular criteria in selecting suitable STAPP candidates are valuable areas for further exploration. The goal of continued work would be not merely to refine and modify selection techniques, but also to clarify the parameters of the group most suited for STAPP—a group that may be larger than currently recognized.

APPENDIX: CRITERIA FOR SELECTION OF PATIENTS

Beth Israel Hospital   *Psychiatric Clinic*
Harvard Medical School

Patient's Name _____ Evaluation Number _____

Address _____

Interviewer _____ Date _____

Type of Interview: __ Evaluative   __ Administrative   __ Research

Please check *Yes* or *No* on each question. Do not check both or put question mark in the middle.

	Part A	Yes	No
1.	Can the patient circumscribe his/her chief complaint or assign top priority to one out of several difficulties? (The above question should be answered after the evaluator has helped the patient define his/her chief complaint.)	—	—
	a. Is the chief complaint a symptom?	—	—
	If so, please underline: anxiety, depression, obsession, compulsion, conversion, phobia, other _____		
	b. Is the chief complaint a problem in interpersonal relations?	—	—
	If so, with whom? Please specify _____		
2.	As a result of systematic history taking can you identify at least *one meaningful relationship* in the patient's childhood? (This implies an ability on the part of the patient to make a sacrifice for another person, or to give up a part of his/her pleasure for a loved one. Meaningful means "give and take altruistic" relationship.)	—	—

Yes   No

3. Can the patient interact flexibly with the evaluator by expressing feelings appropriately during the interview?   ____ ____

4. Is the patient psychologically minded?
   (This question attempts to assess the patient's psychological sophistication as well as a general level of above average intelligence. In answering this question please keep in mind both of the above factors. Excellence in work or educational performance should be helpful factors in answering this question.)   ____ ____

5. Does the patient show adequate motivation for *change*? (This does not imply a motivation for symptom relief or for psychotherapy. The patient must be tired of his/her problems, and be willing to make an effort to alter his/her neurotic behavior.)   ____ ____
   a. Can the patient recognize that the symptoms are psychological in origin?   ____ ____
   b. Is the patient honest in reporting about himself?   ____ ____
   c. Is the patient willing to participate actively in the evaluation?   ____ ____
   d. Is the patient introspective and actively curious about himself?   ____ ____
   e. Does the patient really desire to change and not simply to have the symptoms removed?   ____ ____
   f. Are the expectations of the results of the treatment *realistic* (i.e., not grandiose, magical, etc.)?   ____ ____
   g. Is the patient willing to make a reasonable and tangible sacrifice? (Example: See the therapist at a mutually convenient time, pay a reasonable fee, etc.)   ____ ____

Part B

6. Is there an *oedipal problem* (triangular, genital, heterosexual) which has been clearly established during the evaluation, can explain primarily the patient's psychodynamics, can become the focus for the psychotherapy, and if resolved eliminate the patient's difficulties?   ____ ____

7. If your answer to question 6 is No, please specify if in your opinion there is another focus on which the psychotherapy could concentrate, such as, for example, a loss of a loved one or another.

_____

_____
_____

Part C

8. Please predict all specific changes that will constitute a successful therapeutic outcome for this individual patient. (For example: absence of phobia, depression, etc., improved relations with wife, no need to depend on father or mother to support patient, improved relations with boss, boyfriend daughter, etc.,

better work or educational performance, better relations with men or women.) *Please specify several criteria.* _____

_____

_____

9. Please indicate your recommended therapy by underlining one of the following: (1) STAPP, (2) brief psychotherapy (other kinds), (3) long-term dynamic psychotherapy, (4) brief supportive psychotherapy, (5) long-term supportive psychotherapy, (6) supportive psychotherapy with medication, (7) behavior modification, (8) group therapy, (9) hypnotherapy, (10) crisis support, (11) crisis intervention, (12) couples therapy, (13) relaxation techniques, (14) other.

Part D   Yes   No

10. Does the patient:
    a. Show adequate self-esteem?   ____   ____
    b. Have the potential to show adequate self-esteem?   ____   ____
11. a. Have the ability to solve his/her emotional problem?   ____   ____
    b. Have the potential to solve his/her emotional problem?   ____   ____
12. a. Have the ability to understand himself/herself?   ____   ____
    b. Have the potential to understand himself/herself?   ____   ____
13. Is the patient in a state of emotional crisis?   ____   ____
14. Is he/she under the influence of external stress?   ____   ____

Part E

15. Is the patient able to form a therapeutic alliance?   ____   ____
16. Do you like the patient?   ____   ____
17. Will the patient's symptoms improve?   ____   ____
18. Will the patient's interpersonal relations improve?   ____   ____
19. Do you predict that therapy will be successful?   ____   ____
20. Please rank your overall impression of the patient as a candidate for STAPP on a scale from 0 to 100 _____
    (0% = bad   100% = good)

Part F

Diagnosis _____

_____

_____

REFERENCES

Alexander, F. Psychoanalytic contributions to short-term psychotherapy. In Lewis Wolberg (Ed.), *Short-term psychotherapy.* New York: Grune & Stratton, 1965, pp. 84–126.

Avnet, H. How effective is short-term therapy? Appraisals of mental health after short-term ambulatory psychiatric treatment. In Lewis Wolberg (Ed.), *Short-term psychotherapy*. New York: Grune & Stratton, 1965, pp. 7–22.

Balint, M., Ornstein, P. H., & Balint, E. *Focal psychotherapy*. Philadelphia: Lippincott, 1972.

Barten, H. *Brief therapies*. New York: Behavioral Publications, 1971.

Bellak, L., Hurvich, M., & Gediman, H. *Ego functions in schizophrenics, neurotics, and normals: A systematic study of conceptual, diagnostic, and therapeutic aspects*. New York: Wiley, 1973.

Bellak, L., & Small, L. *Emergency psychotherapy and brief psychotherapy*. New York: Grune & Stratton, 1965.

Bellak, L., & Small, L. The choice of intervention. In Harvey Barton (Ed.), *Brief therapies*. New York: Behavioral Publications, 1971, pp. 42–61.

Burke, J. D., Jr., White, H. S., & Havens, L. L. Which short-term therapy? Matching patient and method. *Archives of General Psychiatry*, 1979, *36*, 177–186.

Cummings, N. A. Prolonged (ideal) versus short-term (realistic) psychotherapy. *Professional Psychology*, 1977, *8*, 491–501.

Davanloo, H. *Basic principles and techniques in short-term dynamic psychotherapy*. New York: Spectrum Publications, 1978.

Malan, D. H. *A study of brief psychotherapy*. New York: Plenum, 1963.

Malan, D. H. *The frontier of brief psychotherapy*. New York: Plenum Medical, 1976.

Mann, J. *Time-limited psychotherapy*. Cambridge, Mass.: Harvard University Press, 1973.

Marmor, J. Short term dynamic psychotherapy. *American Journal of Psychiatry*, 1979, *136*, 149–155.

Sifneos, P. E. Psychoanalytically oriented short-term dynamic or anxiety provoking psychotherapy for mild obsessional neurosis. *The Psychoanalytic Quarterly*, 1966, *40*, 271–282.

Sifneos, P. E. Two kinds of psychotherapy of short duration—selection for anxiety provoking and anxiety suppressive. *American Journal of Psychiatry*, 1967, *123*, 1069–1074.

Sifneos, P. E. Learning to solve emotional problems: A controlled study of short-term anxiety-provoking psychotherapy. In Ruth Porter (Ed.), *The role of learning in psychotherapy*. Boston: Little, Brown, 1968, pp. 87–99.

Sifneos, P. E. *Short-term psychotherapy and emotional crisis*. Cambridge, Mass.: Harvard University Press, 1972.

Sifneos, P. E. *Short term dynamic psychotherapy evaluation and technique*. New York: Plenum Medical, 1979.

Small, L. *The briefer psychotherapies*. New York: Bruner-Mazell, 1971.

Wolberg, L. R. The technique of short-term psychotherapy. In Lewis Wolberg (Ed.), *Short-term psychotherapy*. New York: Grune & Stratton, 1965, pp. 128–200.

Wolberg, L. R. *The technique of psychotherapy* (2d ed.). New York: Grune & Stratton, 1967.

CHAPTER EIGHTEEN

An Adaptation of Ego Function Assessment Techniques to the Phenomenology of the "Schizophrenic Experience"

DORIS MATHERNY MODLY

The ideas discussed in this paper were generated during a short-term therapeutic contact of a nurse therapist with a client, John, hospitalized for diagnostic purposes on a psychiatric inpatient unit. The twice-weekly therapy sessions extended over 8 weeks. The goal for the sessions set by the client were to "talk to somebody and prove once and for all that I am not sick so that I should be left alone." This goal was congruent with the therapist's goal, which was to contribute to the diagnostic profile of the client. Techniques of intervention were based on data obtained about the client through the use of Bellak's Ego Function Assessment Guide. Changes were noted on the Ego Function Profile. Continuous adherence to the objective

Adapted with permission of Charles B. Slack, Inc., Medical Publisher, and the Journal of Psychosocial Nursing and Mental Health Services from An Adaptation of Ego Function Assessment Techniques during Transactions with a Schizophrenic Existence, by Doris Matherny Modly, *Journal of Psychosocial Nursing and Mental Health Services*, Mar. 1979, *17*(3), 16–20.

ego function assessment tool did not always seem feasible given the taciturn nature of the client. An experiential assessment based on Mendel's (1974) phenomenological view of schizophrenia complemented the scientific, objective approach. The purpose of this paper is to discuss the rationale and the process of adapting the two rather different theoretical concepts that guided therapeutic interventions of the nurse therapist in the interactions with the person leading a schizophrenic existence.

In the discussion of the phenomenological theory of schizophrenia, Mendel (1974) states that the responses that a human being living a schizophrenic existence evokes in others frequently have little to do with what is going on in him or her or with his or her needs. The response seems to reflect a combination of the needs of the profession to which the intervener belongs and the views held by the intervener of what it is to be human. Critically, Mendel adds that these interventions will thus have little to do with the needs of the one living this schizophrenic existence. The latter statement might be considered to be rather harsh even though the danger of this possibility has been exemplified all too frequently in many of the helping professions when too strict adherence to theories, principles, and intervention strategies prevented innovative and creative approaches. On the other hand, adherence to one or another theoretical framework that can be quantitatively justified can have an advantage in an age of increased emphasis on accountability to the client for the quality of intervention outcomes. For this reason it would seem that the selection of an assessment and treatment modality best suited to the client or the combination of two or more theoretical frameworks that serve as a basis for the intervention would be the mode of choice in therapeutic nursing approaches.

The feasibility of such an approach was tried by the writer in her work with a 25-year-old male client who was hospitalized for the second time within a year because of progressive inactivity and withdrawal from human contacts. He was eventually diagnosed as falling into the diagnostic category of simple schizophrenia even though much of his behavior was characteristic of a borderline schizoaffective disorder.

The theoretical frameworks from which the client was viewed and on which interventions were based were those of both Bellak's concept of the schizophrenic syndrome as a manifestation of quantifiably impaired ego functions and the phenomenological theory of schizophrenia as discussed by Mendel, who views schizophrenia as a way of life. A combination of these two rather different views was found to be complimentary in the process of therapeutic interactions, as will be evident later.

Bellak (1974) formulated the "egopsychological multiple factor psychosomatic theory of schizophrenia," wherein schizophrenia is seen as a syndrome caused by different etiological factors, all of them sharing as the final common manifest paths, severe disorders of ego functions. Ego functions are theoretical constructs based on observations and on patient's reports of their experiences. The ego constructs should be defined in terms of a number of functions that refer to adaptively relevant actions and reactions of the individual person. (Bellak quotes Hegel's concept of *"Umschlag von Quantitäte zu Qualitäte"* to justify his view of quantified ego functions as a measure of qualitative differences in the client's behavior.) Ego function assessment is particularly useful since it allows for a graphic, quantified presentation of ego strengths and weaknesses, or in other words, the adaptive potential of the client.

A systematic ego function assessment of John would have been extremely difficult to carry out immediately after his admission because of the reluctance he displayed in verbalizing his thoughts and feelings and because of his categorical denial of any problems. He had at that point withdrawn from all human contact, except his brother, but was able to care well for his own personal needs. He did not work for monetary gain and lived on money from an endowment fund left for him by his father. He spent most of his time "mediating." On hospital admission it soon became evident that ego function assessment would have to be done on the basis of observable behavior. For this reason the assessment phase was extended over six to eight interviews. During these sessions an attempt was made systematically to evaluate the 12 ego functions delineated by Bellak on the basis of the information gleaned in the context of the therapeutic encounter by the therapist, who indulged John's frequent nonverbal revelations of pain, joy, and indifference, his distancing, and his moving closer through verbal and nonverbal maneuvers.

The evaluation of John's ego functions was based on material gathered during the first six to eight interviews, interviews with the psychiatrist, and notations on his chart. On the basis of these, the following picture emerged: the lowest ratings were in the areas of Object Relations (6), Defensive Functioning (6), and Mastery–Competence (5). The strengths that emerged were: Thought Processes (10), Reality Testing (10), and Autonomous Functioning (9). (See Figure 18.1.)

The graphic picture was congruent with what was expected by those who were in contact with him. He was actively participating only when asked. He never interacted voluntarily with either staff or the patients on the unit yet he never refused to meet with those who saw him for therapeutic reasons. He was rather passive, unable or unwilling to talk about his feelings and masked his aggressive impulses, which surfaced only on occasion during competitive games in which he frequently engaged and which he performed very well. He frustrated his opponents during these games by suddenly pulling back and not performing well any longer. As much as all concerned tried to convince him of the opposite, he staunchly refused to "compromise his integrity" and to do what he did not see as necessary, such as actively to seek employment or to become involved in the mainstream of life. He claimed that only one relationship was important to him, his relationship with his family, his brother and mother. The longer one knew him the more evident it became that there was something amiss, that John was on the edge of an abyss and that the strength of those areas of more intact functioning were holding him back from the fall.

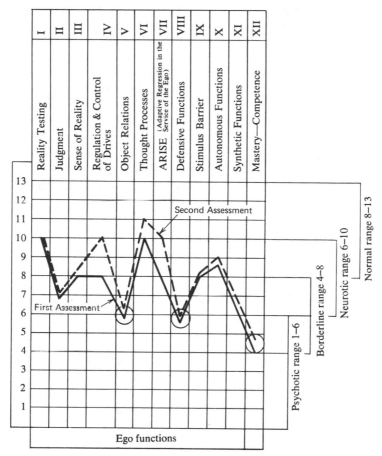

Figure 18.1. Ego Function Profile.

The construction of the ego function graphic was quite helpful for two reasons: the therapist was not as easily caught up in the world of the schizophrenic existence. The ego function assessment was scientifically tested by Bellak and thus considered by the nurse therapist a reliable assessment tool that gave the assessment process objectivity. Second, Bellak's formulations of therapeutic interventions for the strengthening of the weak ego functions guided the working phase of the relationship. Emphasis was placed on the development of a therapeutic relationship with the nurse. Particular attention was given to any potential difficulties that might arise out of the one-to-one relationship—transference, countertransference, resistance, and eventually difficulties around termination.

Group participation was encouraged as optimal distance or closeness could be modulated more easily in the group setting. Areas of mastery and competence, and thus issues of low self-esteem, could also be addressed in the group.

In the context of the individual treatment, John's withdrawal specifically emerged as an attempt to control hostile, aggressive impulses. Exploration of the behavior pattern and semantic and constructive stage interpretations of the dynamics of these behaviors were undertaken once the therapist–client relationship attained the needed stability and ego functions were strengthened. Difficulties in the area of thought processes and sense of reality were addressed through reviews and reconstructions of his present and past life. As more information was gathered, changes from the initial assessment could be noted and recorded, thus giving a clearer picture of the highest, lowest and characteristic levels of functioning (see Figure 18.1).

According to the phenomenological theory of schizophrenia (Mendel, 1974) there are three primary categories of observed existential difficulties of the schizophrenic life-style. These are the failure of "historicity," which is considered the basic difficulty; the failure of anxiety management; and the failure of interpersonal relationships. The failure of historicity underlies all other difficulties, and it leaves the person in a vacuum of the present without recourse to the experiences of the past or the hopes of the future.

The nurse therapist in her interactions with John placed great emphasis on the transactions that occurred between them. During the time that data were gathered for the ego function assessment the nurse therapist attempted to understand and empathize with the patient's experiential world. The patient's difficulty with "historicity" initially impeded the therapist's attempts to involve him in any type of problem defining and problem resolution. The therapist concentrated on establishing historicity through the structure and reliability of the relationship.

The prolonged time needed for ego function assessment resulted in repeated contacts with the patient. The increased opportunities for observation and empathic understanding contributed to the development of a therapeutic relationship between therapist and patient. The combined use of the two orientations—namely, the objective evaluation of ego functions and the experiential assessment of the schizophrenic existence—provided an effective framework for the nurse therapist's interventions in this short-term therapy setting. The blending of the two approaches based on two different conceptualizations about the patient's difficulties also served the function of helping the therapist to remain objective, creative, and innovative during the long hours of working with a client who lives in a schizophrenic life-style.

REFERENCES

Bellak, L., Hurvich, M., & Gediman, H. *Ego functions of schizophrenics, neurotics, and normals.* New York: Wiley, 1973.

Mendel, W. M. A phenomenological theory of schizophrenia. In A. Burton, A. I. Lopez-Ibor, & W. Mendel, *Schizophrenia as a life style.* New York: Springer, 1974.

PART THREE

EFA for Clinical Assessment

CHAPTER NINETEEN

The Drug of Choice

HARVEY MILKMAN AND WILLIAM A. FROSCH

If a man, "whose talk is of oxen," should become an opium eater, the probability is that . . . he will dream about oxen . . . the phantasmagoria of his
dreams . . . is suitable to one of that character . . . (DeQuincy 1907).

Although most drug users have experienced a variety of psychotropic
agents, many experience a prolonged and distinct preference for a particular
drug. Using Bellak and Hurvich's (1969) Interview and Rating Scale for Ego
Functioning, "preferential" users of heroin ($N = 10$) or amphetamines ($N =
10$) were interviewed under conditions of abstinence and intoxication with
their respectively chosen drug. Normals ($N = 10$) were interviewed twice
while abstinent. Data were analyzed, qualitatively and quantitatively to answer: (1) how do preferential users differ from normals and each other under
abstinent conditions, (2) how do they differ under conditions of intoxication,
(3) how does the drug user differ within himself under conditions of abstinence and intoxication?

Kramer's notion of preferential use was applied and supported (Kramer,
Fischman, & Littlefield, 1967). In a sample of more than 30 drug admissions
to Bellevue Psychiatric Hospital, more than 75% stated a specific preference

---

We are grateful to the *Journal of Psychedelic Drugs* for permission to use material for this
chapter. This material was previously published as The Drug of Choice by Harvey Milkman and
William Frosch, *Journal of Psychedelic Drugs*, Jan.–Mar. 1977, 9(1), 11–23.

for either heroin or amphetamine. All subjects had experienced both drugs, but the majority stated a strong preference and prolonged involvement with either heroin or amphetamine. The criteria for drug dependence were intravenous administration and minimal level of use in the past month (amphetamines more than nine times; heroin more than five times). The criteria for "normal" were nonpsychiatric history and screening, complete avoidance of intravenous use of psychotropic drugs, and minimal use of alcohol, marijuana, and so on. All subjects were white, male, middle class, 20–30 years of age, and nonpsychotic. Each heroin user was interviewed while abstinent and under the influence of 15 mg morphine, given intramuscularly, in a clinical setting. Amphetamine users were interviewed while abstinent and intoxicated with 30 mg (oral) dextroamphetamine sulfate, also in a clinical setting. Normals were used as a control and interviewed twice while abstinent. Abstinence was determined by self-report and urine analysis. Interviews were spaced 1–2 weeks apart and taped; the interviewer was blind to subject types and conditions of intoxication. The results pertain to a specific type of drug-using population (white, middle class) but may also be applicable to minority groups.

AN IMPRESSIONISTIC OVERVIEW

Impressionistic scanning of the population suggests distinct relationships between personality style and drug preference. Patterns of differences emerge around the management of self-esteem with visible manifestations in styles of relating to the self, others, and the environment. Although both groups have relatively poor personal relationships and vocational adjustment, the amphetamine user copes with this by a consciously inflated sense of self-worth. He often views himself as endowed with special sensitivity and unusual capacity for personal growth and social contribution. He may call attention to his physical appearance with elaborate costumes, hair styles, and jewelry. Decorations may be exhibitionistic and socially alienated. The swastika and the German cross are not uncommon.

The heroin user is far less conspicuous in appearance. Hair styles are conventional; clothing is shabby; tattoos and needle marks are shielded by long-sleeved shirts. He consciously views himself with contempt; his aspirations are limited to self-maintenance. The heroin user's mood of depression and despair is contrasted with the amphetamine user's denial of depression and compensatory optimism.

The amphetamine user is characterized by active confrontation with his environment. While the heroin user feels overwhelmed by low self-esteem, the amphetamine user utilizes a variety of compensatory maneuvers. He reassures and arms himself against a world perceived as hostile and threatening via physical exhibition of alienated symbols of power and strength. Identification with radical political groups further serves the need for active expression of hostility. Promiscuity and prolonged sexual activity may be the behavioral expression of needs to demonstrate adequacy and potency. High-level artistic and creative aspirations are usually unrealized self-expectations, bordering on delusional grandiosity. Such beliefs often lead to compulsive and unproductive behavior. Active participation in hand crafts, music, drawing, or physical labor is striking in nearly all of the amphetamine users studied. To maintain his tenuous sense of self as a potentially productive individual, the amphetamine user deploys many defenses. Denial, projection, rationalization, and intellectualization are characteristically observed. Equilibrium is maintained at the cost of great expenditures of psychic and physical energy.

In contrast, conscious of his self-contempt and chronically depressed, the heroin user seeks to avoid confrontation with his surroundings. His major preoccupation is survival. Rarely identifying with people or causes, he believes that satisfaction is achieved through self-indulgence. Like the amphetamine user, he perceives the environment as hostile and threatening but maintains equilibrium via withdrawal and passive expression of hostility. His parasitic relationship to the community is rationalized by perceiving himself as a victim. For the heroin user, interpersonal communication is characterized by an initial front of honesty and openness in the service of opportunism. When the façade is relinquished, the user appears introverted, distrustful, and lacking in conviction. In contrast to the amphetamine user, thinking is more concrete and personalized, and defensive structures are more primitive and fragile. Under stress, repression is easily disrupted, permitting the emergence of self-derogation, hostile fantasy, and impulsive acting out.

A QUANTITATIVE ANALYSIS

Each subject participated in two semistructured interviews and was rated in accord with Bellak and Hurvich's Interview and Rating Scale for Ego Functioning (1969). Scoring yields a composite quantitative index of "general adaptive strength," as well as specific scores for degree of impairment in each of 11 specified ego functions: (1) Autonomous Functioning, (2) Synthetic–Integrative Functioning, (3) Sense of Competence, (4) Reality Testing, (5) Judgment, (6) Sense of Reality, (7) Regulation and Control of Drives, Affects, and Impulses, (8) Object Relations, (9) Thought Processes, (10) Defensive Functioning, and (11) Stimulus Barrier. The scale for Adaptive Regression in the Service of the Ego and the scale for Superego were dropped from our study because of insufficient reliability in our population. (Scores for Stimulus Barrier are not indicated in Figures 19.1, 19.2, or 19.3 because rating criteria for this variable provided solely qualitative measures of "high," "medium," or "low.") The scale also provides measures for Sexual and Aggressive Drive strengths. Ratings are calculated on a 13-point

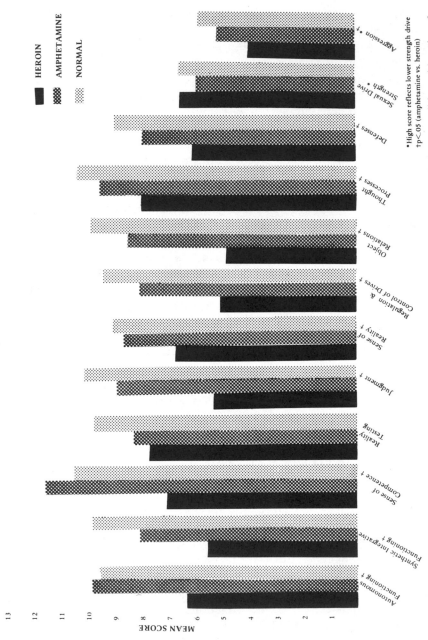

Figure 19.1. Mean ego function ratings for amphetamine S's, heroin S's, and normal in the abstinent condition with ratings for sexual and aggressive drive strengths.

system with each ego function subscale (e.g., Reality Testing) constructed such that a low rating indicates maladaptive functioning and a score of 9 or higher indicates the normal range. Scales for Drive Strengths differ in that a middle score of 7 is considered adaptive while low scores reflect excessive Drive Strength and high scores reflect insufficient Drive Strength.

The test data were submitted to analyses of variances for comparison of heroin and amphetamine users, under abstinent and intoxicated conditions, with a control group of unintoxicated normals. Figure 19.1 compares mean ego function ratings for heroin, amphetamine users, and normals under the abstinent condition and shows subnormal ego function ratings, in both drug-using populations, in most categories. With the exception of Reality Testing, amphetamine users exhibited significantly higher ego strength than heroin users, whether or not they were intoxicated. There were no statistically significant differences between normal and amphetamine users, and Sexual Drive Strength did not show significance under any of the comparisons made. Figures 19.2 and 19.3 compare mean ego function ratings within specific drug groups, under conditions of abstinence and intoxication. In most cases ego functioning was lower in the intoxicated condition with significant differences observed for three variables.

Although, relative to heroin users, ego functioning is more adaptive in amphetamine users when both groups are in the intoxicated condition, one cannot unequivocally extend this finding outside of the laboratory situation. Experimental doses of 30 mg and 15 mg for amphetamine and heroin users, respectively, may not be comparable in effect to average "field" doses of 310 mg and 100 mg. Even at our reduced dose range and relatively small sample size ($N = 10$), the results suggest a trend, in both groups, for ego functioning to be negatively affected by the utilization of their respective drugs. In Figure 19.2, 6 of the 10 means observed for heroin users are lower in the intoxicated condition. Eight of the 10 means observed in Figure 19.3 for amphetamine users are lower in the intoxicated condition. There are four cases in which ego functioning is significantly lower in the intoxicated condition: Regulation and Control of Drive, Affect, and Impulse (for both groups), Judgment (for amphetamine users), Sense of Competence (for heroin users). A nearly significant result is observed for Reality Testing (this function is lower for both groups in the intoxicated condition). It is expected that under conditions of higher dosages and increased sample size, greater impairment of ego functioning may be observed and more significance obtained.

SPECIFIC EGO FUNCTIONS

Autonomous Functioning is assessed according to the degree of impairment of apparatuses of primary autonomy (functional disturbances of sight, hearing, intention, language, memory, learning of motor function) and secondary autonomy (disturbances in habit patterns, learned complex skill,

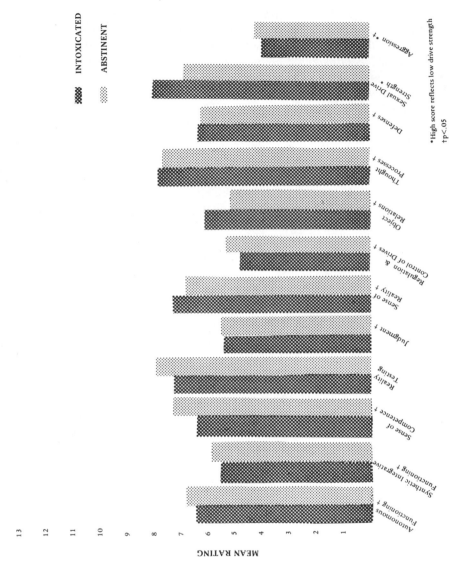

Figure 19.2. Mean ego function ratings for heroin users in abstinent and intoxicated conditions with scores for sexual and aggressive drive strength ($N = 10$).

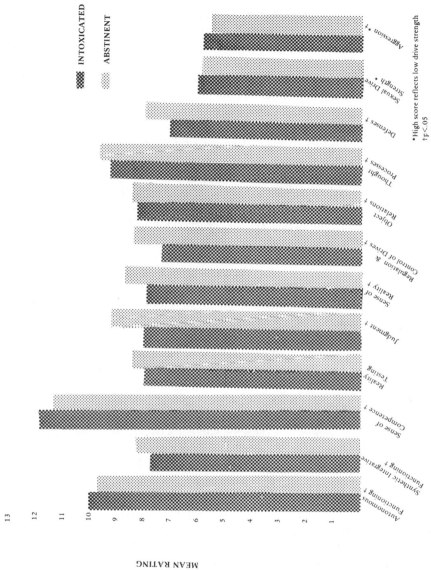

Figure 19.3. Mean ego function ratings for amphetamine users in abstinent and intoxicated conditions with scores for sexual and aggressive drives ($N = 10$).

257

work routines, hobbies and interests). While amphetamine users are relatively unimpaired in this area, heroin users are subject to moderately high interference, by conflict, of their apparatuses of primary and secondary autonomy. Interview material revealed specific problems in concentration, the manifestation of which is relative difficulty in carrying out routine tasks and engaging in skilled behaviors.

Synthetic–Integrative Functioning is rated on the basis of degree of integration of potentially incongruent attitudes, values, affects, behaviors, and self-representations—the ability actively to relate psychic and behavioral events. Although there were no measurable effects of intoxication, amphetamine users were found to be significantly more adept than heroin users independent of intoxication. Figure 19.1 shows respective mean scores of 5.6, 8.1, and 9.8 for heroin, amphetamine users, and normals in the abstinent condition. According to Bellak (Bellak & Hurvich, 1969), Synthetic–Integrative Functioning is the factor that correlates most highly with total ego strength, and the data suggest a continuum from heroin to amphetamine to normal subjects. The heroin user is seen as an individual with no consistent life goals and with serious identity conflicts. There is no adequate organization in daily life, although simple activities may be carried out effectively. Psychological mindedness is virtually absent. For the amphetamine user, identity problems are less severe. Identifications with political or artistic groups remain moderately stable. Purposeful, planned activities can be carried out, but he is usually a step or two behind in meeting the obligations of everyday life and completing what he has agreed to do. There is some psychological-mindedness but active efforts to relate different areas of experience are only moderately successful.

Sense of Competence is based on the subject's overt, conscious statement of his feelings of adequacy. No attempt was made at assessing the underlying dynamics for this statement (e.g., unconscious denial of helplessness). Scores reflect the person's expectation of success or the subjective side of actual performance (how he feels about how he does and what he can do). The data show amphetamine users as having a significantly higher Sense of Competence across both interview conditions. It is noteworthy that although there is no significant drug effect for amphetamine users on this variable, the obtained mean (11.9) is higher in the intoxicated condition (Figure 19.3). While amphetamine appears to bolster feelings of adequacy, heroin seems to have the opposite effect. The amphetamine user denies feelings of helplessness and inadequacy, while the heroin user is prone to accept feelings of hopelessness and despair. These findings are consistent with clinical impressions of the amphetamine user as grandiose with regard to self-expectations, while the heroin user is concerned with survival and self-maintenance.

Reality Testing considers the subject's ability to distinguish inner and outer stimuli; his accuracy of perception, including orientation to time and place; his psychological mindedness or "reflective awareness." The data show no significant differences between heroin and amphetamine users across both interview conditions. There is, however, a nearly significant drug effect within groups (Figures 19.2 and 19.3). This result suggests that heroin and amphetamine users tend to preserve a higher level of Reality Testing in the abstinent condition. Abstinent drug users may be given to occasional perceptual errors and coarse misinterpretations of inner and outer reality but possess a considerable degree of self-recovery, leading to objectivity. Amphetamine users tend to have a predisposition toward projection and rationalization while heroin users utilize more primitive defenses of denial and repression. In both cases, drug intoxication seems to lower the thresholds of Reality Testing and increase the user's potential toward perceptual distortions and relative out-of-touchness. In most subjects, hallucinations and delusions occur only under extreme conditions such as prolonged amphetamine intoxication or the ingestion of psychedelic drugs.

Judgment evaluates the subject's anticipation of the consequences of intended behaviors (legal culpabilities and social censure, disapproval or inappropriateness) and the extent to which manifest behavior reflects the awareness of these consequences. Amphetamine users show significantly more adaptive judgment than heroin users across both interview conditions. Although drug intoxication does not significantly impair the judgment of heroin users in this situation, amphetamine users show a significant decrement in their judgmental capacity while under the influence of amphetamine (Figure 19.3). The heroin user's judgment is so defective that he repeatedly encounters danger in health, work, and interpersonal relationships. Usually he can verbally anticipate the consequences of his actions but manifest behavior rarely reflects this awareness. For the amphetamine user, poor judgment usually occurs in fairly encapsulated or conflict-related areas. In cases of drug involvement, amphetamine users are more prone to utilize their ability to anticipate the consequences of their actions. It is common, for example, for the amphetamine user to take massive doses of vitamins to compensate for the physical deterioration known to accompany amphetamine use.

Sense of Reality rates the extent to which external events are experienced as real and as being embedded in a familiar context; the extent to which the body and its functioning are experienced as familiar and unobtrusive; the degree to which the person has developed individuality and self-esteem. The data show significant differences between heroin and amphetamine users across both interview conditions. The heroin user appears as an individual of quasi-stable sense of identity dependent on outside sources. When external signals and cues are absent, identity can become poorly integrated. Occasional derealization and depersonalization are observed with some unrealistic feelings about the body. In most cases self-esteem is low. The amphetamine user is less dependent on environmental feedback and depersonalization-like phenomena are more likely to occur under unusual conditions: falling asleep, drugs, radical environmental changes. The heroin user's need for external regulation of self-esteem is seen as a potent factor in the relative success of the therapeutic community. Peer pressure is generated to support nonaddictive behavior. For an individual lacking in a sense of independent identity, the group ideal is easily adopted, and until the user returns to his former community, his drug taking and criminal activity may be curtailed.

Regulation and Control of Drive, Affects, and Impulses refers to the directness of impulse expression and the effectiveness of delay and control mechanisms; the degree of frustration tolerance and the extent to which drive derivatives are channeled through ideation, affective expression, and manifest behavior. Amphetamine users score significantly higher than heroin users under intoxicated and abstinent conditions. Both groups display significantly less Regulation and Control of Drive, Affects, and Impulses in the intoxicated condition (Figures 19.2 and 19.3). The significant drug effect for this function is particularly interesting because it suggests that under intoxication both groups might be expected to have less impulse control and present a greater danger to themselves and/or the community. The heroin user appears as an individual given to sporadic rages, tantrums, or binges. Periods of overcontrol may alternate with flurries of impulsive breakthroughs. This may be observed dramatically when the user voluntarily submits himself to extended periods of increased environmental structure, in drug programs, where impulse expression is minimized. Temporarily the user appears to have adequate impulse control. Suddenly and without warning, however, impulses gain the upper hand and the user is seen on a self-destructive binge. Disciplinary action is taken and once again impulses are quieted through self-regulation, authoritative, and peer pressures. The cycle tends to repeat. For the amphetamine user, impulse expression is less direct, pervasive, and frequent. Aggressive behavior is more often verbal than physical and fantasies predominate over unusual behavior. Manifestations of drive-related fantasies are seen in quasi-artistic production, such as "speed freak" drawings where primitive and threatening fantasies are portrayed through massive expenditures of compulsive energy. The amphetamine user may sit for hours drawing frightened faces, decapitated bodies, and so on.

Object Relations takes into account the degree and kind of relatedness to others; the extent to which present relationships are adaptively patterned upon older ones; the extent of object constancy. Amphetamine users are significantly more effective in Object Relations than heroin users, across abstinent and intoxicated conditions. It is interesting to note that for heroin users, the obtained mean for this function is higher in the intoxicated condition (Figure 19.2). Perhaps in this dose range, heroin tends to reduce anxiety and allows for a smoother and more relaxed communication between people. This notion supports Hartmann's observation that "there is an attempt to overcome the lack of affectionate and meaningful Object Relations through pseudo-fusion with other drug takers during their common experience" (Hartmann, 1969). The heroin user is generally detached from people while under stress and strives for nurturant relationships, of a dependent nature, leading to stormy or strained attachments. The amphetamine user, although more successful in Object Relations, tends to become involved in relationships with strong, unresolved Oedipal elements. Castration concerns tend to manifest themselves in unusual and extreme sexual behaviors such as Don Juanism and homosexuality. Underlying concerns about masculinity and adequacy are expressed through compulsive sexual activity and a boasting attitude of sexual prowess and potency. Relationships may, however, endure for long periods of time, although they rarely have the stability and sustaining power of the idealized marital situation.

Thought Processes describes the adequacy of processes that adaptively guide and sustain thought (attention, concentration, anticipation, concept formulation), the relative primary–secondary process influence on thought. Amphetamine users are significantly higher on this variable in both abstinent and intoxicated conditions. The heroin user is viewed as somewhat distractable with intruding thoughts resulting in disruptive communication. There is some vagueness and lack of specificity in memory and, under stress, thinking becomes concrete. Communication is best achieved on a direct, down-to-earth basis with little room for the user to interpret hidden meanings. Evaluative statements are likely to be interpreted as absolutes (i.e., "he thinks I am good" or "he thinks I am bad"). In most cases thinking is logical and well ordered. The amphetamine user is far more abstract in his mode of conceptualizing. Occasionally, thinking is disrupted by tangentially related but irrelevant thoughts. His level of distractability is less severe than the heroin user's and he appears to have the capacity to recover quickly and respond appropriately. Although thinking is for the most part logical and well ordered, it may at times become so abstract that direct communication is difficult.

Defenses measure the extent to which defenses adaptively or maladaptively influence ideation and behavior; the extent to which these defenses have succeeded or failed (degree of emergence of anxiety, depression, or other dysphoric states). Amphetamine users are significantly higher on this variable in both abstinent and intoxicated conditions. Clinically, the heroin user appears to be relatively primitive in his defensive structure, repression and denial being massively deployed and withdrawal a predominant mode. Under stress, repression is easily disrupted and emergence of anxiety and depression are readily observed. Defensive functioning may become minimal, as evidenced by recurrent outbursts of inner- and outer-directed aggression. The amphetamine user is characterized by a variety of defensive maneuvers. He is more successful in preventing the emergence of anxiety and dysphoric affect but is similar in his sacrifice of Reality Testing (Figure 19.1). Denial, projection, rationalization and intellectualization are typically observed.

Stimulus Barrier indicates the subject's threshold for, sensitivity to, or awareness of stimuli impinging upon various sensory modalities; the nature of responses to various levels of sensory stimulation in terms of the extent of disorganization, withdrawal or active coping mechanisms employed to deal with medium or low Stimulus Barriers. Amphetamine users have significantly higher Stimulus Barriers than heroin users in the abstinent condition. Examination of the raw data revealed that six of ten amphetamine users interviewed were rated high on this variable and nine of ten heroin users were rated low. The data tend to support Ellinwood's formulations, explaining a biological predilection for certain drugs (1967). Although it may be argued that long-term involvement with particular drugs may have specific effects on stimulus thresholds, Stimulus Barrier is considered to be the most constitutionally based ego function (Bellak & Hurvich, 1969). The data suggest that amphetamine users, with biologically high thresholds for excitatory stimulation, are seeking homeostasis through self-medication. Amphetamine, a central nervous system stimulant, seems to put the user into closer touch with environmental stimuli that might otherwise be unavailable because of constitutionally based high Stimulus Barriers. Conversely, the heroin user may have a predisposition toward excessive vulnerability to environmental stimuli. He seeks to raise stimulus thresholds, allowing him to function more adaptively in a world of relatively painful and extreme stimulation.

Sexual Drive Strength includes overt sexual behavior (frequency and intensity), associated and substitute sexual behavior, fantasies and other ideation, dreams, symptoms, defenses, and controls. There are no statistically significant differences between heroin and amphetamine users and normals in Sexual Drive Strength in either intoxicated or abstinent conditions. Examination of the mean scores for heroin users (Figure 19.2) indicates a mean rating of 7.8 in the intoxicated condition and 6.6 in the abstinent condition. For this variable, the higher rating reflects a decrease in drive strength. Though not statistically significant, this observation is consistent with subjective reports of decreased sexual drive while under the influence of heroin. It is speculated that the lack of sexual involvement reported by most heroin users is more related to direct drug effects, feelings of inadequacy, and a compensatory style of withdrawal from Object Relations than to a constitutional deficiency in sexual drive strength. Similarly, the reports of excessive promiscuity and compulsive sexual activity given by amphetamine users may be related to a style of active confrontation with underlying fears of helplessness and inadequacy.

Aggressive Drive Strength assesses overt aggressive behavior, associated and substitute aggressive behavior, fantasies and other ideation, dreams, symptoms, defenses, and controls. Heroin users have significantly higher aggressive drive strength than amphetamine users across both interview conditions. There is no apparent difference between normals and amphetamine users on this variable. The heroin user is seen as an individual whose overt acts of aggression are considerably more intense and frequent than average. The presence of physical assaultiveness and multiple suicide gestures is common. Hostile punning and witty repartee are often observed. It is speculated that the relative success of residential treatment programs is

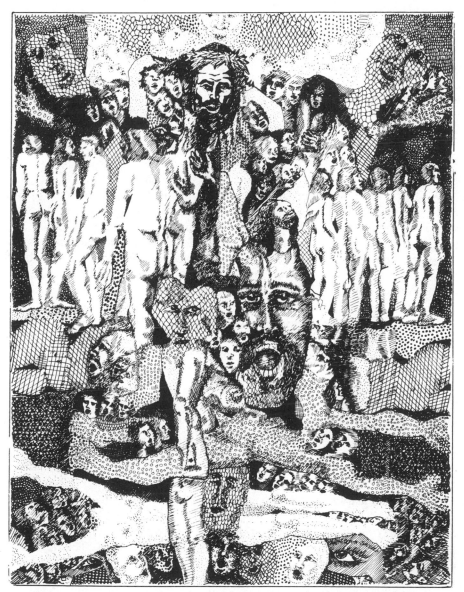

Figure 19.4.   Portrayal of amphetamine user's primitive and threatening fantasies.

related to this phenomenon. Intensive confrontation in group therapy, a major treatment modality in drug programs, provides an outlet for excessive aggressive energy. Violent verbal expressions are often encouraged and readily tolerated, thus reducing the user's tendencies toward repression and withdrawal. This approach seems to be effective in decreasing the heroin user's potential for overt violence of an inner- and outer-directed nature. For the amphetamine user, aggressive energy appears to be less excessive and is channeled more adaptively. Periodic breakthroughs of violence occur, but with the exception of amphetamine psychosis, these expressions are usually not as frequent or intense as the heroin user's. Fantasies of violence are usually expressed verbally and sometimes find their expression through identification with radical political groups. Artistic productions often reflect bizarre and destructive ideation (Figure 19.4).

DISCUSSION

While it is acknowledged that drug preference is regulated, to some presently unknown extent, by social fads and customs, the focus of our discussion is on the role of personality in the determination of drug choice. Although observations were made while male users were under abstinent and somewhat intoxicated conditions, it must be recalled that our subjects had all been heavy drug users for several years. It is, therefore, difficult to know if our findings represent a factor in the etiology of the pattern of drug use or the result of such drug use and its imposed life patterns. However, quantitative analyses and clinical impressions provide a framework for conceptualizing possible psychological differences between preferential users of heroin and amphetamine. Some speculate that these differences are related to early, predrug patterns of childhood experiences.

Having once experienced a particular drug-induced pattern of ego functioning, the user may seek it out again for defensive purposes as a solution to conflict or for primary delight. This seeking out of a special ego state will be related to the individual's previous needs for the resolution of conflict or anxiety. If a particular drug-induced ego state resolves a particular conflict, an individual may seek out that particular drug when in that conflict situation. This will result in preferential choice of drug.

Weider and Kaplan (1969) define the altered ego state induced by opiates, alcohol, barbiturates, and other sedative drugs as "blissful satiation." As Savitt (1963) points out, the elation produced by these drugs has been stressed disproportionately to the sleep or stupor that follows. The transient euphoria preceding the stupor may be related both to the decreased pressure of the drives, sexual and aggressive, and to the sense of gratification of needs. The user "seeks desperately to fall asleep as a surcease from anxiety and the drug provides obliteration of consciousness. Well expressed in the vernacular, the addict 'goes on the nod'."

The heroin user who characteristically maintains a tenuous equilibrium via withdrawal and repression bolsters these defenses by pharmacologically inducing states of decreased motor activity, under responsiveness to external situations, and reduction of perceptual intake. "State of quiet lethargy . . . [is] . . . conducive to hypercathecting fantasies of omnipotence, magical wish fulfillment, and self-sufficiency. A most dramatic effect of drive dampening experienced subjectively as satiation may be observed in the loss of libido and aggression and the appetites they serve'' (Weider & Kaplan, 1969).

Though, as expected, the dramatic effects outlined earlier were not brought on by our low-level, experimental dose, the observed data point in a parallel direction. Elevated scores for Object Relations and Sense of Reality suggest greater relaxation and less pressure from the drives. Though not significantly lower, the mean score for Sexual Drive Strength points to a dampening of sexual appetite. Weider and Kaplan further point out that this style of coping is reminiscent of Narcissistic Regression Phenomena described by Mahler (1967), as an adaptive pattern of the second half of the first year of life. It occurs after the specific tie to the mother has been established and is an attempt to cope with the disorganizing quality of even her brief absences. It is as if the child must shut out affective and perceptual claims from other sources during the mother's absence. This formulation is consistent with earlier remarks by Fenichel (1945). Addicts are "fixated to a passive-narcissistic aim" where objects are need-fulfilling sources of supply. The oral zone and skin are primary and self-esteem is dependent on supplies of food and warmth. The drug represents these supplies. Addicts are intolerant of tension and cannot stand pain or frustration. In one study, the notion of low pain thresholds is supported by the observation that 9 of the 10 heroin users interviewed received a "low" rating for Stimulus Barrier. Drug effects alleviate these difficulties by reproducing the "earliest narcissistic state." The specific need gratification of the passive-narcissistic regression reinforces drug-taking behavior.

The overall decrement in ego functioning and the pressures of physiological dependency set the groundwork for a vicious cycle. The heroin user must increasingly rely on a relatively intact ego to procure drugs and attain satiation. Ultimately, he is driven to withdrawal from heroin by the discrepancy between intrapsychic needs and external demands. Hospitalization, incarceration, or self-imposed abstinence subserve the user's need to resolve his or her growing conflicts with reality.

In contrast to heroin and other sedative drugs, amphetamines have the general effect of increasing functional activity. Extended wakefulness, alleviation of fatigue, insomnia, loquacity, and hypomania are among the symptoms observed. Subjectively there is an increase in awareness of drive feelings and impulse strength as well as heightened feelings of self-assertiveness, self-esteem, and frustration tolerance. Though not statistically significant, our observations support most of these generalizations. Amphetamine intoxication produced in our subjects elevated scores on Autonomous Functioning and Sense of Competence. Interview material suggests a feeling of heightened perceptual and motor abilities accompanied by a stronger sense of potency and self-regard.

As in the case of heroin, the alterations induced by amphetamine intoxication are syntonic with the user's characteristic modes of adaptation. This formulation is in agreement with the observations of Angrist and Gershon (1969) in their study of the effects of large doses (up to 50 mg/hr) of amphetamine. "It appears that in any one individual, the behavioral effects tend to be rather consistent and predictable. . . . Moreover these symptoms tended to be consistent with each person's personality and 'style.' "

The energizing effects of amphetamine serve the user's needs to feel active and potent in the face of an environment perceived as hostile and threatening. Massive expenditures of psychic and physical energy are geared to defend against underlying fears of passivity. Weider and Kaplan (1969) suggest that the earliest precursor to the amphetamine user's mode of adaptation is the "practicing period" described by Mahler (1967). This period "culminates around the middle of the second year in the freely walking toddler seeming to feel at the height of his mood of elation. He appears to be at the peak of his belief in his own magical omnipotence which is still to a considerable extent derived from his sense of sharing in his mother's magic powers." There is an investment of cathexis in the "autonomous apparatuses of the self and the functions of the ego, locomotion, perception, learning."

Our subjects' inflated self-value and emphasis on perceptual acuity and physical activity support the notion that amphetamine use is related to specific premorbid patterns of adaptation. The consistent finding that ego structures are more adaptive in the amphetamine user than they are in the heroin user suggests that regression is to a later phase of psychosexual development.

Reich's (1960) comments on the "etiology of compensatory narcissistic inflation" may provide further insight into the personality structure of amphetamine users. "The need for narcissistic inflation arises from a striving to overcome threats to one's bodily intactness." Under conditions of too frequently repeated early traumatizations, the primitive ego defends itself via magical denial. "It is not so, I am not helpless, bleeding, destroyed. On the contrary, I am bigger and better than anyone else." Psychic interest is focused "on a compensatory narcissistic fantasy whose grandiose character affirms the denial." The high-level artistic and political aspirations witnessed in our subjects appear to be later developmental derivatives of such infantile fantasies of omnipotence. Although the amphetamine user subjectively experiences increments in functional capacity and self-esteem, biological and psychological systems are ultimately drained of their resources. As in the case of heroin, our study points to an overall decrement in ego functioning under the influence of amphetamine. The recurrent disintegration of mental and physical functioning is a dramatic manifestation of the amphetamine syndrome.

Most recent workers (Hekimian & Gershon, 1968) have typically focused on the seemingly indiscriminate use of a variety of psychotropic agents. Multiple drug abuse or "status-medicamentosis" (Wahl, 1967) has been well documented. By viewing the problem from the perspective of the preferred drug used, we have defined differences between users, but also have noted many basic similarities. An underlying sense of low self-esteem is defended against by the introduction of a chemically induced altered state of consciousness. The drug state helps to ward off feelings of helplessness in the face of a threatening environment. Pharmacological effect reinforces characteristic defenses that are massively deployed to reduce anxiety. Drugged consciousness appears to be a regressive state that is reminiscent of, and may recapture, specific phases of early child development.

ACKNOWLEDGMENTS

We thank Ann Drossman for the difficult job of interviewing drug subjects. We thank Judith Lepore-Schreiber for her representative drawing.

REFERENCES

Angrist, B., & Gershon, S. Amphetamine abuse in New York City—1966 to 1968. *Seminars in Psychiatry*, 1969, *1*, 195–207.

Bellak, L., & Hurvich, M. A systematic study of ego functions. *Journal of Nervous and Mental Disease*, 1969, *148*, 569–585.

DeQuincey, T. (1907). *Confessions of an English opium-eater*. New York: Dutton, 1907.

Ellinwood, E. H. Amphetamine psychosis: I. Description of the individuals and process. *Journal of Nervous and Mental Disease*, 1967, *144*, 273–283.

Fenichel, O. *The psychoanalytic theory of neurosis*. New York: Norton, 1945.

Hartmann, D. A study of drug-taking adolescents. *Psychoanalytic Study of the Child*, 1969, *24*, 384–397.

Hekiman, L. J., & Gershon, S. Characteristics of drug abusers admitted to a psychiatric hospital. *Journal of the American Medical Association*, 1968, *205*, 125–130.

Kramer, J. C., Fischman, V. S., & Littlefield, D. C. Amphetamine abuse: Pattern and affect of high doses taken intravenously. *Journal of the American Medical Association*, 1967, *201*, 305–309.

Mahler, M. On human symbiosis and the vicissitudes of individuation. *Journal of the American Psychoanalytic Association*, 1967, *15*, 740–760.

Reich, A. Pathological forms of self-esteem regulation. *Psychoanalytic Study of the Child*, 1960, *15*, 215–232.

Savett, R. A. Psychoanalytic studies on addiction. Ego structure in narcotic addiction. *Psychoanalytic Quarterly*, 1963, *32*, 43–57.

Wahl, C. W. Diagnosis and treatment of status medicementosus. *Diseases of the Nervous System*, 1967, *28*, 318–322.

Weider, H., & Kaplan, E. H. Drug use in adolescents: Psychodynamic meaning and pharmocogenic effect. *Psychoanalytic Study of the Child*, 1969, *24*, 399–431.

CHAPTER TWENTY

Assessment of Ego Functioning in Studies of Narcotic Addiction

CATHERINE TREECE

Although personality correlates of drug use, abuse, and dependence have been widely studied, they have not generally been investigated within a coherent theoretical framework that has wide acceptance and clinical applicability across both psychiatric and psychological fields. Earlier studies, such as that of Chein, Gerard, Lee, and Rosenfeld (1964), demonstrated the value of a comprehensive and broadly based study of personality and addiction using psychoanalytic concepts. However, drug use in the United States has evolved considerably beyond the problem of ghetto adolescent narcotic use that Chein et al. studied. Multiple drug use patterns and diverse socioeconomic and sociocultural populations are now a standard feature of the drug scene.

This diversification has resulted in drug abuse, once an esoteric clinical specialty, becoming a primary target for clinical concern and theoretical interest. Recent psychoanalytic approaches to substance dependency have produced a rich clinical and theoretical literature in which the focus has been increasingly on formulating an understanding of drug use from the point of view of its function in relation to structural and adaptive ego capacities.

However, investigative research has lagged behind clinical and theoretical developments. This paper reviews some of the issues pertinent to research in this area and describes several new studies whose aim has been to undertake the assessment of ego functioning in relation to narcotic use and dependence.

ISSUES IN CURRENT PSYCHOANALYTIC THEORIES OF DRUG DEPENDENCE

The earlier psychoanalytic literature on drug dependency has been well reviewed (see Khantzian, 1974; Yorke, 1970; Rosenfeld, 1964). These reviewers unanimously emphasized the need for reformulation of theory in light of more contemporary understanding of ego functioning, particularly regarding adaptive aspects. They also emphasized the limited generalizability of the case study approach and the need for a broader base of empirical data from which to proceed.

The current literature has begun to fill these gaps. There appears to be a fairly broad consensus about those aspects of ego functioning most critically related to drug dependency. These include management of affects and impulses, other defensive functions, self-esteem, narcissism, object relations, and a broad range of issues that may, for convenience, be grouped under the general heading of judgment. Differences in theoretical perspective and in the nature of specific clinical observations brought to bear in formulating theoretical propositions account for some apparent differences of opinion or emphasis in the literature; but consensus often breaks down around basic issues and assumptions about the nature of drug dependency itself.

One area of controversy centers around the problem of etiology and causality in drug dependence. While most writers share the assumption that severe ego pathology is among the necessary etiological factors in chronic drug dependency in our culture, this position has been challenged by Zinberg (1975). He points out that the presenting clinical picture of the addict is too affected by the drug use itself to allow valid inferences to be made about predrug personality dynamics.

Most clinicians, indeed, recognize that the interactive nature of cause and effect in drug use results in a clinical condition that reflects both predisposing factors and the social and physiological consequences of the drug use. However, there is also considerable diversity of opinion regarding preexisting ego pathology, as to how specifically particular pathological processes are related to particular drug use patterns.

At one end of this spectrum are those who emphasize that the drug of choice is dynamically determined and is related to distinctive patterns of ego deficit. Wieder and Kaplan (1969), for instance, hypothesized that particular drugs are sought out for their capacity to produce ego states characteristic of earlier developmental stages. Khantzian (1974) and Wurmser (1974) have each proposed that narcotics have specific ameliorative effects on intolerable affect states, particularly rage, and also emphasize the etiological importance of narcissistic disorders among their drug-addicted patients. Milkman and Frosch (1973) developed hypotheses regarding differences in defensive style between narcotic users and amphetamine users. Hendin (1974), in studying college students using heroin, observed recurring themes around the use of narcotic effects to manage crises in close personal relationships.

Other authors focus on individual differences in drug effects and the way this may be related to preexisting ego pathology. Krystal and Raskin (1970) described a wide range of drug and ego function interactions, and Radford, Wiseberg, and Yorke (1970) likewise emphasized individuality of drug and ego function interactions and suggest that specific effects of drugs on ego functioning will depend on the personality structures involved. Greenspan (1977) similarly suggests that individual variation in drug effects, as well as in the morbidity of a drug abuse pattern, will vary in relatively specific ways, depending on the timing of preexisting developmental deviations.

The long-term effect of narcotic addiction is an even more controversial and unresolved problem than cause or specificity. In the short term, the effects of a drug are observed to serve a number of adaptive functions, most often the reduction of emotional distress. Disagreement arises around whether the drug use produces long-term ego changes, and the extent to which such changes involve deterioration of function, or are ameliorative of defective ego functioning. Issues of cause and effect are joined in the problem of determining whether the ego states of long-term drug users have changed sufficiently to obscure the predrug developmental picture.

Zinberg (1975) argues against such a focus on predrug ego factors; he suggests that the effects of cycling in addiction from low to high to low again can serve to keep drive tension high, while a variety of social forces also increase dependence on the environment. The net effect of these dual forces impairs relative autonomy from both internal and external forces, thus initiating a regression involving increasingly rigid defenses. Although Zinberg does not consider this outcome inevitable, he considers it to depend more on the specific circumstances in which the addiction evolves than on the specific preexisting ego weaknesses.

Wieder and Kaplan (1969) suggested that narcotics could provide a "prosthetic effect" in which the drug acted to counter certain ego defects; however, they conclude that drug use is essentially a regressive adaptation and that the predisposing ego pathology is ultimately always increased in a regressive circular spiral. Krystal and Raskin (1970) appear to hold a similar position, describing drug use as an "attempt at self-help that fails." Khantzian (1974), though, in general agreement with this view, also points out that overemphasis on the regressive aspects overlooks the potential and actual improvement in ego functioning that may result from specific psychotropic effects of narcotics, for instance, by reducing aggressive responses. Wurmser (1972), making a similar point, has observed that some patients use narcotics in periods of narcissistic crisis to ward off ego regression. Radford et al. (1970) noted the long-term adaptive function of drugs in their case studies and concluded that, at least in those particular cases, the narcotic use appeared to have constituted a compromise resolution that prevented more serious ego pathology from developing.

THE ADAPTIVE VIEWPOINT AND ADDICTION THEORY

The ego is a conceptual abstraction central to the psychoanalytic theory of personality. Broadly defined, it is considered to be the more or less integrated set of functions within the psychic apparatus that regulate the interrelationships of various psychic components and the relationships between the organism and the outside world. Hartmann succinctly called it the "organ of adaptation."

Regardless of specific theoretical differences among clinicians, it is not difficult to find a consensus that in order to understand drug use compulsions it is necessary to understand the key ego processes involved. The reason for this involves one undisputed feature common to drugs that are abused: They alter feeling states. Since a large part of the definition of ego in its various functions involves the regulation of feeling states, drug effects can be said to mimic or preempt the role of these corresponding internal mechanisms. Freud himself, much concerned with drug addiction at a certain point in his career, made the point that drugs may exaggerate or mimic naturally occurring processes (cited in Rado, 1926).

To be sure, a wide variety of external events effect internal changes through processes of stimulus and response. What is unique about psychotropic drugs is that they produce their effects from within, as if they shared common functional channels. Furthermore, feeling states are only the most obvious and agreed on parallels between drug effects and ego functions, and many others have been suggested. The degree of variability of drug effects, however, should caution against an overly simplistic interpretation of this apparent parallelism. The effects of a drug on ego processes will no doubt depend on the state of the ego structures encountered.

What is most controversial, as was indicated in the preceding review, is not that drug use affects ego functions, or even that ego functioning can in turn determine drug effects; rather, differences of opinion occur over the extent to which these effects are sought out to correct and assist existing weaknesses and inadequacies, how specifically "matched" the drug effects and ego deficits are, and under what circumstances drugs have a more permanent structural effect, whether undermining or supportive.

Some of the circularity of cause and effect that leads to seemingly opposing theoretical positions in the literature may be resolvable by a consideration of the concept of adaptation. Klein (1976) defined adaptation as the optimum "fit" between internal strivings and environmental opportunities and limitations. The various functions that comprise the ego are the way this fit is obtained. When one area of the ego is functioning inadequately, this puts a strain on the overall adaptive capacity and alters the balance of adaptive demand. Adaptation is conceived as a dynamic process that must continually shift and respond to alterations in the internal and external environments, and to conflicts between them. Thus, it is possible to speak of a successful adaptation that has maladaptive consequences or of an inadequate adaptation that has some positive adaptive benefits.

Chein et al. (1964) applied this point some years ago by noting that if the experience of a drug's effect produces an adaptive benefit, even if only temporarily, the likelihood of further use increases. If this benefit has involved a change in the equilibrium of psychic functioning and if the process is repeated frequently, a new equilibrium will be established. In this new equilibrium the desire for the feeling states or other effects now attributed to the drug use has become incorporated into the ego's adaptive apparatus.

The process of adaptation thus appears to be a useful way of conceptualizing the meaning of psychological as well as physiological dependence on narcotics. Abstinence would produce a new set of internal adaptive requirements with a corresponding disequilibrium in the balance of ego functioning. This would be a vulnerable, even regressive state, manifested clinically in the altered moods and symptoms associated with "giving up" a drug. Issues of loss, mourning, and fear of being unable to manage, inextricably mixed up with the physiology of withdrawal, would all be a part of this.

If the original adaptive benefit was experienced in relation to a particular set of external stresses, such as pain from a physical illness, then it would be less likely to become a part of the individual's permanent adaptive repertoire and withdrawal would more likely be tolerated without intense fear.

However, when the adaptive benefit experienced (consciously or unconsciously) has involved a significant alteration in the internal environment, the drug use has more likely become involved in the defensive structure building activity of the ego itself. The prerequisite to such involvement could be either defective defensive structures in general or a specific synergy between preferred defenses and narcotic effect; both hypotheses are compatible with this formulation. In either case withdrawal and "giving up" implies a much greater disequilibrium and potential for regression.

Some of the recalcitrance of addiction may be accounted for by the possibility that under certain circumstances the defensive and other adaptations that sustain the addiction have developed a sort of secondary autonomy from the original motives that led to the addiction in the first place. Likewise, it could be hypothesized that a series of transformations analogous to the processes leading to structuralization of other character defenses and symptoms takes place over time. Thus, for instance, the experienced need for a drug and the belief in its effectiveness can persist in the face of obvious evidence to the contrary. The sensation of craving, the conviction that resolution is at hand, in respon;e to a defensive signal, provides the defensive function.

This proposition, that affects or ideas are sometimes transformed into drug craving, provides a way of accounting for a number of otherwise puzzling aspects of addiction. For example, a distinction between possible direct adaptive effects of pharmacological action, and secondary or acquired adaptive effects, could explain the lack of any clear correlation between the potency or amount of narcotics taken and the occurrence or persistence of addiction per se.

The relatively recent transition in psychoanalytic formulations about addiction from a predominantly drive and conflict orientation to a greater emphasis on developmental and adaptive aspects has provided a fresh perspective from which to consider the processes involved in drug use, dependency, and addiction. The recent psychoanalytic literature offers a variety of formulations, each of which accounts for many of the clinical observations and research findings about narcotic use and addiction. Although the ramifications of an addiction "model" based on the adaptive viewpoint have only been sketched briefly, it is meant to demonstrate how these divergent positions might be viewed within a common, perhaps simplified, framework, thus enabling specific hypotheses to be developed, compared, and systematically investigated. The adaptive point of view stresses the ego structures as the point of mediation between internal and external stimuli to experience, and thus appears particularly appropriate to the study of drug use.

NARCOTIC USE "STYLE" AND ADAPTATION

Much of the psychoanalytic theory about drug use and addiction has evolved from clinical case-oriented work. Quantitative studies have generally focused on description of drug-using populations, but rarely within a psychoanalytic framework. Surprisingly little research has been done that actually attempts to test clinical hypotheses about drug-using individuals.

The formulation of a general model that can integrate clinical propositions based on different populations and differing theoretical emphasis, can be, as was noted earlier, a useful first step toward resolving some of the controversies about the nature of addiction. Various theoretical formulations can provide clinically useful insights into the addictive process; however, to serve as a research tool, theoretical propositions must also be able to generate specific operational hypotheses.

A small study undertaken a few years ago by this author (Treece, 1977) illustrates one way that the adaptive perspective can be used to test a particular hypothesis. This was a study investigating the relationship between narcotic use and anxiety management among a group of incarcerated women. For this study the perceived adaptive benefit from narcotics was inferred from a subject's reported reaction to initial experimentation with these drugs. Out of 60 women interviewed, 41 had experiences with narcotics. All had had ample opportunity in their communities to use drugs and thus "test" their reaction to them. At the time of the study, though, they were (with minor exceptions) free of drug or withdrawal effects.

Four groups were defined based on differing reported responses to narcotic use experiences. Seven of the women were "triers" who had felt relatively indifferent to narcotics and had no particular interest in further use. Five were "polyusers," whose narcotic use was part of extensive multiple drug use, but not the most preferred or most sought out drug. Five other women were "controlled users," who preferred narcotics over all other drugs but actively monitored their use to avoid addiction. Finally, 24 women had used drugs extensively and were "addicts," that is, they had experienced definite withdrawal symptoms and craving when they stopped using, and this had usually occurred several times.

Data to assess anxiety management were obtained using simple self-report questionnaires (unpublished). The prediction was that the four groups would differ on one or more characteristics of anxiety management. Analysis of the data confirmed this prediction and several interesting and statistically significant results emerged.

These results were interpreted in terms of a typology of "anxiety management styles" each of which was associated with one of the four "narcotic use styles." For both the addicts and the controlled users, narcotics was the preferred drug; in terms of the adaptive viewpoint, this was interpreted as the relatively greater "fit" for these subjects between narcotic effect and internal adaptive need: that is, high anxiety. Both of these narcotic preferring groups reported abnormally high levels of anxiety, anxiety symptoms, and general affective discomfort. The difference between these two groups was that for the addicts, but not for the controlled users, this high anxiety was associated with feeling out of control and feeling intensely vulnerable to loss of control.

The triers and the polyusers both reported very low levels of anxiety and other affective symptoms, but the polyusers (like the addicts) felt highly out of control with respect to feelings, needs, and impulses. Thus, the two low-anxiety groups were also the two for whom narcotics was not a high-preference drug. On the other hand, both of the groups who felt highly impulsive (i.e., the polyusers and the addicts) were the two who reported compulsivity in their drug use. The pattern of the triers, whose impulsivity scores were so low as to suggest denial, probably reflects an intensely rigid defensive pattern; in reality some of these subjects were among the most impulse ridden in the sample. Their rejection of narcotics appeared partly related to their need to maintain a self-image of high control. When they did have a drug preference, it tended toward the stimulants that appeared to support their need for active power and control.

Although the samples were small, the results were strongly supportive of the hypothesis that anxiety management and patterns of narcotic use are systematically related. This in turn is consistent with psychoanalytic formulations that stress the specific role of narcotics in affect management.

In this context one other study that explicitly compares controlled and compulsive narcotic users is worth noting, since this type of comparison is very rare in the literature. This is a study just being completed by Zinberg and Harding at the Department of Psychiatry (Harvard Medical School), The Cambridge Hospital in Cambridge, Massachusetts.* These investigators followed 61 controlled narcotic users and 30 compulsive users for a 2-year period, thus documenting considerable stability for the two different use patterns. Although this was not primarily a study of ego functioning, they do report that compulsive users were repeatedly assessed to be more "distanced from affects" compared to the controlled users. On the surface this appears contradictory to the results of the prisoner study, although the difference might lie in the fact that the Zinberg and Harding sample was actively using, while the Treece sample was unable to obtain drugs.

METHODOLOGICAL ISSUES AND ADDITIONAL RESEARCH FINDINGS

The desirability of having some standard methods of assessing ego functions, so that studies by different investigators can be compared and integrated, is readily illustrated by the two studies discussed earlier. Indeed, the problem of "measuring" intrapsychic structure and activity in general has been a major technical impediment to testing psychoanalytically oriented theories. Even where long-term intensive and sophisticated clinical data are available, the reduction or translation of such data to a manageable but meaningful form that lends itself to statistical analysis is a stumbling block.

It is, therefore, of interest to review some additional recent studies of drug addiction that have made use of some relatively new methods developed to assess ego functioning.

One recent study was done at the Addiction Research Foundation, Yale University, in New Haven, by Kleber, Weissman, and Rounseville.† These investigators compared data from several instruments on three groups: applicants for narcotic addiction treatment, applicants for a CETA program, and acutely disturbed patients on an inpatient unit.

The Loevinger Scale (1967) is based on a model of stages of ego develop-

* The study, titled "Controlled Narcotic Use" was supported by National Institute on Drug Abuse Grant No. DA 01360-05 (Investigators, Norman Zinberg, M.D. and Wayne Harding, Ph.D.).

† From "The Significance of Psychiatric Diagnosis in Opiate Addiction," Final Report to NIDA for Contract No. 271-77-3430, March, 1981, by H. Kleber et al. The ego assessment portion of the study was under the direction of Sidney Blatt, M.D., and carried out by Alan Sugerman, Ph.D.

ment; in the New Haven study the 97 addicts tested averaged at a "level of ego development" equivalent to that found among normal adolescents; there was no difference in average level between the addicts and the 29 CETA applicants, though there was a fairly wide range of scores in both groups.

On the Ego Function Assessment (EFA) scales of Bellak, Gediman, and Hurwich (1973) (described elsewhere in this volume), the average scale scores for 77 addicts were very close to those obtained for the original comparison group of "neurotics" on which the EFA scales were standardized; this was in contrast to the CETA group whose scale scores closely resembled the original Bellak et al. "normals." The largest decrement in ego functioning among the addicts was on the Judgment scale, which was rated as more impaired than that of the neurotics. Also in contrast to the neurotics, but in a healthier direction, was the relatively high average score for Sense of Reality of the Self and of the World.

The New Haven group also used a number of measures, both new and standard, from the Rorschach test. As with the Loevinger Scale, little difference was found between 77 addicts and the CETA subjects. However, compared to the inpatient sample, the addicts were significantly less impaired, with two important exceptions: the addicts showed greater affective lability and a lower developmental level of object concepts. Interpreted overall, the Rorschach data was said to suggest that the most prominent disturbances of the addicts as a group were their poor capacity to contain and modulate affective experience and their poor capacity to establish meaningful and appropriate interpersonal relationships.

Having assessed the addict sample as a group, the investigators further subjected all three sets of ego data for the addict sample to a cluster analysis to identify likely subgroups. Three groups emerged in the analysis. The largest group manifested those characteristics already noted in the general findings regarding difficulties in affect modulation and object relations. Of the two smaller groups, one was characterized by a disturbance in thought process and another was distinguished because of a lowered level of activity, thus perhaps a depressed group.

A second recent study was done at the Department of Psychiatry (Harvard Medical School) in Cambridge, by Long, Khantzian, and Treece.* These investigators assessed ego functioning in a group of 54 mixed sedative-hypnotic and narcotic users, most of whom had a history of narcotic addiction. This group was actively using drugs three times a week or more and was not seeking treatment.

The Cambridge group also used the Loevinger scale. The results for this drug population were similar to those obtained by New Haven for the addiction treatment applicants. The largest percent of subjects (33%) scored at a

* From "Ego Functioning in Drug Users and Addicts," Final Report to NIDA for Grant No. 5 RO1 DA 01828-01, 1980. The project director and author of the report was Jancis F. V. Long, Ph.D.

level comparable with normal adolescents, with the rest distributed above and below this level.

Long et al. also used the Bellak et al. EFA scales; their results again showed a drug-using sample to be most similar to the neurotic comparison group and significantly lower, on the average, compared to the normals group. The major difference between the Cambridge and New Haven results on the Bellak scales was the greater decrement in Judgment for the latter.

A self-report instrument assessing relative preference for certain defensive styles, the Defense Mechanism Inventory (Gleser & Ihilevich, 1969) showed the drug-using sample to have a specifically higher preference for the defense of "turning against others" compared with several other normal and patient comparison groups; this result was particularly strong for women. On a self-report scale of impulsivity (the same scale used in the prison study), the drug-using sample averaged at a level equal to that for an unselected prison sample, which is lower than that for addict prisoners alone but considerably higher than "normals."

Assessing the results overall, including considerable interview data that was not quantified, the Cambridge investigators emphasized the prominence of severe anxiety, a sense of helplessness with regard to affect and impulses, and poor object relations as the most salient disturbances observed in the group as a whole. With regard to object relations, two apparent types of adaptive function for narcotics and other drugs were noted. In one, narcotics appeared to serve adaptively to help *maintain* relationships and "normal" social functioning. In the second, the drugs appeared to compensate for the *absence* of meaningful relationships. This distinction was sharper among newer users, with the differences blurring among the more chronic addicts.

This latter observation is related to the strong statistical association reported in the same study, between chronicity of narcotic use and the severity of impairment on several of the ego measures, including the EFA scales, particularly in the areas of Judgment, and the sense of being out of control, as reflected on the impulsivity self-report. In addition, chronicity of narcotic use and the amount of current use, when analyzed together in relation to the overall average of EFA scale scores, each *independently* as well as cumulatively contributed to lower ratings of ego functioning.

STANDARDIZED MEASUREMENT: THE EFA SCALES

Both studies summarized earlier, from Cambridge and from New Haven, and a third study by Milkman and Frosch (1975, and in a separate chapter of this volume) have all made use of the EFA scales to study ego functioning in narcotic-using populations. This offers a rare opportunity in the field to compare results directly across studies.

In a recent review of psychiatric rating scales, Spitzer and Endicott (1975) noted that there have been only a few attempts at developing rating scales for the evaluation of impairment that use psychoanalytic concepts. Of these, the EFA scales of Bellak et al. (1973) offer the most comprehensive effort that has proved feasible and appropriate for the type of study under consideration here. The EFA scales are based on a definition of ego as a "number of functions that refer . . . to adaptively relevant actions and reactions of the individual person" (p. 71). Of the various ways the construct of ego has been conceptualized and operationalized, this one is closest to the concepts of mainstream ego psychological thinking. The scales have the advantage that they can be used with a nonpatient, nonresidential population, that they have been standardized to some extent, and that they include a detailed interview, rating protocol, and scoring system to facilitate use by various investigators.

In all three of the studies under consideration the investigators followed the interview and scoring protocols as described by Bellak et al., except that each group eliminated one or more of the total of 12 scales that were problematic for one reason or another. In the following discussion, therefore, only the nine scales common to all three are included.

In Figures 20.1–20.3 various results from the three studies have been displayed in graph form. In these figures the EFA scale scores have been retained on a 13-point scale as used by each of the studies, but rounded to the nearest half point.

In Figure 20.1 the 10 normal control subjects from Milkman and Frosch, the 29 CETA control subjects from New Haven, and Bellak et al.'s 25 original "normals" are shown and compared against the original 25 outpatient "neurotic" sample of Bellak et al. What is striking in this figure is the close similarity among the three "normal" samples and their similar distance from the "neurotics." Although none of the investigators suggested that their interviewers were blind to the fact that they were interviewing normal controls, such similar results for groups of raters working independently is encouraging and supports the validity of the "normal" standard for the scales.

Figure 20.2 shows the results for the Cambridge and New Haven narcotic samples contrasted with the EFA normal and neurotic standardization groups. This comparison is also quite remarkable in the similarity of the drug user results, though again rater bias has not been ruled out.

Figure 20.3 shows the Milkman and Frosch narcotic samples in the intoxicated and abstinent conditions, contrasted with the neurotic and schizophrenic standardization samples of Bellak et al. (1973). The two sets of narcotic user scores were quite similar except that Regulation and Control of Impulses and Affects and Sense of Competence were significantly lower in the intoxicated conditions than in the abstinent condition; Reality Testing was also suggestively lower in the intoxicated condition. On most of the scales the Milkman and Frosch narcotic users were rated lower than the other two narcotic samples shown in Figure 20.2. The most extreme differences between the Milkman and Frosch narcotic users and the neurotics was

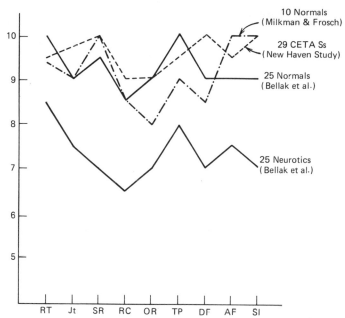

Figure 20.1. EFA scores for three control groups. RT, Reality Testing; Jt, Judgment; SR, Sense of Reality of the World and of the Self; RC, Regulation and Control of Drives, Affects, and Impulses; OR, Object Relations; TP, Thought Processes; DF, Defensive Functioning; AF, Autonomous Functioning; SI, Synthetic–Integrative Functioning.

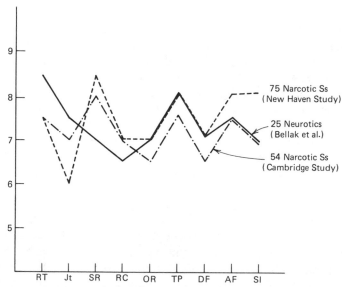

Figure 20.2. EFA scores for two narcotic user samples. RT, Reality Testing; Jt, Judgment; SR, Sense of Reality of the World and of the Self; RC, Regulation and Control of Drives, Affects, and Impulses; OR, Object Relations; TP, Thought Processes; DF, Defensive Functioning; AF, Autonomous Functioning; SI, Synthetic–Integrative Functioning.

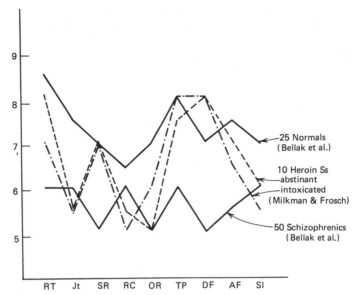

Figure 20.3. EFA scores for Milkman & Frosch sample. RT, Reality Testing; Jt, Judgment; SR, Sense of Reality of the World and of the Self; RC, Regulation and Control of Drives, Affects, and Impulses; OR, Object Relations; TP, Thought Processes; DF, Defensive Functioning; AF, Autonomous Functioning; SI, Synthetic–Integrative Functioning.

for the two scales of Regulation and Control of Impulses and Affects, and for Object Relations, on which the narcotic users were rated almost as impaired as the schizophrenic standardization group.

These comparisons help to highlight the most general and consistent findings to emerge from the three studies. The most prominent decrement noted by the New Haven investigators was the low average scale score for Judgment among their narcotic users applying for treatment. Judgment was rated very low for both intoxicated and nonintoxicated narcotic users in the Milkman and Frosch sample as well. In the Cambridge sample, the Judgment score for the narcotic user sample was only slightly lower than for the neurotic group; but it was Judgment that was the scale most strongly correlated with chronicity of narcotic use in a negative direction.

The most severely impaired functions reported by the Milkman and Frosch study for narcotic addicts were those of Object Relations and Regulation and Control of Drives, Impulses, and Affects. Although these functions were not rated as low for narcotic users on the EFA scales by the other two studies, both of the latter studies did emphasize both object relations and lability or impulsivity in affect management as the major deficits in functioning associated with narcotic use, taking all of their results into account.

Taken together, these results are very consistent and indicate that they may be considered quite generalizable with respect to other comparable narcotic-using populations. Such discrepancies as there were on the EFA scales specifically would be due to a combination of "error"—that is, differences in scoring among the different investigators and "real" differences, particularly to differences in drug use history and current status.

A comparison of the results of these three studies using the EFA scales also highlights the value of having a method of assessing ego functioning that is based on widely accepted definitions of ego function; the results are immediately meaningful to a broad audience, particularly to clinicians. The EFA scales have not yet undergone the kind of extensive evolutionary development and standardization as have some other basic measures in psychological research, such as the Wechsler IQ Scales, or as the descriptive psychiatric rating scales like the Research Diagnostic Criteria, or even the DSM-III. However, having a standard set of ego function rating scales meets such an important need in the field of psychoanalytic ego psychology, and since the EFA scales appear to have met such initial success and acceptance, their further evolution is almost inevitable and certainly highly desirable.

A FACTOR ANALYTIC STUDY

In another study at the Cambridge Hospital, for which this author was responsible, along with Edward J. Khantzian,* the assessment of ego functioning was approached somewhat differently.

This project was primarily a diagnostic study comparing narcotic users in various settings. However, the investigators also sought to develop a foundation for the later testing of some psychoanalytic hypotheses about addiction. Rather than attempt a broad coverage, they concentrated on a few specific areas of ego function. Thus, four of the EFA scales were selected to be combined with several experimental scales being piloted in the study.

The four EFA scales selected were Object Relations, Sense of Reality of the World and of the Self, Thought Processes, and Regulation and Control of Drive, Affect, and Impulse. These four scales are comprised of a total of 13 subscales. Rather than use the summary assessment for each complete scale, as was done in the other studies, the subscale scores were retained as discrete variables. The method for assessing the EFA scales was also varied somewhat for this study. Thus, a special interview protocol designed to meet the requirements of the whole study was substituted for the Bellak et al. interview. Further, some of the specific definitions for certain scale stops were modified and amplified somewhat, both to make them conceptually more consistent with a character disorder spectrum (in contrast to the schizophrenia–neurosis spectrum) and to make reliability easier to achieve.

* The study was titled "Implications of Psychiatric Diagnosis for Narcotic Dependence Treatment, NIDA Contract No. 271-77-3431. Material for this paper was based on the Final Report to NIDA, January, 1980, and from several unpublished manuscripts.

In doing this the investigators ran the risk of losing comparability with other studies using the scales, but the final results suggest that these deviations did not substantively alter the essential identity of the EFA scales.*

Fifty-seven subjects from the larger study, and 23 ego variables in all, including the EFA subscales, were subjected to a factor analysis. The best solution produced six factors, which are listed in Table 20.1, along with the major variables contained in each factor. The EFA subscales are listed separately from the experimental variables and inspection of the table shows that the four EFA scales were each clearly identified by the factor analysis. The subscales "hung together" according to their identity with specific scales.†
Since by definition in this analysis the factors were statistically independent, this result provides empirical support for the conceptual identity of the scales.

In addition to the four factors that are identified with the four EFA scales (in some cases supplemented by the experimental variables), there were two other factors. One of these (differentiation) appeared to involve discriminations with regard to inner experience and external objects. A sixth factor (hysteria [?]) was rather puzzling and seemed to reflect a particular character style more than an ego function as such.

The six ego factors were tested in several ways prior to analyzing their relation to drug use in the subjects. The sample was a diverse group, including 31 patients in methadone maintenance treatment, 9 patients from a drug-free residential facility, and 17 individuals from the drug-using community at large, all of whom reported extensive narcotic use. These three subsets of subjects were compared on the set of ego factors and no differences were found. Thus, the sample could be treated as a whole. Additional analysis established that the factors were independent of race, years of education, and family socioeconomic status. Differentiation and sense of reality were slightly correlated with age and there was a slight sex difference in which women tended to score higher (in a healthier direction) than men, especially on closeness. IQ was also unrelated to all but the differentiation factor, for which a small correlation existed. Finally, the ego factors were evaluated in relation to the formal diagnosis for personality disorder as defined by DSM-III. Two of the factors, regulation and control and closeness, significantly discriminated between subjects who met the criteria for a personality disorder from those who did not.

* The mean of the subscale scores for each of the four EFA scales was compared with those of the other two narcotic using samples shown in Figure 20.2. The group means were again very similar, the one exception being that in this sample Thought Processes were closer to normal than to neurotic.

† Factor 1 has been called regulation and tolerance of closeness since this seemed to reflect the main variables in the factor and to distinguish it from differentiation, which also appeared in a factor related to object relations. The second factor is called regulation and control, implying identity with the EFA Scale of Regulation and Control of Drives, Affects, and Impulses. However, it should be noted that in this context it is primarily a measure of the regulation of anger.

Table 20.1. *Primary Variables for Six Factors of Ego Function*

EFA Variables	Experimental Variables

Factor 1: Regulation and Tolerance of Closeness

Object Relations Stop a—degree and kind of relatedness to others (factor loading = .82)

Object Relations Stop d—maintenance of object constancy (factor loading = .79)

Object Relations Stop c—others perceived as independent entities (factor loading = .73)

Object Relations Stop b—primitivity–maturity of object relations (factor loading = .73)

Sense of Reality Stop c—stable sense of self (factor loading = .60)

Regulation and Control Stop b—effectiveness of delay and control (factor loading = .47)

Capacity for Intimacy (factor loading = .74)

Acceptance of Anger in Self (factor loading = .47)

Factor 2: Regulation and Control

Regulation and Control Stop a—directness of impulse expression (over/under control) (factor loading = .74)

Regulation and Control Stop b—effectiveness of delay and control (factor loading = .55)

Anger Leads to Behavioral Activation (factor loading = .56)

Factor 3: Differentiation

Objectivity in Description of Important Others (factor loading = .85)

Capacity for Empathic Concern (factor loading = .74)

Complexity of Object in Description of Important Others (factor loading = .59)

Capacity to Discriminate Own Anxiety (factor loading = .59)

Factor 4: Thought Processes

Thought Processes Stop b—ability to conceptualize (factor loading = .81)

Thought Processes Stop c—primary/secondary process in communication (factor loading = .81)

Thought Processes Stop a—memory, concentration, attention (factor loading = .57)

283

Table 20.1. *(Continued)*

EFA Variables	Experimental Variables

Factor 5: Sense of Reality

Sense of Reality Stop c—stable sense
of self (factor loading = .72)
Sense of Reality Stop b—body and
behavior belong to self (factor loading = .66)
Sense of Reality Stop a—external
events real and familiar (factor loading = .65)
Sense of Reality Stop d—clear ego
boundaries (factor loading = .61)

Factor 5: Hysterical (?)

Acceptance of Own Fear (factor load-
ing = .75)
Awareness of Physiological Aspects of
Affect (factor loading = .73)
Involvement with Magical Power (fac-
tor loading = .63)

Five of the nontreatment subjects had reported never having been ad-
dicted to narcotics, despite an extensive history of use. When compared to
the rest of the subjects who had addiction histories, these five averaged
significantly higher (i.e., healthier) on the same two factors, closeness and
regulation and control, as differentiated between subjects with and without
formally diagnosable personality disorders.

Although this result was exciting, it rested on a very small group of
subjects. The factors were next analyzed in relation to three additional features of the subject's drug histories: an intensity index of heaviest narcotic
use, an index that summarized the overall intensity of involvement with the
other drugs and alcohol, and the number of years of involvement with narcotics (chronicity). Using multivariate statistical techniques, the results
again implicated regulation and control and closeness, and in one case,
differentiation.

Differentiation was strongly but exclusively associated with chronicity of
narcotic use. Closeness was associated with the extent of heaviest involvement with narcotics (regardless of chronicity). And regulation and control
was strongly related to both intensity and chronicity of narcotic use, and
(from a separate analysis) also showed some relationship to intensity of
recent and current use.

In the case of both closeness and regulation and control, when the overall intensity of all *other substance use* was taken into account, both factors were as much related to this overall drug use as to narcotic use specifically.

One additional analysis from a different portion of the study will also be mentioned here, as it adds one more dimension to the ego assessment picture. Nicholson and Treece (1981), using a scale of narcissistic development modeled after the EFA scales, found that methadone maintenance patients who continued to be polydrug users while in treatment showed a greater degree of narcissistic disturbance compared with methadone patients who were satisfied with methadone alone.

To put these results into perspective in relation to the studies reviewed earlier, it can be noted that the two areas of object relations and management of affect, in their broadest connotations, have repeatedly emerged as the areas of functioning most consistently and strongly associated with heavy narcotic involvement. A third area in the present study appears to involve the capacity for cognitively based differentiation as it is elaborated in the interpersonal and affective spheres. The fact that this cognitive capacity was related only to chronicity of narcotic use parallels the finding regarding the EFA Judgment scale in the other Cambridge study by Long et al. Judgment and differentiation may thus mirror a common underlying phenomenon and point to a third, perhaps less well defined, area of ego functioning associated with narcotic addiction.

The finding that regulation and control (particularly as related to anger, as it was assessed in the present study) was associated with all the drug use variables assessed is consistent with the prison study, which associated emotional and behavioral impulsivity with compulsivity of drug use, and with the Milkman and Frosch results that Regulation and Control suffered a decrement in the intoxicated condition.

DISCUSSION

These excerpts from recent research projects have been presented to illustrate some recent trends in the difficult quantitative investigation of psychoanalytically based theories of substance dependence, particularly as viewed from the perspective of adaptation.

Much of the research in this field remains fairly simplistic as investigators grope for the methods that adequately reflect their conceptual framework. Indeed, it is to be hoped that research on addiction and ego function may, in elaborating its own methodologies, contribute as much to ego psychology as to the understanding of drug use itself.

Notwithstanding, the recent developments reviewed indicate a fruitful meeting of recent methodological developments (such as the EFA scales) with increasingly sophisticated psychoanalytic perspectives on the adaptive significance of drug dependence. Clearly, the move toward specifying dimensions of drug use is already producing interesting results. Research has moved from generalizations about addiction and associated ego impairment to analyzing discriminated aspects of ego functioning in relation to different aspects of substance use, including drug effects, context, and styles of use. Indeed, it already seems odd that research on addiction for so long stayed stuck on trying to explain the addict per se rather than viewing drug use as a continuum of behaviors. Such a viewpoint reflected an implicit model of addiction in which the drug itself was viewed as the locus of compulsion, or, equally untenable, the addictive personality.

One dimension of drug use that has been the subject of considerable speculation is that of the specificity of "drug of choice" and its relation to impairments in ego function. A central confounding factor in all the studies presented here is that in a street population claiming to be "dope addicts" the amount of actual narcotic use over time relative to a variety and quantity of other substances is always open to question and difficult to estimate accurately. All of these other street and pharmaceutical drugs have acute and chronic effects on many aspects of functioning. Thus, when groups of addicts are compared with other groups, it is the net effect of all the drug use that goes into the group differences. In those studies that made some attempt to control for the other drug use, the polydrug use tended to account for large shares of the group differences. Thus, it is clearly necessary in further studies to take greater account of this multiple drug use even among ostensible narcotic addicts. Indeed, it is likely that the degree of preference for a particular drug, in contrast to indiscriminate drug using, is in itself a key dimension in the relationship between drug use and ego function.

Having reiterated the limitations of these studies, we can now turn to an overview of the findings and note the implications of the progress that has been made to date. The research reported here repeatedly emphasized affect management and object relations, and some aspect of judgment, as central areas for focus in understanding narcotic and other drug use. Clinically, of course, these areas of development and functioning are highly interrelated. Difficulties with impulse control, anxiety tolerance, management of aggression, and developmental distortions that impair identity and interpersonal satisfaction and intercourse are central developmental issues that bear on the definition of character disorder itself.

One important point documented by the recent research is that the longer an individual has been involved with narcotics (not necessarily continuously) and the more intense the heaviest periods of use, the more severe (on the average) are the pathological manifestations of the character disorder. Severity of character disorder appears to distinguish not only casual and controlled users from compulsive users, but also short-term and milder addicts from chronic addicts.

That addiction per se is not *inevitably* associated with serious ego pathology was most dramatically demonstrated by the Vietnam experience, where a majority of the men neither showed serious psychopathology nor continued their addiction after return to the States (Robins, 1980). Likewise, most acute pain patients treated with narcotics do not develop a classic addiction and do not demonstrate major ego distortions. In such cases, the adaptation model suggests that narcotics may provide a temporary adaptive benefit in relation to extraordinary demands on the ego's capacities, combined with unusual "environmental opportunities." In the case of certain character disorders, by contrast, the adaptive requirement is generated from within, perpetuated perhaps by the failure to develop alternative resolutions through maturing ego functions.

It is not possible to say, based on the evidence at hand, whether this link between greater psychopathology and chronicity is a function of the mechanism of compulsion as such, of narcotic and other drug use per se, or of the sheer persistence of drug seeking in the face of increasing risk, financial hardship, and pressure from social sanctions that inevitably multiply over time. The probability that greater desperation is a factor in these findings echoes Vaillant's (1970) comment that the addict "is a person with a paucity of gratifying alternatives rather than a man whose instinctual needs are readily answered by heroin" (p. 497).

The fact that most *chronic* addicts show evidence of severe character disorder does not, of course, imply that all individuals with character disorder are equally at risk for addiction. This seems to be the strongest argument for some kind of specificity hypothesis. In the prison study there were a number of intriguing clues about this point that suggest further study. Out of 60 subjects interviewed, only 7 were "naive" in that they had really no exposure to narcotics. Less than half the remaining 53 were addicts, even though most had no compunctions about engaging in illegal activities, and most could readily be characterized as having serious character disorders. A certain number of these subjects had already made "commitments" to another substance, prior to encountering narcotics. Thus, one hypothesis involves the chance factor of what substance is available at the time certain adaptive needs are great and alternatives meager. Wurmser (1977) postulated that an "addictive search" compels certain people to seek some exogenous source of relief for narcissistic crisis. Thus, whatever provides the experience of relief, however transient, may be grasped in a special way.

A different kind of specificity was suggested by those subjects who rejected narcotics because they preferred to be "in control." A few of these subjects preferred stimulants, which parallels the differences reported by Milkman and Frosch (1975) in defensive style between narcotic-preferring and amphetamine-preferring users. Such clear-cut preferences are not always apparent, however; and, as was noted earlier, the degree of specificity in drug choice may itself indicate differences in defensive structures.

Regarding the question of etiology, then, the research presented here is still a long way from resolving the problem, though it does provide grist for the mill. Some of the consequences of addiction can be understood in terms similar to those of other character disorders that involve unappetizing or socially alienating behavior. Social reactions, the need for secrecy, the fear that someone will take away that which has become a needed part of oneself, for instance, can also be seen in cases of anorexia nervosa or of exhibitionism. In other words, the idea that character distortions generate feedback experiences and secondary defensive and adaptive needs that interact with and complicate further development leads to complexities of formulation but is not unfamiliar. However, exactly what features of specific drugs themselves make addiction a special and unique type of compulsion will continue to be unraveled for some time to come.

The role of psychotherapy, or counseling, in drug treatment programs remains a controversial subject. Currently, in many treatment programs, even where counseling is provided, it is rarely used in a manner involving specific theoretical frameworks and specific therapeutic techniques. Too often these terms are used in the most general sense, and there is little structured guidance to the therapeutic endeavor.

This is an area where input from research and clinical expertise based on an ego psychological approach is most immediately needed. For example, treatment efforts on behalf of addicts have at times taken into account the apparent need among many patients for social supports and controls. The self-help movement in the 1960s reflected cognizance within the ex-addict community of the social needs of addicts struggling to remain abstinent. Thus, many programs such as the so-called concept houses as well as some professionally run half-way houses, *required* a high degree of social interaction and involvement on the part of their clients. From our point of view, however, too many of these efforts had a fatal flaw, which helps to explain their demise in popularity. The intrapsychic and social reasons underlying the perceived needs of these addicts were not really addressed.

Methadone programs often offer a sort of de facto social network, though some have also instituted "drop-in centers" and other efforts in recognition of the need for social normalization. Here again, however, there is a tendency for a social network based solely on shared deviancy to become institutionalized.

The historical association between narcotic addiction and antisocial behavior, though certainly valid often enough, unfortunately led treatment of addictive disorder out of the mainstream of psychoanalytically oriented study and treatment. Further elaboration of treatment implications here is beyond the scope of this paper. Suffice to say, now that ego psychology has advanced to a point where antisocial behavior can be integrated into the larger body of knowledge about disturbed narcissistic development and other aspects of severe character disorder, it need no longer remain the stepchild of the field.

REFERENCES

Bellak, L., Hurvich, M., & Gediman, H. D. *Ego functions in schizophrenics, neurotics, and normals: A systematic study of conceptual, diagnostic, and therapeutic aspects.* New York: Wiley, 1973.

Chein, I., Gerard, D. L., Lee, R. S., & Rosenfeld, E. *The road to H: Narcotics, Delinquency, and Social Policy.* New York: Basic Books, 1964.

Gleser, G., & Ihilevich, D. An objective instrument for measuring defense mechanisms. *Journal of Consulting and Clinical Psychology,* 1969, *33*(1), 51–60.

Greenspan, S. I. Substance abuse: An understanding from psychoanalytic developmental and learning perspectives. In J. D. Blaine & D. A. Julius (Eds.), *Psychodynamics of drug dependence.* National Institute on Drug Abuse Research Monograph Series, No. 12, May 1977, pp. 73–87. Washington, D.C.: U.S. Government Printing Office.

Henden, H. Students on heroin. *The Journal of Nervous and Mental Disease,* 1974, *156*(4), 240–255.

Khantzian, E. J. A preliminary dynamic formulation of the psychopharmacological action of methadone. *Proceedings of the Fourth National Conference on Methadone Treatment.* San Francisco, January 1972, pp. 371–374.

Khantzian, E. J., Mack, J. E., & Schatzberg, A. F. Heroin use as an attempt to cope: Clinical observations. *American Journal of Psychiatry,* 1974, *131*(2), 160–164.

Klein, G. S. *Psychoanalytic theory: An exploration of essentials.* New York: International Universities Press, 1976.

Krystal, H., & Raskin, H. A. *Drug dependence: Aspects of ego function.* Detroit: Wayne State University Press, 1970.

Loevinger, J. The meaning and measurement of ego development. *American Psychologist,* 1967, *21,* 195–206.

McLellan, A. T., Luborsky, L., Woody, G. E., & O'Brian, C. P. The generality of benefits from alcohol and drug abuse treatment. In L. S. Harris (Ed.), *Problems of drug Dependence 1980.* The Committee on Problems of Drug Dependence, Inc., NIDA Research Monograph Series, No. 34, February 1981, pp. 123–130. Washington, D.C.: U.S. Government Printing Office.

Milkman, H., & Frosch, W. A. On the preferential abuse of heroin and amphetamines. *The Journal of Nervous and Mental Disease,* 1973, *156*(1), 242–248. (Also in this volume.)

Nicholson, B., & Treece, C. Object relations and differential treatment response to methadone maintenance. *Journal of Nervous and Mental Disease,* 1981, *169,* 424–429.

Radford, P., Wiseberg, S., & Yorke, C. A study of "mainline" heroin addiction. *Psychoanalytic Study of the Child,* 1972, *27,* 156–180.

Rado, S. The psychic effects of intoxicants: An attempt to evolve a psychoanalytical theory of morbid cravings. *International Journal of Psychoanalysis,* 1926, *7,* 396–407.

Robins, S. *The Vietnam drug user returns.* (Special Action Office Monograph, Series A, No. 2.) Washington, D.C.: U.S. Government Printing Office, 1974.

Rosenfeld, H. A. The psychopathology of drug addiction and alcoholism (A critical review of the psychoanalytic literature). In H. A. Rosenfeld, (Ed.). *Psychotic states: A psychoanalytic approach* New York: International Universities Press, 1965.

Spitzer, R., & Endicott, J. Psychiatric rating scales. In D. Freedman et al. (Eds.), *Comprehensive textbook of psychiatry,* Vol. II Baltimore: Williams & Wilkins, 1975.

Treece, C. Narcotic use in relation to selected ego functions among incarcerated women. (Doctoral dissertation, Boston University, 1977.) Dissertation Abstracts International, Vol. 4, 1977. (University Microfilms No. 77-21-621.)

Vaillant, G. E. The natural history of narcotic drug addiction. *Seminars in Psychiatry*, 1970, *2*(4), 468–498.

Vaillant, G. E. The natural history of alcoholism. Cambridge, Mass.: Harvard University Press, 1982.

Wieder, H., & Kaplan, E. Drug use in adolescents. *Psychoanalytic Study of the Child*, 1969, *24*, 399–431.

Wurmser, L. Psychoanalytic consideration of the etiology of compulsive drug use. *Journal of the American Psychoanalytic Association*, 1974, *22*(4), 820–843.

Wurmser, L. Mr. Pecksniff's horse? (Psychodynamics in compulsive drug use). In J. D. Blaine & D. A. Julius, (Eds.), *Psychodynamics of drug dependence*. National Institute on Drug Abuse Research Monograph Series, No. 12, 1977, pp. 36–72. Washington, D.C.: U.S. Government Printing Office.

Yorke, C. A. A critical review of some psychoanalytic literature on drug addiction. *British Journal of Medical Psychology*, 1970, *43*, 141–159.

Zinberg, N. E. Addiction and ego function. *Psychoanalytic Study of the Child*, 1975, *30*, 567–588.

— CHAPTER TWENTY-ONE ———————

The Use of Ego Function Analysis for the Screening of Civil Service Applicants

**LOUIS N. GRUBER, J. ROBERT BARNES,
JAMES A. KNIGHT, AND MICHAEL J. MADIGAN**

INTRODUCTION

Applicants for police recruit and certain other positions in the New Orleans civil service routinely undergo psychological screening. About one-fourth of these were referred for psychiatric evaluation during a 4-year period. The psychiatrists were to rate these applicants as "suitable" or "unsuitable" for the jobs, using any method they chose. Any applicant found to be "unsuitable" was dropped from further consideration, but could reapply for the position after 6 months. The present report concerns 36 applicants who, for various reasons, were interviewed more than once.

We were struck by a finding with these "repeaters" that we noted on more than one occasion: The individual reapplied for a civil service position after previously passing the psychiatric evaluation, and then having severe behavior difficulties on the job. Looking back at the previous psychiatric evaluation we might find something like this: "He is extremely guarded, won't say much about himself, but I can't really find any good reason to reject him."

Feeling that valuable data were being elicited but not utilized in such interviews, we determined to find a more systematic evaluation method. We also hoped that a study of these evaluation "repeaters" might tell us something about the reliability—and limitations—of psychiatric evaluations. By using Ego Function Assessment (EFA) for the evaluations we also hoped to examine the process in some detail.

METHOD: EGO FUNCTION ASSESSMENT

Bellak et al.'s clinical interview (Bellak et al., 1973) is a procedure that can take full advantage of the clinician's observational skills and ability to pursue significant points in more depth. We selected EFA for the civil service evaluations after evaluating and rejecting a number of interview techniques and rating scales as too cumbersome, superficial, or limited in scope to the severe pathologies.

As it assesses a wide range of functioning, from severe disturbance to extreme psychological well-being, we felt that EFA could be extended and adapted to our cohort. We found it to be a particularly penetrating examination of the personality structure that can elicit subtle degrees of psychopathology even in persons who are well defended and are trying to present themselves in a favorable light (viz., for employment). The interview assesses enduring patterns and styles of functioning in addition to the current mental state. Furthermore, findings can be reported as numerical profiles without divulging intimate personal data. However, since much of the original work on EFA has dealt with the diagnosis of schizophrenia, we found the suggested questions and rating stops largely aimed at a psychiatric population. In the interests of expanding the use of the interview to its potential range, we developed our own interview and rating manuals. This adaptation of EFA enabled us to give accurate ratings to subjects who by and large fell within the normal range and yet manifested subtle degrees of psychopathology.

In developing the revised interview manual we structured the questions so as to facilitate the conceptualization of ego functions as integrative tasks. For example, the way in which inner and outer reality (Reality Testing) or action and reflection (Judgment, Regulation, and Control) are synthesized could be assessed as to their varying degrees of smoothness, grace, and adaptiveness. In addition, questions could be framed in such a way as to give no indication of the "right" or "normal" answer.

We also simplified the instrument, by giving only a single composite score for each ego function, to reflect the subject's current functioning. To the rating manual of Bellak et al. we added our own clinical examples, as we became familiar with the range of typical responses to our questions.

Because of time constraints we limited our examinations to those ego functions that seemed most relevant to the jobs in question. Therefore, the assessment of ARISE, Stimulus Barrier, Autonomous Functioning, and Synthetic–Integrative Functioning was frequently omitted. A fairly thorough evaluation could be performed in the 1-hour interview time allotted, with a scoring of five to eight ego functions. EFA was not experienced by most applicants as either invasive or stressful. Many commented that they found the questions intriguing and enjoyed the opportunity to talk about themselves in this way.

DESCRIPTIVE REPORTS AND EFA

Since the standardized interview using EFA was gradually implemented by us over a 2-year period, many of the earlier reports were in narrative form alone. As we developed our modified manual with clear behavioral examples, we found that these verbal reports could themselves be rated on anywhere from two to five ego functions, thus putting them in a form that allowed all the evaluations to be compared statistically. We tested this procedure by scoring 40 interviews from the verbal reports. Of these, 26 were selected at random, with the restriction that any applicant could only be used once. Profiles derived by one of us (LNG) from the verbal reports were compared to those obtained directly from interview material, using product-moment correlation. The correlation between these two sets of profiles was high ($r = 0.91$, $df = 24$, $p < .01$), suggesting that all the evaluations could be compared, including those not originally reported with EFA.

We examined all the interviews in terms of suitable–unsuitable decision, clinical descriptive features, and EFA profiles. We also analyzed the performance of the individual psychiatrists to see if their evaluations were truly comparable.

SUBJECTS (GENERAL)

In 1978–1979, 375 evaluations were conducted by three of the authors. Three hundred sixty-two evaluations had been performed in the past 2 years by a psychiatrist not involved in the study, and included some applicants who were subsequently to fall into our "repeater" group.

The applicants were predominantly young black men, 20–30 years of age, of lower socioeconomic class background. Many looked on civil service positions as a way of improving their economic status. Most applicants saw themselves as having achieved in spite of great obstacles, but wished they had gone further in school. Many had worked in various "security" or police-related jobs and a few related a life-long obsession with law enforcement work.

The applicants did not consider themselves to be psychiatrically ill, and most were considered to be functioning within a normal if not ideal range of adaptation. Certain psychopathologic features were frequently noted in the descriptive reports, however. The most prominent were: extreme defensiveness; hypomanic features; mild paranoid features; and subtle thinking disorders. A few subjects showed anxiety, depression or a variety of other characterological features. Although these clinical features were striking when present, they were hard to define and compare on the whole, and were also not consistent between interviews. Therefore the remainder of the discussion will focus on suitability–unsuitability and EFA scoring.

In the group of 375 applicants interviewed, there was no correlation between suitability–unsuitability and the age, sex, or race of subjects. Married, divorced, and separated individuals were significantly more likely than never-married to be found suitable ($\chi^2 = 16.22$; $df = 6$, $p < .01$). There were no differences between examiners on any of these parameters. Individuals with more than one interview had a significantly lower chance of being found suitable. Thus, 61% of applicants on a first interview were considered suitable, while only 40% were accepted on a second, third, or fourth interview ($\chi^2 = 33.5$; $df = 6$, $p < .00001$).

SUBJECTS SEEN MORE THAN ONCE ("REPEATERS")

The 36 "repeaters" accounted for 86 interviews. Some of these returned for evaluation after being found "suitable" and then failing on the job. These are the failures of psychiatric evaluation. Others were consistently rejected by the psychiatrists but continued to reapply for the same or other civil service positions. Still others were reevaluated for incidental reasons: applying for two different jobs; failing the preemployment polygraph test; unable to accept position; hiring freeze after subject was found suitable; and so on. Five subjects were initially rejected but on reapplication were felt to show "growth" or "maturation" and were then found suitable.

On the basis of the ratings, we divided our 36 subjects into three categories:

1. U-U, those found "Unsuitable" on all interviews
2. U-S, those found "Unsuitable" on some interviews, "Suitable" on others
3. S-S, those found "Suitable" on all interviews

Table 21.1 gives an overall survey of the 36 applicants interviewed more than once, their division into groups, and the mean EFA scores for each group. The mean disagreement between EFA score ratings (between interviews) is also included.

The table shows that exactly half the subjects were consistently rated as either suitable or unsuitable by all examiners. The remaining subjects were rated differently on different occasions. Examination of the mean EFA

Table 21.1.   Tabular Summary of the Cases

	S's	%	Interviews	%	Mean EFA Scores	Mean Disagreement
U-U	13	(36)	30	(35)	4.16	0.4
U-S	18	(50)	45	(52)	4.68	0.6
S-S	5	(14)	11	(13)	5.08	0.3

scores for these three groups suggests that the examiners were in fact discriminating between three groups of applicants: a well-functioning group who are consistently found suitable; a poorly functioning group who are consistently found unsuitable; and a large intermediate group of applicants in whom suitability is hard to decide. An analysis of variance shows these groups to be significantly different ($F = 15.6$, $df = 2$, $p < .05$).

We wished to know if any single component of EFA would be useful in discriminating suitable from unsuitable applicants. Among the five ego functions most often scored (i.e., Judgment, Sense of Reality, Regulation and Control, Thought Processes, and Defensive Functioning) we noted that Defensive Functioning showed the closest interrater agreement and seemed most likely to reflect pathological functioning. As defined by Bellak et al. (1973) Defensive Functioning is a complex construct that includes the protective limitation of awareness (and the adaptive cost thereof), as well as the effectiveness of such operations in warding off unpleasant and dysphoric feeling states. Thus, this function reflects "defensiveness" as seen in the interview, defensive style as reported by the subject, and the manifestations of the failures of defense such as anxiety and depression.

We found that mean scores for Defensive Functioning did clearly distinguish among our three outcome groups of "repeaters." The mean scores for Defensive Functioning for the U-U group was 3.96, for the U-S group 4.62, and for the S-S group 4.8. Again, an analysis of variance indicated that these scores could significantly discriminate "suitable" and "unsuitable" applicants ($F = 295$, $df = 2,33$; $p < .01$.). This finding lends statistical support to the clinical impression that Defensive Functioning can be a sensitive indicator even in subjects who are not otherwise very forthcoming (e.g., the individual who "never" gets anxious or upset, "never" worries, etc.).

RELIABILITY

We studied interrater reliability in the following way: for each of our 36 applicants we compared mean EFA scores for the last (most recent) and next to last interviews. The computed correlation coefficient, $r = 0.745$ ($df = 34$, $p < .01$), was higher than that attained by Bellak et al. for "normals," which seems remarkable for interviews conducted by different examiners at intervals of weeks to months.

We also examined the mean disagreements between interviews in scale points (see Table 21.1). Disagreement between examiners on mean EFA scores ranged from zero to 1.8 scale points, with a mean of 0.43. Decisions as to suitability were generally made within a range of 0.5–1 scale point. The distance from 4 to 5, in particular, often represented the difference between noticeable difficulties in coping and a mild "psychopathology of the average." When a number of functions are scored within this range, the decision as to suitability may indeed be difficult. Thus, when interviewers differ in their ratings by more than 0.5 scale points, and do so within this critical range, different decisions may well be reached. Perhaps this is an area where further refinement of the instrument can result in better discriminations.

Skilled examiners evaluating the same individual may also reach different conclusions because of subtle differences in strategy, interpretation, or philosophy. The use of a systematic technique such as EFA may help to reduce these differences or at least make them more accessible to study. In our own group we found, for example, a systematic tendency on the part of two examiners to reject any applicant interviewed previously ($\chi^2 = 12.85$; $df = 3$; $p < .01$). We assume that the discrepancies between examiners can be addressed and corrected so as to improve reliability. For this purpose the examiners continue to observe each others' interviews, compare their findings, and refine the interview and rating manuals.

DISCUSSION

Psychiatrists not only make refined behavioral observations but also use these observations to make important and determining decisions. While the psychiatric interview can generate persuasive data about an individual, its reliability and predictive value remain unproved (Harris et al., 1963). Following Meehl (1954), many workers have compared intuitive interviewing skills to the rigid application of statistical formulas, generally favoring the latter. While the clinician may devise the best evaluation strategy for a particular client, he may not follow his own strategy consistently (Hammond and Summers, 1972). Even skilled interviewers may tend to deny psychopathology in subjects who are likable or charming, or in those who seem to show "insight" or "growth."

Furthermore, the traditional mental status examination as commonly performed includes many questions and "tests" of doubtful validity (Rapp, 1979). Inordinate emphasis may be placed, for example, on the interpretation of proverbs or "similarities" or on the highly subjective appraisal of the patient's "associations." Many of these traditional procedures, designed for the very ill or regressed patient, add little to the assessment of partially treated, compensated, or subtle cases.

The authors in the present study were also subject to such factors as the needs of civil service, experiences with police officers, feelings about crime in their own community, and so on. These problems are particularly relevant when making fairly subtle discriminations as in our large intermediate group of applicants (the U-S group). In reviewing the reports we often found descriptive indicators of psychopathology, yet the examiner was reluctant to make a global judgment of "Unsuitable." Some of these applicants were accepted with reservations and later reappeared after doing poorly on the job.

In summary, our study represented a preliminary effort to improve the reliability of our psychiatric evaluations. Our findings suggest that the psychiatric interview can be a more reliable investigative tool than commonly thought, when conducted in a systematic, semiquantitative manner, using EFA. With a modified interview we found that we could adapt and extend the use of EFA to a relatively high-functioning, well-defended group of individuals, in the upper ranges of ego functioning. EFA appeared to generate reliable data between three different examiners overly fairly long intervals of time. We hope that with ongoing use, we will continue to improve the reliability of our evaluations, to delineate inconsistencies and systematic biases by our psychiatric interviewers, and to approach the whole evaluation process in a more objective and systematic manner.

ADDENDUM

We would like to supplement our remarks by treating one aspect of the EFA technique in a little more detail. Of the functions assessed by EFA, we found Reality Testing particularly difficult to evaluate in intact individuals who pride themselves on their grasp of reality. In clinical work it is an area of function that is often not even assessed in those patients who do not show obvious difficulties, such as hallucinations. In the course of our civil service study, we observed that Reality Testing is more accessible to questions that have no obvious "right" or "wrong" answers and that address process (How?) rather than outcome (e.g., Voices). The scale was not only helpful in evaluating our civil service applicants, but also extremely informative in the clinical assessment of patients with partly compensated, concealed, or subtle psychotic disturbances.

Four simple questions can be used to address the discrimination between inner and outer reality. The questions are asked as a set, and in the same precise way each time, so that the answers are comparable. The examiner can push for elaboration of the answers as needed:

1. How do you go about deciding if something really happened, or if you imagined it?
2. Suppose you were walking down the street and you heard someone call your name, but you didn't see anyone. How would you react?

3. Suppose you heard it again?
4. Have you noticed anything strange recently about the radio or TV programs?

Interpretation

These questions address the process by which an experience is checked to determine its origin. The process typically begins at a level out of awareness; only when uncertainty persists are increasingly active and conscious efforts required to locate the source of the experience. "Healthy" individuals know that the discrimination between inner and outer reality is reliable but not infallible and can enjoy challenging it, as in fantasy, drama, and perceptual illusions. The well-integrated individual may respond by repeating the question, or show some mild surprise, amusement, or thoughtfulness. Such a person's answers will reflect some kind of testing, checking, investigating, or hypothesis formation. If the experience continues, greater efforts will be made to explain it, but only to a point that does not interfere with other adaptive functions.

Mildly pathologic responses are characterized by discomfort or annoyance with the questions, defensiveness, or answers that are inflexible or dogmatic, or show selective perceptions (e.g., "I just know," "What's real is real," "I never imagine things").

Severe impairment (psychotic level response) may be characterized by dismay, confusion, or helplessness; admission that the individual does not know how to test his experiences; refusal to attempt such testing; or description of actual psychotic experiences.

Question 4 can elicit indicators of psychotic decompensation because radio, television and movies represent a sort of public fantasy—an intermediate area between inner and outer reality. Patients in the early stages of psychosis, who are beginning to lose the discrimination between the two realities, will often reply that they are receiving direct personal messages from these media or that the programs are specifically directed at themselves. This is an important clinical sign, easily elicited.

The reality testing questions may seem baffling or amusing to the normal individual, but to one who has been psychotic they strike close to home. Patients are often amazed at the examiner's acumen in asking these questions and are then more open to discussing strange experiences. To lose one's grasp on reality is a frightening experience. Many patients continue to be concerned about reality testing in spite of clinical remission. With modern, rapid treatment, patients may quickly "seal over" and deny symptoms, and "thought disorders" may no longer be evident. The persistence of tenuous reality testing may be an important guide to continuing treatment. Although the questions are posed in theoretical terms, these patients respond with vivid personal accounts of psychotic experience.

Clinical Validation

As a preliminary clinical check on the validity of the questions, we obtained answers to the first three questions from a group of 10 "normals" (subjects found suitable for civil service positions) and 10 psychiatric outpatients with a documented past history (or current complaints) of psychotic experience (i.e., delusions or hallucinations). Most of these patients were asymptomatic and socially intact at the time of examination. Most of them would meet DSM-III criteria for schizophrenia or paranoid disorders, in remission.

Answers to the questions were rated blindly by three experienced interviewers, faculty members in the L.S.U. Department of Psychiatry who were not familiar with the questions or with EFA. These raters were able to discriminate the responses of the "psychotic" from the "normal" individuals with a mean accuracy of 82%.

Scoring

Scoring norms from Stops 3 through 6 are given in Table 21.2 showing how we rate the answers to our four questions. These are modified from Bellak et al. (1973), with clinical examples from our own experience.

Table 21.2. Rating Stops for Reality Testing

Stop	Description
6	*S*. is comfortable, shows some thoughtful silence or mild amusement, and gives answers that reflect testing, checking, investigation, or the entertaining of many hypotheses.
5	*S*. is mildly defensive, uncomfortable, or annoyed with the questions, or shows rather limited efforts to investigate, few hypotheses.
4	Answers reflect rigid construction of reality, selective perceptions, inability to entertain more than one hypothesis, or need to be absolutely in touch with things (e.g., "I just know," "What's real is real" or "Just ignore it").
3	*S*. may be aware that he or she sees or hears things that are not there but knows that others do not . . . OR distortions and misinterpretations of reality under provoking circumstances . . . OR *S*. may be quite upset when unable to discriminate realities or may give up (e.g., "I wouldn't know what to do!" or "I'd go see a Doctor!").

REFERENCES

Bellak, L., Hurvich, M., & Gediman, H. K. *Ego functions in schizophrenics, neurotics, and normals: A systematic study of conceptual diagnostic and therapeutic aspects.* New York: Wiley, 1973.

Hammond, K. R., & Summer, D. A. Cognitive control. *Psychological Bulletin,* 1972, 79(1), 58–67.

Harris, M. R., Fisher, J., & Epstein, L. J. The reliability of the interview in psychiatric assessment for job placement. *Comprehensive Psychiatry,* 1963, 4(1), 19–28.

Meehl, P. E. *Clinical versus statistical prediction: A theoretical analysis and a review of the evidence.* Minneapolis: University of Minnesota Press, 1972.

Rapp, M. S. Reexamination of the clinical mental status examination. *Canadian Journal of Psychiatry,* 1979, 24(8), 773–75.

CHAPTER TWENTY-TWO

Ego Functioning and the Vocational Rehabilitation of Schizophrenic Clients

JEAN A. CIARDIELLO, MYRA E. KLEIN, AND SHAWN SOBKOWSKI

Despite the vocational rehabilitation efforts of the past 20 years, reports in the literature have shown that as many as two-thirds of discharged chronic mental patients remain unemployed (Evje et al., 1972). In 1965 the research unit of the Veterans Administration conducted one of the most extensive studies of the vocational rehabilitation of the chronically mentally ill. Over 3600 schizophrenic patients under 60 years of age who had been discharged from hospitals 6 months earlier were questioned. Two-thirds reported working 1 month or less, and only 14% had worked five months or more (V.A., 1965). Addressing a similar question experimentally, Griffiths (1974) tested the effectiveness of vocational rehabilitation by randomly assigning 56 schizophrenic subjects to treatment and control groups. After 15 months, assessments revealed no significant differences between those who had participated in the vocational rehabilitation program and those who had not. Based on these results, Griffiths (1974) concluded that rehabilitation had no detectable effects on schizophrenic subjects. Even within sheltered workshops, schizophrenic clients were two to three times less likely to be placed in competitive employment than individuals with other disabilities (Ciardiello, 1981a). The National Institute of Handicapped Research (1979) concluded that "although mentally disabled clients make up the largest number of cases eligible for vocational rehabilitation services, they have the least probability of success before and after rehabilitation" (p. 1).

Although it is clear that rehabilitation programs serving schizophrenic clients have had a great deal of difficulty meeting their vocational objectives, the reasons for this lack of success are unclear. Several variables have been identified as predictive of rehabilitation outcome. Watts and Po-Kwan (1976) and Griffiths (1974) found that low self-esteem was one of the best predictors of vocational rehabilitation outcome and was invariably associated with unemployment in former psychiatric patients. Feared loss of disability benefits (Gunn, 1975), motivation to work (Searls et al., 1970; Griffiths et al., 1974), realism of vocational choice (Patterson, 1957; Searls et al., 1970), the inconsistency between aptitude patterns and available employment opportunities (Ciardiello, 1981a), and certain biographical data have also been cited as significant variables in the vocational rehabilitation of schizophrenic persons.

Past failures to rehabilitate schizophrenic clients vocationally and the results of rehabilitation outcome research underscore the need to understand more about the ways in which the schizophrenic disability impairs vocational functioning and frustrates the efforts of rehabilitation programs to return disabled persons to the work force. A better understanding of the vocational functioning of schizophrenic persons has important implications for the rehabilitation process. If critical variables can be identified, an assessment strategy can be devised to determine which clients are most likely to benefit from specific program interventions and which interventions are most likely to facilitate their vocational success.

EGO FUNCTIONING

In general terms, Freud conceptualized ego functioning as reflected in an individual's ability to love and to work. According to Freud's structural theory of personality, the ego is the central integrating core of the personality, mediating between the inner demands of the id and superego and outer demands from the environment. Therefore, successful work selection and performance can be seen as requiring a complex set of ego functions that effectively integrate the self and the world of work.

Bellak and Loeb (1969), Federn (1952), and many others who are psychoanalytically oriented, view schizophrenia as primarily an ego dysfunction. When early ego development has been seriously impaired, the result is often a schizophrenic syndrome characterized by regressive and restitutional symptoms that often include depersonalization, passivity, disordered thinking, delusions, and hallucinations. Although these symptoms can be controlled to some extent in some patients with the use of chemotherapy, the important functions of the ego rarely escape severe impairments. The changing realities of the work world often place strenuous demands on the ego to achieve high levels of adaptive, integrative, and autonomous functioning. These stressors present a challenge to the normal ego, and it seems likely that the impaired ego of the schizophrenic person would experience a great deal of difficulty coping with vocational demands (Ciardiello & Bingham, 1982).

Hartmann (1950) noted that although ego weaknesses are characteristic of schizophrenic patients, specific ego functions are differentially affected. The vocational difficulties of schizophrenic persons can be clarified by relating specific ego functions to their roles in work selection and performance. For instance, flexibility and adaptability is important in work because even the most routine jobs do not remain unchanged over time. Supervisors come and go, machinery is modernized, schedules change, new products are assembled, and the reactions and requests of customers vary. Rigid adherence to former thought patterns and failure to adapt to the requirements of a new job situation can seriously hinder work performance. Thus, adaptive regression in the service of the ego (ARISE) can have important implications for vocational functioning, particularly in variable work environments. Individuals whose ARISE capability is poor would be more likely to succeed in a work environment in which there were few changes and least likely to succeed in variable work settings. A low ARISE capacity would also suggest that the person would have difficulty making realistic vocational choices that took new information about themselves or an occupational alternative into account. Similarly, other specific deficits in ego functioning have some predictable vocational consequences. In brief, inadequate reality testing often results in delusions and/or hallucinations that can make it almost impossible for the individual to concentrate on work tasks. Poor judgment is likely to lead to inappropriate responses to supervisors and co-workers, and inaccurate estimations of the time and resources needed to complete a work assignment. The ability to follow directions, benefit from feedback, and work cooperativity with others is often impaired by exaggerated or inadequate boundaries resulting from disturbances in the individual's sense of reality of the world and of the self. Various dimensions of autonomous functioning—attention, concentration, memory, learning, perception, motor functioning, language skills, habit patterns and intention—are the essential aspects of work itself. The remaining ego functions—object relations, impulse control, thought processes, defensive functioning, stimulus barrier, synthetic functioning, and mastery–competence also can be seen to have important and often obvious effects on work performance and selection.

When the employment difficulties of schizophrenic individuals are viewed in terms of specific ego functioning patterns, a clearer and more comprehensive theoretical picture of their vocational strengths and weaknesses begins to emerge. However, there are several important empirical questions that are unanswered: (1) Do schizophrenic persons who are employed have higher levels of ego functioning than those who are unemployed? (2) Are certain specific ego functions more important than others in the successful vocational rehabilitation of schizophrenic individuals? (3) Do schizophrenic individuals with higher levels of ego functioning report less psychiatric symptomotology and higher levels of general and vocational functioning than individuals exhibiting lower levels of ego functioning? These questions were investigated in the following preliminary study of ego functioning and the vocational rehabilitation of schizophrenic clients.

PROCEDURE

As part of a 3-year research project that focused on the vocational assessment and rehabilitation of the chronically mentally ill, 30 schizophrenic clients enrolled in a psychosocial rehabilitation program were interviewed for 3 or 4 hours over several sessions by specially trained, master's-level psychologists. All the subjects had been diagnosed as schizophrenic (by clinical records and a reevaluating clinician) and the predominant subtypes were chronic undifferentiated (57%) and paranoid (33%); 40% were female and 60% male; the mean age was 32 years; 90% were white and 10% were black; 63% had some paid work experience (usually program assisted) during the 6 months prior to the interview and 43% were employed for some time during the month of the assessment.

In part, the interview consisted of a detailed employment history, Bellak's (1973) Ego Functioning Scale, the SCL-90 (Deragotis, 1977), and the Katz Social Adjustment Scale (Katz and Lyerly, 1963). The Ego Functioning Scale is a structured interview developed by Bellak et al. (1973) for the clinical assessment of ego functions. Each subject was given four global ratings from 1 to 7 (with half points) for each of the 12 dimensions of ego functioning. Scoring was done from the recorded interviews and current, characteristic, highest and lowest levels of ego functioning were rated for each dimension. The SCL-90 is a 90-item, self-report symptom inventory developed by the Clinical Psychometrics Research Unit of Johns Hopkins University to measure the psychological symptom patterns of psychiatric and medical patients. The Katz Social Adjustment Scale was developed in conjunction with the forerunner of the SCL-90 to assess those aspects of general functioning in the "normal" adult world that did not fall within the traditional notion of psychiatric symptoms. The two Katz scales used were the Activities of Daily Living (ADL) and Leisure Time Activities (LTA) Scales. The reliability and validity of each of these instruments for schizophrenic subjects are well documented. In addition, psychometric monitoring of these instruments during the course of the project supported their reliability and validity for research purposes (Ciardiello & Turner, 1980).

The data were analyzed using regression techniques to test the relationships among the variables of interest and a discriminant function analysis was used to determine if current ego function ratings could be used to classify schizophrenic subjects as presently employed or unemployed.

RESULTS AND DISCUSSION

Scores for 30 schizophrenic subjects on each of the 12 dimensions of characteristic ego functioning ranged from 2 to 6, with most scores falling between 4 and 5, with a grand mean of 4.2 and a standard deviation of 1. Compared to Bellak's (1973) group of 50 schizophrenic subjects, the present sample showed lower overall levels of ego functioning and less variability in their scores. Intercorrelations among the 12 scales were significant in almost every instance and higher than those reported by Bellak et al. (1973). These differences probably reflected the facts that Bellak's sample consisted of acute schizophrenic inpatients, whereas the subjects in the present investigation were chronic outpatients attending a rehabilitation day program.

High scale score intercorrelations indicated that each of the ego function scales was not operating independently. To identify the independent dimensions of ego functioning for chronic schizophrenic subjects, the 12 scale scores were factor analyzed using a varimax rotation and the principal components method. Although the sample size was small, it met Cattell's (1966) recommended criteria of a 2.5 subject-to-variable ratio (30 : 12). Results of the factor analysis are reported in Table 22.1. Three factors were identified that explained 79% of the variance in the ego function scores. The first factor explained 62% of the variance and consisted of 8 of the 12 scales. Factor I overlapped Factor II by sharing loadings for the Reality Testing, Judgment, Sense of Reality, and Autonomous Functioning scales; Factors II and III shared the Defensive Functioning scale; and Factors I and II overlapped on ARISE. The scales shared by Factors I and III, supported the notion of Rapaport (1951) and others that reality testing, judgment, and sense of reality can be considered aspects of autonomous functioning. The overlap in scales can also be attributed to the chronicity of the sample, and greater differentiation of ego functions would be expected in individuals who had not suffered from severe and chronic ego impairments.

Examining the factor structures, the three conceptual dimensions of ego functioning are not evident unless the factors are viewed in terms of their general functional consequences. Which factor or set of ego functions reflects a schizophrenic individual's ability to love and which factor is related to his or her ability to work? The ego functions in Factor I combined reality orientation, autonomous, adaptive, and integrative functions, as well as mastery–competence, which are essential for survival in the work world. While Factor III included reality orientation and autonomous functioning, it

Table 22.1.   Factor Analysis of Characteristic Ego Function Scores for 30 Schizophrenic Clients

Ego Function Factor	Factor Loadings	Eigen Values	Explained Variance (%)
I. Reality Testing	.698	7.45	62
Judgment	.696		
Sense of Reality	.546		
Thought Processes	.815		
ARISE	.594		
Autonomous Functioning	.676		
Synthetic Functioning	.767		
Mastery–Competence	.825		
II. Regulation and Control	.801	1.25	10
ARISE	.517		
Defensive Functioning	.536		
Stimulus Barrier	.803		
III. Reality Testing	.616	.82	7
Judgment	.627		
Sense of Reality	.684		
Object Relations	.802		
Defensive Functioning	.746		
Autonomous Functioning	.408		

Note: Loadings of .400 or greater were used to determine factor inclusion.

also included object relations and defensive functioning. Thus, Factor III included the ego functions that seem to be related to successful social adjustment.

The second factor was made up of regulation and control of impulses, affects and drives, ARISE, defensive functioning, and stimulus barrier. The common element that seems to link this set of ego functions is that they can provide protection against threats to the individual from within and from without. Some of these adaptations and defenses include: the person's ability to tolerate anxiety, depression, and frustration and to regulate sexual impulses; and the ability to use defense mechanisms adaptively so that anxiety is warded off without symptom formation. Maintaining an effective stimulus barrier protects the individual against trauma and aversive external stimulation; and the ARISE capability allows the schizophrenic person to recover from temporary regressions and use them adaptively, instead of becoming uncontrollably psychotic. In essence, Factor II ego functions work together to deal with internal and external threats so that they do not result in psychiatric symptoms.

Summarizing the face validity of these three ego functioning factors for schizophrenic clients, Factor I included ego functions related to vocational functioning, Factor II consisted of defensive ego functions that inhibit the formation of psychiatric symptoms, and Factor III was made up of ego functions that appear to have important roles in social adjustment. To test the face validity of these factors and to determine their construct and con-current validity, factor scores were used to discriminate employed and un-employed schizophrenic clients; and ego function factor scores were correl-ated with measures of psychiatric symptom distress (SCL-90) and social adjustment (Katz).

As expected, Ego Function Factor I was successful in correctly classify-ing 84% of the schizophrenic subjects as employed for any length of time during the 6 months prior to the assessment. Wilks' Lambda for the discrimi-nant function analysis was .60 and was significant at the .0002 level. Current ego functioning scores for individual scales were also used to discriminate between schizophrenic subjects who had any paid work experience during the month of the assessment. Two specific ego function scores were found to achieve greater than chance discriminations. Autonomous functioning (Wilks' Lambda = .70, $p < .002$) and ARISE (Wilks' Lambda = .63, $p < .002$) correctly classified as currently employed or unemployed a total of 70% of the cases. The results of these three discriminant function analyses are reported in Table 22.2.

It is not surprising that autonomous functioning was found to be an impor-tant variable in work performance. Autonomous ego functions such as habit patterns, skills, routines, interests, learning, intentionality, and motility have central roles in work and, as Bellak et al. (1973) noted, impaired auton-omous functioning may result in difficulty in carrying out one's usual job or the complete inability to work. The importance of ARISE in work perfor-mance has been previously illustrated; however, there are two aspects of ARISE that may make it particularly relevant in understanding the voca-tional adjustment of chronic schizophrenic clients. Using the broad, adap-tive sense of ARISE, this ego function not only permits greater flexibility in meeting the demands of a job, but also gives the individual creative alterna-tive strategies to deal with the schizophrenic disability itself, so that it is less

Table 22.2. *Discriminant Function Analysis Using Ego Functioning Scores to Discriminate the Employment Status of 30 Schizophrenic Clients*

Significant Ego Function Variable	Wilks' Lambda	Sig.	Rao's V	Sig.	Change in V	Sig.
Factor I	.60	.0002	18.48	.00001	18.48	.00001
Autonomous Functioning	.70	.002	11.89	.001	11.89	.001
ARISE	.63	.002	16.14	.001	4.25	.039

likely to interfere with vocational functioning. In other words, the individual with a high ARISE score is not only better able to adapt to the demands of work, but is also better able to adjust to the disabling effects of schizophrenia. A related idea, suggested by Bellak et al. (1973), was that adaptive regressions in the service of the ego may also serve to maintain a flexibility of ego functions themselves, so that autonomous ego functioning is not disrupted under stress. Ego impairments tend to be more discrete when the structure of the ego is less rigid and there are a number of different ways and ego functions available to meet the demands of everyday life. This type of successful adjustment to mental illness and ego adaptability is exemplified by a schizophrenic worker whose sense of reality warns that his impulse control is very poor on a given day. Good judgment tells him that if he goes to work he will become uncontrollably angry with his boss and the consequences may be unemployment and/or hospitalization. Successful functioning was maintained by seeing absence from work as an adaptive way to deal with poor impulse control and requesting that his supervisor allow him to take a vacation day. In this case ARISE was useful in adjusting to work and preventing his anger from overrunning his other ego functions resulting in further decompensation.

Turning to Factor II, previous studies (Ciardiello & Turner, 1980; Ciardiello et al., 1981) failed to demonstrate significant relationships between psychiatric symptomatology and vocational functioning. These findings were consistent with the finding of the present study that seven of the nine SCL-90 subscales were correlated significantly with ego function Factor II and only two subscales (Paranoid Ideation and Psychoticism) were correlated significantly with Factor I. For chronic schizophrenic subjects, vocational functioning was a separate dimension of ego functioning that was independent of the ability to deal with internal and external threats without symptom formation. The correlation matrix in Table 22.3 illustrates the significant negative relationships between Ego Function Factor II and SCL-90 subscales; correlation coefficients ranged from $-.45$ for the Anxiety scale to $-.29$ for Psychoticism.

Psychoticism ($-.29$), Interpersonal Sensitivity ($-.29$), and the Katz Social Adjustment Scale ($-.40$) correlated significantly with Ego Function Factor III. Since this was a chronic schizophrenic sample, it is not surprising that psychoticism was related to each of the three ego function factors. The significant correlations with the interpersonal scale of the SCL-90 and the Katz Social Adjustment Scale supported the hypothesis that Factor III reflected those aspects of ego functioning that are important in the social adjustment of chronic schizophrenic clients. Although Factor III was found to be functionally independent of the other factors, it overlapped on four ego functions (Reality Testing, Judgment, Sense of Reality, and Autonomous functioning) with Factor I. Again, this finding is consistent with the significant relationship between employment status and scores on the Katz ADL scale (Ciardiello, 1981b). Therefore, social and vocational functioning in

Table 22.3.   Correlations between Ego Function Scores and the SCL-90/Katz for 29 Schizophrenic Clients

SCL-90/Katz Scales	Ego Function Factor I	Ego Function Factor II	Ego Function Factor III
SCL-90			
Somatization	−.27	−.22	.06
Obsessive-Compulsive	−.23	−.36	−.18
Interpersonal Sensitivity	−.18	−.38	−.29
Depression	−.18	−.43	−.24
Anxiety	−.22	−.45	−.28
Hostility	−.21	−.40	−.09
Phobic Anxiety	−.21	−.41	−.08
Paranoid Ideation	−.33	−.23	−.20
Psychoticism	−.29	−.29	−.29
KATZ			
Activities of Daily Living (ADL)	−.01	−.00	.40

Note: Italic values are significant at the .05 level.

schizophrenic clients have certain ego functions in common, as well as ego functions that appear to be unique to each.

In general, significant relationships were found between Ego Function Factor I and employment status; Factor II and the SCL-90 scales; and Factor III and the Katz Social Adjustment Scale. Although there was some overlap in ego functions, the three factors were found to be functionally independent. These findings suggest that chronic schizophrenic clients use a different set of ego functions in work than are needed to maintain mental health. Possibly this differential use of ego functions explains previous findings that some schizophrenic clients reported considerable psychiatric symptomotology, but remained employed. Since Factors I and III shared several ego functions, the different roles of these functions in the social and vocational rehabilitation of schizophrenic clients was less clear. However, if the three factors identified in this study are found to be reliable and valid in other studies with chronic schizophrenic subjects, then perhaps the factor overlap can be viewed as reflecting the multipurpose nature of ego functions and possibly some compensatory functioning that results from chronic ego impairment.

CONCLUSIONS AND IMPLICATIONS FOR REHABILITATION

Three different sets of ego functions have been identified as having important and differential impacts on the mental health and functioning of chronic schizophrenic clients. If these three characteristic ego function factors are found and validated by others studying comparable subjects, there are several ways that ego function assessment can be useful in the rehabilitation process.

Assessing a client's ego strengths and deficits using Bellak et al.'s (1973) Ego Functioning Scale will generate a profile that can be used in individual rehabilitation planning. Program interventions can be focused to address specific ego function deficits, particularly those that are interfering with the ability to work. Bellak et al. (1973) outlined strategies for improving each of the 12 ego functions. Bellak and Black (1960) have emphasized that the ego functions of psychotic persons in the community can be substantially improved by devising interventions and experiences that make maximal use of ego strengths to remediate ego deficits. For instance, an autonomous function, like an interest in automobile mechanics, can be used to improve object relations by meeting others with the same interest and working together to repair a car.

According to the results of the present study, several ego functions (Factor I) were related to successful vocational functioning. Higher levels of autonomous functioning and ARISE were found to be associated with employment for most schizophrenic clients. Therefore, these two ego functions have particular importance in the vocational rehabilitation process and should be the focus of program interventions geared to returning clients to the work force. Along with Factor I scores, clients' scores on the autonomous functioning and ARISE scales can also be used as measures of work readiness.

In addition to identifying the ego functioning patterns of clients, jobs can also be analyzed in terms of the varying degrees to which specific ego functions are required. It seems likely that schizophrenic clients have a greater chance to achieve vocational success in those jobs that place demands on their ego strengths, rather than their weaknesses. Therefore, congruence between the ego functioning profiles of jobs and clients is an important consideration in work selection. Similarly, vocational rehabilitation programs that offer sheltered employment are often able to structure jobs so that they are consistent with an individual's pattern of ego functioning. For instance, a schizophrenic client with poor object relations, some impairment in autonomous functioning, and good judgment and reality testing can probably be successfully employed as a night security person at a warehouse.

Ego function assessments can also serve as a guide to the selection of prevocational activities that will improve ego functioning and work readiness. Whether clients are work ready or not, program interventions that improve certain sets of ego functions of schizophrenic clients can be expected to improve their mental health, social functioning, and ability to engage in the activities of daily living. Gains in ego functioning not only improve a schizophrenic clients' chances to achieve vocational success, but also enhance functioning in other life roles and, thus, improve the general quality of their lives.

Lastly, ego function assessment can be used to evaluate the progress of individual clients in achieving rehabilitation goals. On a program level, results of the ego function assessment can be used to evaluate the outcome and impact of rehabilitation programs. Ego function assessment also has an important role in future research that evaluates the relative effectiveness of rehabilitation strategies to improve the ego functions of schizophrenic clients. In addition, a reliable and valid assessment of ego functions offers a comprehensive way to conceptualize the vocational difficulties of schizophrenic clients and an effective strategy to evaluate the solutions offered by rehabilitation programs.

ACKNOWLEDGMENTS

This project was funded by research grants from the New Jersey Department of Education, Division of Vocational Education and Career Preparation (SREG 808/116), and the University of Medicine and Dentistry of New Jersey, Community Mental Health Center of Rutgers Medical School. Special thanks to Michael Gara, Ph.D. for his assistance in analyzing the data and to Roberta Waller for her help preparing the manuscript.

REFERENCES

Bellak, L., & Black, B. The rehabilitation of psychotics in the community. *American Journal of Orthopsychiatry,* 1960, *30,* 346–355.

Bellak, L., Hurvich, M., & Gediman, H. *Ego functions in schizophrenics, neurotics and normals: A systematic study of conceptual, diagnostic, and therapeutic aspects.* New York: Wiley, 1973.

Bellak, L., & Loeb, I. *The schizophrenic syndrome.* New York: Grune & Stratton, 1969.

Cattell, R. B. The meaning and strategic use of factor analysis. In R. B. Cattell (Ed.), *Handbook of multivariate experimental psychology.* Chicago: Rand McNally, 1966.

Ciardiello, J. A. Job placement success of schizophrenic clients in sheltered workshop programs. *Vocational Evaluation and Work Adjustment Bulletin,* 1981a, *14*(3), 125–128.

Ciardiello, J. A. *A path model to predict the employment status of psychiatrically disabled clients.* Unpublished doctoral dissertation, Rutgers, The State University, 1981b.

Ciardiello, J. A., & Bingham, W. C. The career maturity of schizophrenic clients. *Rehabilitation Counseling Bulletin,* 1982, *26*(1), 3–9.

Ciardiello, J. A., & Turner, F. D. *Final report of the vocational assessment project* (SREG 808). Trenton, N.J.: Department of Education, Division of Vocational Education and Career Preparation, 1980.

Ciardiello, J. A., Klein, M. E., & Sobkowski, S. *Final report of the vocational rehabilitation project—Part I* (SREG 116). Trenton, N.J.: Department of Education, Division of Vocational Education and Career Preparation, 1981.

Deragotis, L. R. *SCL-90 revised version manual—I*. Baltimore: Johns Hopkins University School of Medicine, Clinical Psychometrics Research Unit, 1977.

Evje, M., Bellander, I., Gibby, M., & Palmer, I. S. Evaluating protected hospital employment of chronic psychiatric patients. *Hospital and Community Psychiatry*, 1972, *23*, 24–28.

Federn, P. *Ego psychology and the psychoses*. New York: Basic Books, 1952.

Griffiths, R. D. Rehabilitation of chronic psychotic patients: An assessment of their psychological handicap, an evaluation of the effectiveness of rehabilitation and observations of the factors which predict outcome. *Psychological Medicine*, 1974, *4*, 316–325.

Griffiths, R. D., Hodgson, R., & Hallam, R. Structured interview for the assessment of work-related attitudes in psychiatric patients: Preliminary findings. *Psychological Medicine*, 1974, *4*, 326–333.

Gunn, R. L. Special problems in work adjustment of the mentally ill. In R. E. Hardy & J. G. Cull (Eds.), *Modifications of behavior of the mentally ill: Applied principles*. Springfield, Ill.: C. C. Thomas, 1975.

Hartmann, H. (Ed.) Comments on the psychoanalytic theory of the ego (1950). In *Essays and Ego Psychology*. New York: International Universities Press, 1964.

Katz, M. M., & Lyerly, S. B. Methods for measuring adjustment and social behavior in the community: I. Rationale, description, discriminative validity and scale development. *Psychological Reports*, 1963, *13*(2), 503–535.

National Institute of Handicapped Research, Department of Health, Education and Welfare, Post-employment services aid mentally disabled clients. *Rehabilitation Brief: Bringing Rehabilitation into Effective Focus*, 1979, *6*(2), 1.

Patterson, C. H. Interests and the emotionally disturbed client. *Educational and Psychological Measurement*, 1957, *17*, 264–280.

Rapaport, D. The autonomy of the ego. *Bulletin of the Menninger Clinic*, 1951, *15*, 113–123.

Searls, D. J., Lowell, T. W., & Miskinins, R. W. Development of a measure of unemployability among restored psychiatric patients. *Journal of Counseling Psychology*, 1970, 223–225.

Veterans Administration. To work again, to live again: The vocational rehabilitation of homebound veterans. Washington, D.C.: Veterans Administration, Department of Veterans Benefits, 1965, VA pamphlet 21-65-1.

Watts, F. N., & Po-Kwan, Y. The structure of attitudes in psychiatric rehabilitation. *Journal of Occupational Psychology*, 1976, *49*, 39–44.

CHAPTER TWENTY-THREE

Ego Function Profiles of Manic-Depressives in Remission

JONETTE MUSZYNSKI SAWYER

Over the years mental health professionals have conceptualized, diagnosed, and treated manic-depressive illness from a variety of theoretical frameworks. Some of the major frameworks have included psychoanalytic, interpersonal, behavioral, and biological models. In recent years the biological framework has become the model of choice in the treatment of manic-depressive illness. The effectiveness of chemotherapeutic agents, particularly lithium carbonate, has provided support for this model (APA, 1975; Prien, 1979).

A survey of the literature suggests that the most appropriate treatment for manic-depressive individuals is a combination of chemotherapy and psychotherapy (Klerman, 1978). Hence, the need for a specific psychological model for the assessment, diagnosis, and treatment of manic-depressive individuals is indicated.

Independent of the biological model is the ego psychological model of manic-depressive illness. Bellak (1952) theorized that, as in schizophrenia, the outstanding factor in manic-depressive illness is a weakness of the ego. Efforts to quantify ego strength culminated in a study that assessed 12 ego functions in schizophrenics, neurotics, and normals (Bellak et al., 1973).

Ego psychology has provided, through the delineation of 12 ego functions, a model for describing an individual's behavior.

The ego function assessment of manic-depressives is in its beginning stages (see Schwindl et al., this volume). It has been suggested that the manic-depressive profile would show less severe disturbances of reality testing and judgment when compared to a schizophrenic sample and reveal little impairment of thought processes. The manic-depressives also would manifest marked fluctuations between highest and lowest level of impulse control and possibly on object relations and defenses (Bellak et al., 1973).

Although many manic-depressives are maintained in remission through the use of chemotherapeutic agents, relatively little is known about the psychological functioning of manic-depressives in remission. Psychoanalytic theorists identified an abnormal dependent character formation in the manic-depressive in remission (Abraham, 1924; Cohen et al., 1954; Freud, 1915). The personality patterns of manic-depressives have been found to demonstrate dependency drives, the orientation of values in terms of what others think, difficulty in dealing with feelings of envy and competitiveness, insensitivity to the feelings of others, social awkwardness, explosive temper, a tendency toward externalization, and the use of denial as a major defense (Gibson et al., 1959; Stone, 1978). Inadequate social adjustment has been shown in studies of the clinical course in manic-depressive illness as well (Bratfos & Haug, 1968; Carlson et al., 1974; Hastings, 1958; Shobe & Brion, 1971; Welner et al., 1977; Winokur et al. 1969).

In contrast, Kraepelin (1921), supported by Lundquist (1945), concluded that manic-depressive illness held a uniform benign prognosis with a complete return to normal functioning between episodes. Recent studies evaluating the effect of lithium carbonate have shown that manic-depressives, when responding well to lithium carbonate, do not want or require psychotherapy during their remissions (Dunner et al., 1978; Fieve & Dunner, 1975; Kerry & Orme, 1979; MacVane et al., 1978).

This study attempted to (1) utilize an ego psychological framework to assess the ego functions of manic-depressives in remission, (2) identify patterns in their ego function profiles, and (3) discuss the potential utility of the ego psychological model in clinical practice. The hypothesis was that the ego function profiles of manic-depressives in remission would demonstrate lowest functioning in the areas of (1) reality testing, (2) judgment, (3) regulation and control of drives, affects, and impulses, (4) object relations, and (5) defensive functioning.

METHODOLOGY

Subjects

The subjects were 22 manic-depressives in remission. A computer printout of all patients served by a community mental health center (CMHC) was obtained. The printout included a population of 53 individuals who were diagnosed as manic-depressive according to the *Diagnostic and Statistical Manual of Mental Disorders,* 2d ed. (APA, 1968). A chart review determined those manic-depressive individuals eligible for admission to the study. The selection criteria included: (1) mania substantiated by the chart documentation of excessive elation, irritability, talkativeness, flight of ideas, and accelerated speech and motor activity, (2) depression substantiated by the chart documentation of severely depressed mood, mental and motor retardation, uneasiness, apprehension, perplexity, and agitation, and (3) exclusion of those individuals diagnosed manic-depressive on a major tranquilizer alone. The inclusion of other depressive disorders (e.g., depressive neurosis, psychotic depressive reaction, and involutional melancholia) was prevented by additional selection criteria for the depressed type of manic-depressive. The depressed type of manic-depressive was admitted to the study if the chart review indicated: (1) the absence of precipitating factors that could be considered under the generality of stress and/or loss, (2) evidence of more than one depression, and/or (3) maintenance on lithium carbonate. Remission was defined as not exhibiting signs of clinical mania or depression requiring inpatient treatment. The sample selection criteria was met by 36 out of 53 manic-depressive individuals. Six subjects refused to participate and seven could not be contacted. The sample included 23 manic-depressive individuals. One subject did not meet the criteria for remission and, therefore, only 22 subjects were utilized in the data analysis.

Instrument

The Abbreviated Clinical Assessment of Ego Functions (ACAEF) is a shortened version of the Clinical Assessment of Ego Functions (Bellak et al., 1973). A structured interview format* was used to assess the current adaptive level of the 12 ego functions. The assessment of the individual ego functions was composed of 10 questions, each of which had three possible answers (1) rarely, (2) sometimes, or (3) often. The value range for the questions was from 0 to 2. A total score of 20 was possible for each ego function, indicating the highest level of adaptive functioning. A score of 0 indicated the lowest level of adaptive functioning.

In addition to the ACAEF, demographic and psychological data were obtained. These included age, sex, race, marital status, religion, educational level, occupation, combined income of all adults in the household, urban/rural dweller, living alone/with others, current psychotherapy, current chemotherapy, length of illness, and history of mental illness in the family of origin.

---

* This procedure is basically a questionnaire. Refer to Part 5 of present volume for a discussion of this method.

Procedure

The ACAEF interview schedule was administered by the investigator to 23 manic-depressive individuals, one of whom did not meet the criteria for remission. Interviews were conducted at the CMHC where the subjects normally receive their care. At the beginning of the interview a detailed explanation of the study was given. If the subject chose to participate, an informed consent form was signed.

The structured interview process was begun by eliciting demographic and psychological data not available in the charts. The ACAEF was then used to elicit and record information. Each interview took between 45 and 60 minutes. Scoring was done following the interview and took another 5 minutes. The total process took between 50 to 65 minutes per subject.

RESULTS AND DISCUSSION

The analysis of demographic and psychological data on the 22 manic-depressives in remission yielded some interesting information. The assessment of educational level showed that only 5% had less than a high school education, while 32% had more than a high school education. Only 9% of the total number of subjects were unable to work due to mental disability.

Out of the total number of subjects, 77% were treated with lithium alone or lithium in combination with another chemotherapeutic agent. All the subjects on medication were seeing a psychiatrist for medication assessment at least once every 3 months.

An assessment of current psychotherapy showed that 36% of the subjects were not involved in psychotherapy, while 64% were involved in individual psychotherapy. The frequency of the individual therapy sessions ranged from once every 2 weeks to once a month. It is interesting to note that none of the subjects were involved in group, family, couples, or other forms of psychotherapy.

A two-way analysis of variance for a randomized block design was used to assess differences in the 12 ego functions. Differences were observed at a statistically significant level ($p < .0001$), implying that there is strong evidence to indicate differences in the scores of the 12 ego functions. Duncan's multiple range test was then used to determine differences in the mean scores of the 12 ego functions. The mean scores from highest to lowest for each of the 12 ego functions are presented in Table 23.1.

The investigator's hypothesis that manic-depressive individuals in remission would demonstrate lowest functioning in (1) reality testing, (2) judgment; (3) regulation and control of drives, affects, and impulses; (4) object relations; and (5) defensive functioning was not found to be statistically significant.

As a group, the manic-depressive individuals in remission interviewed in

Table 23.1.   Ego Function Mean Scores

Ego Function	Mean Score
Reality Testing	18.5
Sense of Reality of the World and of the Self	18.4
Object Relations	16.7
Thought Processes	16.1
Judgment	16.0
Regulation and Control of Drives, Affects, and Impulses	15.6
Synthetic–Integrative Functioning	15.3
Defensive Functioning	15.2
Autonomous Functioning	15.1
Mastery–Competence	13.6
Stimulus Barrier	13.5
ARISE	10.0

Note: Any two scores that are not connected by vertical lines are significantly different.

this study demonstrated highest ego functioning ($p < .05$) in reality testing and sense of reality of the world and of the self, low functioning ($p < .05$) in stimulus barrier and mastery–competence, and lowest functioning ($p < .05$) in adaptive regression in the service of the ego (ARISE). The findings of this study do not appear to totally support the literature on the psychological functioning of manic-depressive individuals in remission (Bellak et al., 1973; Cohen et al., 1954; Gibson et al., 1959; Stone, 1978).*

Deficits in stimulus barrier indicate low thresholds and/or inadequate responses to sensory stimuli. A low score in mastery–competence denotes an inferior degree of active striving to deal with situations, overcome obstacles, and actualize potentials. Low functioning in ARISE signifies an inability to meet life's demands with other than previously learned solutions. These findings lead one to conclude that manic-depressive individuals in remission lack the creativity, flexibility, coping mechanisms, and self-confidence that facilitate meeting the demands and stresses of everyday life.

The data extrapolated from this study appear to have implications for mental health professionals in the assessment, treatment, and evaluation of manic-depressive individuals in remission. The present results can also be integrated into the specific interpretive strategies used in the treatment of

---

* The discrepancy between the present results and Bellak et al's. (1973) earlier speculations are more apparent than real. In fact, the prediction for the manic-depressive profile was that it would reveal less severe disturbances of reality testing and judgment (except in the area of self-blame) and reveal "little impairment of thought processes but marked fluctuations between highest and lowest level on impulse control and possibly on object relations and defenses" (Bellak et al., 1973, p. 337). Elsewhere, it was also suggested that a disturbance in stimulus barrier is crucial for affective disorders (Bellak & Bermeman, 1971, p. 388).

such patients. Bellak et al. (1973) suggested specific treatment interventions for the 12 ego functions. An appreciation of varying ego strengths and weaknesses observed in the profiles of the current population, for instance weaknesses in the areas of stimulus barrier, mastery–competence, and ARISE, might therefore, generate specific therapeutic approaches. The ACAEF could intermittently be readministered to evaluate the effect of treatment interventions on the adaptive level of ego functioning.

This study identified statistically significant strengths and weaknesses in the ego function profiles of manic-depressive individuals in remission. A most important recommendation of this investigation is for the establishment of the reliability and validity of the ACAEF. In addition, a comparison of the ego function profiles of normal, neurotic, manic-depressive, and schizophrenic subjects should be conducted using the ACAEF. Cutoff points for the various levels of functioning need to be established, as well.

The ACAEF is an objective, efficient assessment tool that identifies and quantifies strengths and weaknesses, pinpoints areas where intervention is needed, and is useful in the evaluation of treatment interventions. Once the reliability and validity of the ACAEF is established, the instrument will be a valuable clinical and research tool. The ACAEF will be useful not only in the assessment, treatment, and evaluation of manic-depressive individuals, but also for individuals suffering from other disorders.

SUMMARY

The need for a specific psychological model for the assessment, diagnosis, and treatment of manic-depressive illness was proposed. The purposes of this study were to (1) utilize an ego psychological framework to assess the ego functions of manic-depressive individuals in remission, (2) identify patterns in their ego function profiles, and (3) discuss the potential utility of the ego psychological model in clinical practice.

The sample consisted of 22 subjects diagnosed manic-depressive in remission according to the *Diagnostic and Statistical Manual of Mental Disorders,* 2d ed. A structured interview was conducted to obtain demographic and psychological data and to assess 12 ego functions.

The hypothesis was that the ego function profiles of manic-depressive individuals in remission would demonstrate lowest functioning in (1) reality testing, (2) judgment, (3) regulation and control of drives, affects, and impulses, (4) object relations, and (5) defensive functioning.

The manic-depressive individuals in remission interviewed in this study demonstrated highest ego functioning ($p < .05$) in reality testing and sense of reality of the world and of the self, and were significantly lower ($p < .05$) in stimulus barrier and mastery–competence, and lowest functioning ($p < .05$) in ARISE.

ACKNOWLEDGMENTS

The authors would like to acknowledge the contributions of the following individuals: Faye Gary-Harris, R.N., Ed.D., Associate Professor of Nursing, University of Florida, Gainesville, Florida; Ronald G. Marks, Ph.D., Associate Professor of Statistics, University of Florida, Gainesville, Florida; Gustave Newman, M.D., Associate Professor of Psychiatry, University of Florida, Gainesville, Florida; Douglas I. Starr, Ph.D., Executive Director of the North Central Florida Community Mental Health Center, Gainesville, Florida.

REFERENCES

Abraham, K. A short study of the development of the libido, viewed in the light of mental disorders. In E. A. Wolpert (Ed.), *Manic-depressive illness: History of a syndrome.* New York: International Universities Press, 1977. (Originally published, 1924.)

American Psychiatric Association. *Diagnostic and statistical manual of mental disorders* (2d ed.). Washington, D. C., 1968.

American Psychiatric Association Task Force on Lithium Therapy. The current status of lithium therapy: Report of the American Psychiatric Association Task Force. *American Journal of Psychiatry,* 1975, *132,* 997–1001.

Bellak, L. *Manic-depressive psychosis and allied conditions.* New York: Grune & Stratton, 1952.

Bellak, L. *Abbreviated clinical assessment of ego functions.* Presented at the West Central Florida Human Resource Center Conference on Brief Psychotherapy, Ocala, Florida, March, 1979.

Bellak, L., & Berneman, R. A systematic view of depression. *American Journal of Psychotherapy,* 1971, *25*(3), p. 388.

Bellak, L., Hurvich, M., & Gediman, H. K. *Ego functions in schizophrenics, neurotics, and normals: A systematic study of conceptual, diagnostic, and therapeutic aspects.* New York: Wiley, 1973.

Bratfos, O., & Haug, J. O. The course of manic-depressive psychosis. *Acta Psychiatrica Scandinavica,* 1968, *44,* 89–114.

Carlson, G. A., Kotin, J., Davenport, Y. B., & Adland, M. Follow-up of 53 bipolar manic-depressive patients. *British Journal of Psychiatry,* 1974, *124,* 134–139.

Cohen, M. B., Baker, G., Cohen, R. A., Fromm-Reichmann, F., & Weigart, E. V. An intensive study of 12 cases of manic-depressive psychosis. *Psychiatry,* 1954, *17,* 103–137.

Dunner, D. L., Igel, G. J., & Fieve, R. R. Social adjustment in primary affective disorder. *American Journal of Psychiatry,* 1978, *135,* 1412–1413.

Fieve, R. R., & Dunner, D. L. Unipolar and bipolar affective states. In F. F. Flach & S. C. Draghi (Eds.), *The nature and treatment of depression.* New York: Wiley, 1975.

Freud, S. Mourning and melancholia. In E. A. Wolpert (Ed.), *Manic-depressive illness: History of a syndrome.* New York: International Universities Press, 1977. (Originally published, 1915.)

Gibson, R. W., Cohen, M. B., & Cohen, R. A. On the dynamics of the manic-depressive personality. *American Journal of Psychiatry,* 1959, *115,* 1101–1107.

Hastings, D. W. Follow-up results in psychiatric illness. *American Journal of Psychiatry,* 1958, *114,* 1057–1066.

Kerry, R. J., & Orme, J. E. Lithium, manic-depressive illness, and psychological test performance. *British Medical Journal,* 1979, *1,* 230.

Klerman, G. Affective disorders. In A. M. Nicholi (Ed.), *The Harvard guide to modern psychiatry.* Cambridge, Mass.: Belknap Press of Harvard University Press, 1978.

Kraepelin, E. Manic-depressive insanity. In E. A. Wolpert (Ed.), *Manic-depressive illness: History of a syndrome.* New York: International Universities Press, 1977. (Originally published, 1921.)

Lundquist, G. Prognosis and course in manic-depressive psychosis. *Acta Psychiatrica et Neurologica Scandinavica,* 1945, Supp. *35,* 1–96.

MacVane, J. R., Lange, J. D., Brown, W. A., & Zayat, M. Psychological functioning of bipolar manic-depressives in remission. *Archives of General Psychiatry,* 1978, *35,* 1351–1354.

Prien, R. F. Clinical uses of lithium—Part I: Introduction. In T. B. Cooper, S. Gershon, N. S. Kline, & M. Schou (Eds.), *Lithium: Controversies and unresolved issues.* Amsterdam: Excerpta Medica, 1979.

Shobe, F. O., & Brion, P. Long-term prognosis in manic-depressive illness. *Archives of General Psychiatry,* 1971, *24,* 334–337.

Stone, M. H. Toward early detection of manic-depressive illness in psychoanalytic patients. *American Journal of Psychotherapy,* 1978, *32,* 427–439.

Welner, A., Welner, Z., & Leonard, M. Bipolar manic-depressive disorder: A reassessment of course and outcome. *Comprehensive Psychiatry,* 1977, *18,* 327–332.

Winokur, G., Clayton, P. J., & Reich, T. *Manic-depressive illness.* St. Louis: C. V. Mosby, 1969.

CHAPTER TWENTY-FOUR

Ego Function Assessment of Psychiatric Aspects of Minimal Brain Dysfunction (ADD) in Adults

LEOPOLD BELLAK

Any concept, particularly a new one, usually evokes two different attitudes. One is to find the new idea altogether unacceptable. The other is to overextend the concept and apply it to practically everything. Historically, in psychiatry, both tendencies have occurred with the introduction of ECT,

This chapter utilizes and synthesizes with permission of the respective publishers, previously published material by the author (Bellak, L., Psychiatric states in adults with minimal brain dysfunction, *Psychiatric Annals,* 1977, *7,* 575–589; Bellak, L., A possible subgroup of the schizophrenic syndrome and implications for treatment. *American Journal of Psychotherapy,* 1976, *30,* 194–205; Bellak, L., Schizophrenic syndrome related to minimal brain dysfunction: A possible neurologic subgroup, *Schizophrenia Bulletin,* 1979, *5*(3), 480–489, along with new observations on this subject. We are also grateful to Grune & Stratton, Inc., for permission to use material for this chapter. Some material was previously published as Psychiatric Aspects of Minimal Brain Dysfunction in Adults: Their Ego Function Assessment by Leopold Bellak in: *Psychiatric Aspects of Minimal Brain Dysfunction in Adults,* Edited by Leopold Bellak, Grune & Stratton, Inc., 1979.

phenothiazines, community psychiatry, the concept of schizophrenia, psychoanalysis, and many other schools of thought and therapeutic modalities. The same situation prevails with the concept of minimal brain dysfunction (MBD), which is classified as Attentional Deficit Disorder (ADD) in DSM-III.

HISTORY AND CONCEPT OF MBD

The establishment of MBD as a well-defined concept in children can be arbitrarily dated from a 1966 conference on MBD at the National Institutes of Health (Clement, 1966). Prior to 1966 and up to the present time, MBD has been referred to by various terms that, in fact, designate only some of the symptoms and syndromes now subsumed under the definition of MBD—symptoms such as dyslexia and other learning difficulties.

Orton (1937) and Strauss and Lehtinan (1947) were among the pioneers of MBD in the United States. Early recognition of childhood MBD is suggested by Cantwell (1972) who cites the colorful and well-known German children's story *Der Struwelpeter*. This is a tale written over a century ago by a physician concerning the adventures of an unruly lad who would not cut his hair or his nails, who engaged in all sorts of mischief, and displayed frequent temper outbursts (Hoffman, 1845). As far back as 1940, in the psychiatry department of the Massachusetts General Hospital, under the chairmanship of Stanley Cobb and under the supervision of F. L. Wells, one of the pioneers of clinical psychology in the United States, we were taught to examine all children for left–right dominance, verbal and performance IQs were compared, and special note was taken of mirror writing, letter reversals, and speech difficulties, including stuttering.

Though MBD in children has been written about for many years, most systematically by Wender (1971), and discussed under different names and in different contexts, this syndrome only very recently provoked real interest in regard to its role in psychiatric disorders of adults.

The relationship between MBD in children and adults has been largely overlooked because these symptoms of MBD are most obvious in childhood and indeed decrease or disappear in some by age 12 owing to neurological maturation. It is my impression, however, that even more often they persist into adulthood. People learn to compensate for these difficulties, masking them, or denying that problems such as constantly getting lost when driving are related to difficulties with spatial orientation, and are part of a minimal neurological dysfunction.

The most sophisticated concept and model of MBD (also only in relation to children) has probably been formulated by Arnold (1976). The hydraulic parfait illustrates the concept of symptom production by additive accumulation of pathologies from various etiologies (Figures 24.1, 24.2). This implies

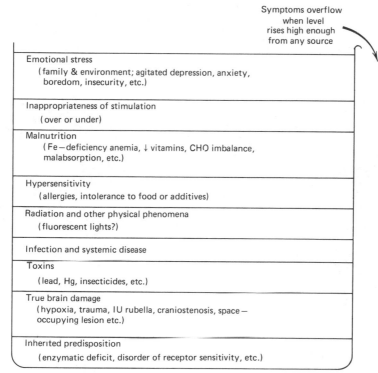

Symptoms overflow
when level
rises high enough
from any source

Emotional stress
   (family & environment; agitated depression, anxiety,
     boredom, insecurity, etc.)

Inappropriateness of stimulation
   (over or under)

Malnutrition
   (Fe—deficiency anemia, ↓ vitamins, CHO imbalance,
     malabsorption, etc.)

Hypersensitivity
   (allergies, intolerance to food or additives)

Radiation and other physical phenomena
   (fluorescent lights?)

Infection and systemic disease

Toxins
   (lead, Hg, insecticides, etc.)

True brain damage
   (hypoxia, trauma, IU rubella, craniostenosis, space—
     occupying lesion etc.)

Inherited predisposition
   (enzymatic deficit, disorder of receptor sensitivity, etc.)

Figure 24.1. Hydraulic parfait model of minimal brain dysfunction. When the level of total pathology rises high enough from any combination of layers, behavior and learning disorder symptoms spill over. Reprinted with permission from *Diseases of the Nervous System* (Arnold, E.: MBD: A hydraulic parfait model, 1967 *37*, 171–173.)

a psychophysiological disorder and also a multidimensional spectrum of etiologies that could be important for treatment plans in individual cases.

The many and diverse manifestations of MBD have certainly led to the abuse of the concept, especially in some school systems, but probably also to unwarranted skepticism concerning its existence and usefulness. In this context it may be useful to compare MBD to the aphasic syndrome. In its sensory and motor form, aphasia represents a similar problem of apparent vagueness, and yet it is a well-established concept in medicine.

In discussing MBD in relation to adult psychiatric patients, it must again be stated that MBD is a multifaceted disorder that interacts subtly and in quite variable ways in different people according to the psychodynamic and structural aspects of their personalities. It does exist, however, as a syndrome that plays an important part in psychiatric disorders of adults. Cognitive functioning—including the registration, storing, and retrieval of experiences—is, of course, affected by any dysfunction in any of the organs

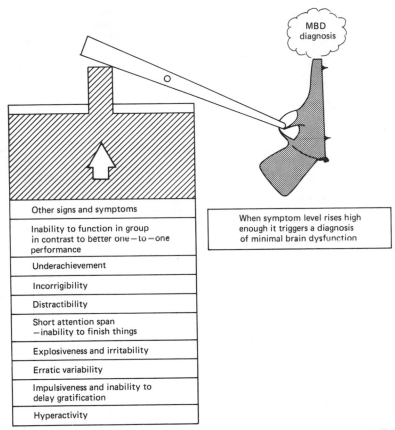

Figure 24.2. Hydraulic parfait concept of relationship between MBD symptoms and diagnosis. Sufficient symptoms in sufficient quantity produce enough pressure to "trigger" a diagnosis. Reprinted with permission from *Diseases of the Nervous System* (Arnold, E.: MBD: A hydraulic parfait model, 1967, *37,* 171–173.)

involving sense perception. The person with MBD suffers such distortions not only in the initial perception of experiences but also in their subsequent recording and recall. Thus, the effects of MBD on adult personality development cannot be disregarded by anyone searching for the experiential factors generally considered basic for psychiatric disorders.

In an early study by Cantwell (1972) it was hypothesized that hyperactive children grow into hyperactive adults. To test the theory, he conducted a systematic psychiatric examination of the parents of 50 hyperactive children and the parents of 50 matched control children. The parents of the hyperactive children had an increased incidence of alcoholism, sociopathy, and hysteria, and Cantwell judged 10% of these parents to have been hyperactive children themselves.

Studies by Borland and Heckman (1976) support Cantwell's findings.

They suggest that many emotional problems result from the persistence of symptoms of hyperactivity into adult life and believe that most social and psychiatric consequences of the disorder relate to its presence in both childhood and adulthood.

In the Borland and Heckman study, hyperactive children and their brothers were followed up 25 years after the initial contact. MBD symptoms had diminished considerably in the patients. Nevertheless, half of the probands had psychiatric problems that affected their socioeconomic status, despite normal intelligence and education. They frequently changed jobs; to them, work was a means of avoiding feelings of restlessness.

A number of longitudinal and adoption studies suggest that MBD persists into adult life, and unfortunately its existence is camouflaged by the application of a variety of diagnostic labels. To test the hypothesis that MBD persisted into adulthood, Wood et al. (1976) identified 15 putative MBD adults on the basis of MBD-like complaints, self-descriptions of MBD characteristics in childhood, and so on. Of the 15, 11 were then given a double-blind trial of methylphenidate hydrochloride, and 8 of them showed a significant response. Other stimulants or tricyclic antidepressants were also tried, and 8 of the 15 showed a good response and 2 a moderately favorable response. The authors of this study concluded that MBD does persist into adult life, with the signs and symptoms lessening or disappearing in the third and fourth decades of life rather than in the teens.

Mann and Greenspan have offered suggestions for the identification and treatment of adult brain dysfunction (1976). Their 20 patients each had the following characteristics: a history of early learning disorder with short attention span, diffuse severe symptoms in adulthood with prominent elements of anxiety and depression, dramatic improvement with the administration of imipramine, and a mental status characterized by rapid speech and many shifts of subject (but without overt indicators of psychotic thinking).

According to Hartocollis (1968) evidence of "soft neurologic signs" is often overlooked in adolescent and young-adult psychiatric patients. Reporting on such a group whose difficulties were not obviously organic but who had responded poorly to treatment, he noticed that there was often an unevenness in psychological test performance—for example, a discrepancy between verbal and performance IQ scores. He found that these patients had a history of frustration, failure to perform up to parental and school expectations, poor results from psychiatric treatment, and evidence of organicity—but the evidence had been overlooked or ignored. Such persons can learn to function with much less frustration once these neurological signs are recognized and a properly structured environment is provided (Hartocollis, 1968).

Many of these authors believe that the concept of MBD may account for a group of adult impulse disorders. The pharmacological techniques useful in treating MBD in childhood therefore provide a rational basis for treating psychiatric patients who have been poorly understood and evidenced treatment-unresponsive symptoms. Adults treated with small amounts of methylphenidate, pemoline, and tricyclic antidepressants showed improvement. Both the low doses of drugs and the patients' rapid response to medication were comparable to experience with the use of these agents in children.

In summary, it may be said that a number of authors who have investigated the possibility of MBD occurring in adults have concluded that it is an etiologic factor in some of the most common and least understood psychiatric disorders.

DEFINING MBD IN TERMS OF EGO FUNCTIONS

MBD needs to be operationally defined in adults as well as in children, and it can be defined by the *systematic assessment of crucial ego functions*.

This is a technique of assessment I have previously described for schizophrenia (another slippery concept!). In a way analogous to Arnold's concept of MBD, I described schizophrenia as a multifactorial psychobiological syndrome of different causes and pathogeneses, sharing as a final common pathway severe but variable disturbances of the functions of the ego (Bellak et al., 1973). I have therefore found it useful to study schizophrenics in terms of their ego function disturbances.

An analogous ego function assessment of MBD may prove helpful in both clarifying the concept and systematizing the descriptions of the syndrome. Assessment of the 12 crucial ego functions can be made in an operational, statistically valid, and reliable way. Although the ego function concept is part of a set of psychoanalytic propositions and is most useful within the entire matrix of psychoanalytic theory, it can also be used simply as a systematic mental status examination by clinicians not psychoanalytically trained.

Ego functions and their components are reported in Table 24.1. The functions can be graphed as in Fig. 24.3, which plots not only the patient's current ego functioning but characteristic optimal and minimal functioning as well. Plotting such curves permits the physician to see at a glance the discrepancy in ego functioning between periods of minimal stress and periods of maximal stress. At the same time, it enables the physician to pinpoint the specific ego functions that are most deviant.

I would like to comment briefly on each of the ego functions listed in Table 24.1—not in the logical order indicated in the table but rather in a descending order of importance insofar as they play a role in most cases of MBD in adults.

DISTURBANCES OF AUTONOMOUS FUNCTIONS IN ADD

Hyperkinesis may be apparent in infancy. Symptoms include restlessness and other problems that will usually bring the child to the attention of a

Table 24.1. Ego Functions and Their Components

Ego Function	Components	Ego Function	Components
1. Reality testing	Distinction between inner and outer stimuli Accuracy of perception Reflective awareness and inner reality testing	7. Adaptive regression in the service of the ego	Regressive relaxation of cognitive acuity New configurations
2. Judgment	Anticipation of consequences Manifestation of this anticipation in behavior Emotional appropriateness of this anticipation	8. Defensive functioning	Weakness or obtrusiveness of defenses Success and failure of defenses
3. Sense of reality and sense of self	Extent of derealization Extent of depersonalization Self-identity and self-esteem Clarity of boundaries between self and world	9. Stimulus barrier	Threshold for stimuli Effectiveness of management of excessive stimulus input
4. Regulation and control of drives, affects, and impulses	Directness of impulse expression Effectiveness of delay mechanisms	10. Autonomous functioning	Degree of freedom from impairment of primary autonomy apparatuses Degree of freedom from impairment of secondary autonomy
5. Object relations	Degree and kind of relatedness Primitiveness (narcissistic, attachment, or symbiotic-object choices) Degrees to which others are perceived independently of oneself Object constancy	11. Synthetic–integrative functioning	Degree of reconciliation of incongruities Degree of active relating together of events
6. Thought processes	Memory, concentration, and attention Ability to conceptualize Primary-secondary process	12. Mastery–competence	Competence (how well the subject actually performs in relation to his existing capacity to interact with and actively master and affect environment) The subjective role (subject's feeling of competence with respect to actively mastering and affecting environment) The degree of discrepancy between the other two components (i.e., between actual competence and sense of competence)

Source: Reprinted with permission from L. Bellak, Psychiatric states in adults with MBD. *Psychiatric Annals,* 1976, 7, 58–76.

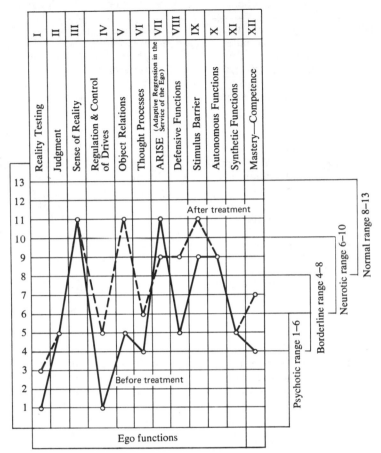

Figure 24.3. Ego function profiles of a schizophrenic before (———) and after (-----) treatment with imipramine (Tofranil). (Reprinted with permission from *The Journal of Nervous and Mental Disorders*, Bellak et al., 1973b.)

teacher by school age. Many of these pertain to language—difficulty in learning to read or write. A neurological examination may reveal the presence of "soft neurological signs."

Adults with MBD may have the same cognitive disturbances, evidenced by difficulties with spatial relationships. They may, for example, often get lost—while either walking or driving. They are likely to have general problems with orientation. Verbal expression may be impaired—if it is only mildly impaired, they may stutter; if the impairment is severe, they may seem aphasic.

Some people with MBD can become disorganized, especially when required to perform under time pressure or sensory overload (personal communications, H. Kravitz, M.D., P. Hartocollis, M.D., Ph.D., and others). A teenage student with MBD, for instance, may have difficulty passing examinations under time pressure but be capable of performance commensurate with high intelligence if the time pressure is removed. In some adult patients with MBD I have observed an increase in anxiety approaching catastrophic levels when they have been subjected to inordinate internal or external pressure.

Such people respond poorly to any kind of overload—time pressure, excessive light or noise, or excessive social contact. The result often is disorganization, with possible disturbances in attention and the shift of thinking from the abstract to the concrete, and may also involve problems of impulse control.

It is important here to keep in mind what I have pointed out elsewhere (Bellak et al., 1973) that ego functions interrelate with each other and that a disturbance in one is likely to have an effect on the functioning of others. In this respect, the ego functions interrelate with each other like the subfunctions of intelligence on the WAIS (Wechsler Adult Intelligence Scale) (Bellak et al., 1973). Nevertheless, they still vary enough to merit separate consideration.

Catastrophic reactions of people with MBD should not be mistaken for schizophrenia, although at times this condition may coexist with the schizophrenic syndrome.

DISTURBANCES OF REGULATION AND CONTROL OF DRIVES

As I have noted, an outstanding characteristic of the child with MBD is a profound disturbance in the regulation and control of drives and impulses. The persistence of this characteristic into adolescence and adulthood has now been documented by several investigators (Cantwell, 1972). Emotional outbursts—including assaultive behavior, restlessness, and inability to hold jobs—are typical manifestations of MBD in the adult. There is suggestive evidence that a high percentage of the people with alcoholism, drug addiction, and other social problems are minimally brain damaged.

People with MBD have a tendency to act out on a neurotic or psychotic level. They act—instead of verbalizing—as verbalization was impaired or failed to develop properly in childhood (Bellak, 1965; Greenacre, 1950).

Many of these patients engage in violent activities to get rid of their tensions or, at other times, use drugs to give them some relief. Marijuana is most common among those used. Overworking and hypomanic-type activity are other aspects of their behavior. Their impulsivity often impairs their judgment. Related to this lack of regulation and control of drives is a tremendous need for constant stimulation; otherwise they suffer feelings of emptiness and depersonalization.

One patient of mine, a highly gifted artist, frequently developed "pie in the sky" projects. It was a close race between his losing interest in them or failing at them. He literally would be with a different woman every day, initially expecting that each one would be "the woman" of his life. Psychotherapy had much to do with teaching him self-observation and self-reporting, making him aware of his constant stimulus hunger. It sensitized him to "signal awareness" when he was about to act out and thus reinforced impulse control. Sometimes it is helpful to permit or to encourage the development of obsessive-compulsive controls as a defense against impulse breakthrough.

DISTURBANCES OF STIMULUS BARRIER

A low stimulus barrier was noted in 25% of the schizophrenics in our original ego function study (Bellak et al., 1973). Although the patients in this study were not examined neurologically, subsequent clinical experience has revealed that adults with MBD, both schizophrenic and nonschizophrenic, are easily overloaded by visual and auditory stimuli.

The same phenomenon as low stimulus barrier has been described by Mednick and Schulsinger and was operationalized as a high arousal pattern on the galvanic skin response (1968). The question of whether or not patients who demonstrate a high arousal pattern also show other signs of MBD warrants future investigation. It is widely agreed that people who demonstrate a low stimulus barrier or high arousal pattern also exhibit a great deal of stimulus hunger (Ludwig, 1975).

Stimulus barrier is of clinical importance in only a relatively small percentage of patients, but when it is important and is recognized, it may play a major role in their psychopathology. As a consequence of the low stimulus barrier their response may be variable. On the one hand, they may show extreme restlessness and the need for a great deal of stimulus input, such as loud music, "psychedelic" effects, and stimulation by drugs. In these instances, external stimuli may help to counteract flooding by internal stimuli. This might be similar to the case of a typical adolescent who drowns out his or her troubles with loud rock music.

Usually, however, a low stimulus barrier will manifest itself in great sensitivity, to noise, to lights, to too active a social scene, or to an oversensitivity to time pressure. Under such circumstances this type of person complains of headaches, actual migraines, and disorganization. Overload is the key word to explain what ails these people, and therapy may have to be concerned with helping them to avoid the overload by treating them with drugs that will increase the stimulus barrier. Diphenylhydantoin (Dilantin) is at times useful, and a wide variety of other anxiolytic and tranquilizing drugs may be of help.

DISTURBANCES OF THOUGHT PROCESSES

Verbalization plays a crucial role in the development of most children after they reach the age of about 30 months. When there is MBD, however, development of language skills is delayed. As Greenacre (1950) has noted, the child who has difficulty in learning is likely to develop motoric acting out in lieu of verbal communication. Problems with verbalization appear to be related to difficulties with thinking. Typically, the person with MBD is more at home with concrete than with abstract thought. Sequential thinking is often impaired—perhaps leading to a very specific difficulty, such as the inability of a highly intelligent adolescent to enumerate the months of the year. The adult schizophrenic with MBD shows not excessive symbolization and overinclusion but rather concreteness of thinking.

In turn, concrete thinking is related to problems in perceptual organization. This phenomenon was originally demonstrated by Goldstein (1939) in his study of perceptual deficits of German soldiers with head wounds in World War I.

Sometimes a patient is referred to me as a schizophrenic because of symptoms of a thought disorder. It occasionally turns out that it is primarily a matter of concrete thinking or disorganized thinking under the impact of anxiety and other pressures in a person suffering from MBD. In that case, psychotherapy designed to decrease the anxiety and the internal pressure is very helpful. The patient also has to be taught how to go about problem solving and learning to speak slowly. Syllable reversals often play an obvious role in this disturbance. Pressured thought occurs and is experienced as unpleasant by the patient, and interferes with tasks. Imipramine or methylphenidate can slow this process down. Patients can be taught "signal awareness," that is, to be made conscious of factors that disturb them and precipitate disordered thought processes.

Some patients suffering from very concrete thinking actually have to be taught self-observation, that is, inner reality testing.

DISTURBANCES OF SENSE OF REALITY AND SENSE OF SELF

Problems with spatial orientation are a hallmark of the adult with MBD as evidenced by difficulties in distinguishing left from right. These are also apparent in situations where the adult is required to have a sense of direction—for example, when reading a map or navigating while driving. The child with MBD has difficulties vis-à-vis spatial orientation that lead to problems in the establishment of clear ego boundaries. Failure to establish clear boundaries, in turn, has an effect on object relations, leading to insufficient individuation and a poorly defined self-image. Freeman et al. (1958) consider this phenomenon to be the basic factor in the development of schizophrenia.

Typically, both children and adults with MBD feel perplexed and can suffer from the uncomfortable sensation of being lost, an experience that may produce high levels of anxiety. Adults with MBD have poorly defined body images and the interactions of this with the other symptoms that arise from impairments in their autonomous functions often make them clumsy.

The difficulties in self and object differentiation interfere with a consolidation of the sense of reality and self and may be manifest in an experience of emptiness. Feelings of depersonalization are frequent and occur as complications in the process of psychotherapy. Dreams are especially informative about disturbances in the sense of self. For instance, one patient often dreamt of herself as an open and empty refrigerator, suggesting both how cold and empty she felt.

In schizophrenics with marked disturbances of body boundaries, the body ego technique originally described by May et al. (1963), may be useful. Severely disturbed patients are engaged in rhythmic exercise, as well as systematic interchanges of touching the body and the floor and other people as a way to increase a feeling of differentiation.

DISTURBANCES OF OBJECT RELATIONS

Secondary to the problems arising from poorly defined self-boundaries are disturbances in the area of object relations. The separation–individuation process can be affected by neurological and cognitive factors, which then can be manifested psychodynamically. Since MBD children are often the subject of ridicule, they frequently become asocial or suspicious of others as they grow older. Their impatience, labile moods, and inability to concentrate further impair their ability to relate to others.

People with difficulties in object relations on the basis of having MBD are examples par excellence of the "porcupine dilemma" (Bellak, 1970). On a cold winter day some porcupines decided to move together to give each other some warmth, only to find that they stung each other with their quills. They moved apart again, and were cold. They moved back and forth until they found the optimal distance at which they gave each other warmth without hurting each other.

People with MBD are like porcupines with a particularly strong need for warmth, and, at the same time, extremely sensitive skin and long, sharp quills. The net result is that they are people who suffer from labile object relations. Among other things, their relationships are interfered with by explosive disruptions of regulation and control of drives and inhibited by their fear of their own perceived potential loss of regulation and control of drives. One young schizophrenic, for instance, was primarily asocial because he felt easily ridiculed and was afraid that his rage might burst out as it had once on a single occasion. He therefore preferred to live in isolation, creating a self-imposed prison.

DISTURBANCES OF MASTERY AND COMPETENCE

MBD adults often exhibit a lack of self-confidence. This emerges as they become aware of the disturbances of autonomous functions, such as in speech, writing, and fine motor coordination (i.e., the use of a needle, hammer, pen, pencil) as well as in performing many functions requiring gross coordination, such as athletic activities.

Failure in school often plays a role in the development of a lack of confidence, and even very intelligent people often carry with them the feeling of being inadequate physically and mentally. On the other hand, some develop overcompensated defenses. In one patient, it led to hypomanic overactivity, with its own resulting pitfalls. In addition, the patient exhibited a constant need for clowning in order to feel accepted.

DISTURBANCES OF THE SYNTHETIC–INTEGRATIVE FUNCTION

By definition, this function is concerned with the synthesis and integration of conflicting emotions, drives, and thoughts so that smooth intellectual performance, appropriate emotion, and coordinated motor activity become possible. MBD patients have a difficult task in this regard, in view of their difficulties with impulse control. Clinically, their problems produce symptoms that are often resistant even to lengthy and skillful psychoanalysis. There seems to be more integrative work that needs to be done than the cerebral integrative–synthetic capacity of the MBD adult permits.

The most colorful example of a lack of synthetic–integrative ego function predates Freud. Pierre Janet (whose term *psychasthenia* is as close as any to the concept of ego weakness in psychoanalytic terms) told the story of the French lady who went to market with the typical net bag, which she stuffed with cabbages, beets, long bread, carrots, and some fruits. As she went along, some of the carrots fell out. She stuffed the carrots back in, and some oranges fell out. In short, her net bag did not have sufficient "synthetic capacity," and many a patient suffers from similar problems. Psychotherapy, of course, can reduce conflicts that dynamically interfere with integration and synthesis.

DISTURBANCES OF ADAPTIVE REGRESSION

This ego function is a complex one to discuss in relation to MBD because of the lowered external and internal stimulus barriers. A person who is suffering from MBD is flooded by internal and external stimuli from the psyche and the environment. In a gifted person with enough synthetic–

integrative function, this low stimulus barrier may lead to substantial artistic and scientific creativity. Such people are more "open" to unconscious and preconscious ideation.

Historical examples of such people probably include Michelangelo, da Vinci, Newton, and Einstein. In the absence of talent, intelligence, and sufficient integrative function, it leads instead to pseudoart, as exemplified by schizophrenic productions or amateurish efforts. In some, obsessive defenses minimize adaptive regression in the service of the ego. In the fortunate, other good ego functions lead to creative Gestalt formations in artistic and scientific fields.

DISTURBANCES OF DEFENSES

Because of the major problem of impulse control, the defenses are often too weak to deal with the conflicts existing among drives, superego, and reality. In extreme cases this may result in psychotic phenomena. In less severe cases it probably accounts for some of the anxiety phenomena that seem resistant to psychotherapeutic intervention, as in some neurotics in whom the diagnosis of MBD has usually been missed.

Some persons with weak defenses (in the sense that they function inadequately) become excessively rigid. As in obsessive-compulsives without MBD, there may be fluctuation from obsessiveness to impulse breakthrough.

Some gifted people with MBD may develop a whole complex compensatory character structure as a defense against various aspects of MBD.

One patient of mine, who had suffered from a severe learning disability and had little formal education, nevertheless is today highly successful as a businessman and is the president of several corporations. He can, for the most part, think only in concrete terms and prepares himself for complicated corporate conferences by developing many concrete scenarios. "If *A* says such and such, and *B* replies with such and such, what will I say?" His thinking is very similar to the way some people work out complex chess moves in a game. In addition to this particular type of thought process, he has learned to overcome his once vicious lack of impulse control by a particularly rigid moral code.

DISTURBANCES OF JUDGMENT

Judgment may often be poor in adults with MBD, even though reality-testing functions are intact. This is because sound judgment is based not only on an accurate perception of reality but also on the ability to regulate the expression of internal drives and impulses so as to meet the demands imposed by reality. In people with MBD, difficulties with the latter may result in defects in judgment that in turn may lead to ill-conceived, violent, or criminal acts. At times, a life history may be characterized by spectacular failures as a result of judgment impaired by impulsiveness—apparently due to MBD. The criminal behavior that can stem from MBD-associated impairments of judgment should be given more attention by those interested in the problems of forensic psychiatry.

Judgment in people with MBD is, of course, most often interfered with by their problems with impulse control. Acting out is typical for them (Bellak, 1965). The need for quick gratification is a critical problem in this area.

DISTURBANCES OF REALITY TESTING

Reality testing is only sometimes affected by excessive drive and impulse push. At times, impulses that are subjectively overwhelming are projected onto external objects, which the MBD adult then reacts to inappropriately.

The adult with MBD may attempt to exert control over factors in the external environment—including people—in a paranoid fashion. In some schizophrenics with MBD, reality testing may be only minimally impaired. In such cases, and in a setting of poor impulse control, these patients may go AWOL from hospitals. I would, in fact, go so far as to say that I would consider MBD immediately in any schizophrenic patient who goes AWOL or shows both sociopathic tendencies and good organizational ability.

MBD IN RELATION TO ADULT CLINICAL STATES: SOME HIGHLIGHTS AND NOSOLOGIC PERSPECTIVES

MBD may be present in a group of people who must be considered psychiatrically normal. Such seemed to be the case in relatives of patients I had occasion to interview. Undoubtedly the interaction of a relatively mild organic disorder with unimpaired or even better-than-average intelligence, as well as fortunate experiential factors, accounts for the existence of this group.

MBD may play a role in a variety of psychiatric conditions and may influence the specific nature of each. In persons suffering from anxiety (psychodynamically understandable as a response to experiential factors but occurring in subjects who also have MBD), the anxiety often seems more extreme and less amenable to psychotherapeutic intervention than would have been expected from their life histories. This holds true especially where free-floating anxiety, acute anxiety attacks, and panic states are concerned.

In *hysteria* combined with MBD, the problem of self-boundaries may be expressed as a more serious disturbance of object relations than one would otherwise expect.

Claustrophobic symptoms may be related to problems with object relations: the fear of being engulfed or smothered may be related to a symbiotic merging on the basis of cognitive developmental problems of MBD.

Depressives often attempt to decrease the stimulus input in order to avoid overload and disorganization. Bellak and Berneman (1971) have suggested a theory that understands both depressive and manic features, as well as the transition between the two, in terms of a utilization of different defense mechanisms to deal with stimulus overload, stimulus hunger, and a low stimulus barrier.* Thus, complete withdrawal and avoidance are seen as an attempt to deal with excessive external stimuli; the increased stimulus hunger of the hypomanic, resulting in a flooding with stimuli, may be seen as an attempt to drown out internal conflicts. The latter phenomenon is exemplified not only by the manic and hypomanic but also by the seeking of "psychedelic" experiences and other kinds of stimulation by adolescents who might otherwise suffer depressions or feelings of depersonalization.

The possible role of MBD in delinquent and criminal behavior has been described by Cantwell (1972), among others.

In patients suffering from the borderline syndrome, MBD often makes a major contribution to poor organization of the self-image. A distorted and primitive self-image will often persist in these patients despite extensive psychotherapy—clearly expressed, for example, in dreams of their being small, helpless, isolated, or swallowed up. Symbiotic relations frequently persist in this group as a result of their continuing problems with self-boundaries, even when there do not seem to be sufficient experiential data to account for them.

Several authors have referred to the relationship between MBD and schizophrenia, and some have described the interaction of MBD and schizophrenia. Tucker et al. (1975) found a strong but not exclusive relationship between neurological impairment and thought disorder as well as between neurological impairments and schizophrenia.

Quitkin et al. (1976) suggest the existence of a subgroup of schizophrenics characterized by "soft neurologic signs." They found that patients diagnosed as "schizophrenic with premorbid asociality," as well as those with "emotionally unstable character disorders," exhibited neurological impairments not found in the rest of the patients. The authors consider CNS impairment a criterion for syndrome validity.

There is suggestive evidence that persons with childhood MBD may be predisposed to schizophrenia as adolescents and adults. Handford (1975) hypothesizes that individuals who experience brain hypoxia prenatally, perinatally, or immediately after birth will be at risk for MBD in childhood and for schizophrenia as adults, possibly resulting from damage to the dopaminergic pathways.

Fish et al. (1965) have analyzed early developmental profiles to identify infants vulnerable to schizophrenia. In one pilot study at a baby clinic, 16

---

* There is no conceptual reason why experiential factors would not sometimes trigger biochemical changes; at other times, pathological metabolic changes could in turn produce psychological changes in patients so predisposed.

infants from families with a high incidence of social and psychiatric disorders were examined periodically from the age of 1 month, and predictions of schizophrenia were made on the basis of uneven neurological development. The children were given psychological examinations at 9–10 years of age, and those originally diagnosed as vulnerable to schizophrenia had significantly higher incidence of disorder than the others. In a study by Fish and Hagin (1972) the visual-motor development of 10 infants whose mothers were schizophrenic was measured from birth to 2 years of age. Psychological evaluation after 10 years revealed a relationship between poor neurological integration in childhood and later emotional impairment.

Neurological findings in identical twins discordant for schizophrenia were discussed by Mosher et al. (1971). In this study some very suggestive evidence was found for a relationship between "soft neurological signs" and schizophrenia. Huessy's findings (1974, 1976) in adult schizophrenics whom he considered hyperkinetic further support this hypothesis.

Powerful although inadvertent support comes indirectly from a study reported by Rosenthal et al. at the National Institutes of Mental Health, in collaboration with a Jerusalem-based group, in which 50 children of schizophrenic parents and 50 controls were examined neurologically in great detail. According to a summary by Mosher and Feinsilver (1973), each group was divided at the median to form subgroups composed of high and low scores. Comparison of the two high-scoring subgroups revealed that the index group had significantly higher scores than the controls. No significant differences were found between the two low-scoring subgroups. However, when the subjects were divided into those above and those below age 11 years, the younger index group had higher neuropathology scores than the older group. These findings suggested that certain abnormal neuropathological traits detectable at younger ages may disappear as puberty approaches. The authors observed that these outward signs of an apparently inherited predisposition to schizophrenia tended to disappear at puberty. Since the general opinion is that maturation at least decreases the manifestations of MBD, it seems very likely that we are dealing with the role MBD played in the offspring of some schizophrenic parents. It is my unsupported theory that these particular "schizophrenic" parents also suffered from MBD.

Hanford's hypothesis that infants with brain hypoxia are at risk for MBD in childhood and schizophrenia in adulthood is similar to my own convictions about the pathogenesis of psychosis in the presence of MBD. Many years ago I began to suspect neurological findings in some schizophrenics. There were histories of unexplained bouts of high fever in infancy that led me to wonder whether or not such occurrences could have resulted in cortical damage and, subsequently, the psychiatric syndromes I was encountering (Bellak, 1949).

Many years later a confluence of data from a factor analytic study with clinical data again brought the question of schizophrenia with MBD to my attention (Bellak et al., 1973a). Members of one factor analytic group of schizophrenics were characterized not only by the signs and symptoms of schizophrenia but also by impulsiveness, a history of having low stimulus barriers, escapes from psychiatric institutions, sociopathy, a paucity of hallucinations, and a variety of MBD phenomena (Bellak, 1976).

The hypothesis that I first published in 1949 (Bellak, 1949)—namely, that the schizophrenic syndrome consists of many etiologic and pathogenic groups—is finally finding increased support. One such subgroup, I believe, is composed of schizophrenics with MBD. Although the cause of the MBD may be attributed to prenatal, perinatal, or postnatal factors, I continue to be impressed with the frequency of the familial occurrence of the dysfunction as it appears in various degrees of neurological and psychiatric disturbance. Undoubtedly, the interaction of MBD and experiential factors plays a role in the spectrum of many psychiatric disturbances.

REFERENCES

Arnold, L. E. MBD: A hydraulic parfait model. *Diseases of the Nervous System*, 1976, *37*, 171–173.

Bellak, L. A multiple-factor psychosomatic theory of schizophrenia. *Psychiatric Quarterly*, 1949, *23*, 738–755.

Bellak, L. The concept of acting out: Theoretical considerations. In L. Apt and D. Weisman (Eds.), *Acting out: Theoretical and clinical aspects*. New York: Grune & Stratton, 1965.

Bellak, L. *The porcupine dilemma*. New York: Citadel, 1970.

Bellak, L., & Berneman, R. A systematic view of depression. *American Journal of Psychotherapy*, 1971, *24*, 384–393.

Bellak, L., Hurvich, M., & Gediman, H. *Ego functions in schizophrenics, neurotics and normals: A systematic study of conceptual, diagnostic, and therapeutic aspects*. New York: Wiley, 1973a.

Bellak, L., Chassan, J., Gediman, H., et al. Ego function assessment of analytic psychotherapy combined with drug therapy. *Journal of Nervous Mental Disease*, 1973b, *157*, 465–469.

Bellak, L. A possible subgroup of the schizophrenic syndrome and implications for treatment. *American Journal of Psychotherapy*, 1976, *30*, 194–205.

Borland, B. S., & Heckman, H. C. Hyperactive boys and their brothers. A 25-year follow-up study. *Archives of General Psychiatry*, 1976, *33*, 663–675.

Cantwell, C. P. Psychiatric illness in the families of hyperactive children. *Archives of General Psychiatry*, 1972, *27*, 414–417.

Ciompi, L., Ague, C., and Dauwalder, J. P. *L'objectivation chargements psychodynamiques: Experiences avec une version simplifée des "ego strength rating scales" de Bellak et al*. Read before the 10th International Congress of Psychotherapy, Paris, July 4–10, 1976.

Clement, S. MBD in children: Terminology and identification. Phase One of a Three-Phase Project. U.S. Department of Health, Education & Welfare. *NINDB Monograph 3* (PHSPR 1415), 1966.

Fish, B., & Hagin, R. Visual-motor disorders in infants at risk for schizophrenia. *Archives of General Psychiatry*, 1972, *27*, 594–598.

Fish, B., Shapiro, T., Halpern, F., et al. The prediction of schizophrenia in infancy: III. A ten-year follow-up report of neurological and psychological development. *American Journal of Psychiatry*, 1965, *121*, 768–775.

Freeman, T., Cameron, J., & McGhie, A. *Chronic schizophrenia.* New York: International Universities Press, 1958.

Goldfarb, W. *Childhood schizophrenia.* Cambridge, Mass.: Harvard University Press, 1961.

Goldstein, K. *The organism.* New York: American Books, 1939.

Greenacre, P. General problems of acting out. *Psychoanalytic Quarterly,* 1950, *19,* 455–467.

Handford, H. A. Brain hypoxia. MBD and schizophrenia. *American Journal of Psychiatry,* 1975, *132,* 192–194.

Hartocollis, P. The syndrome of MBD in young adult patients. *Bulletin of the Menninger Clinic,* 1968, *32,* 102–114.

Heston, L. L. The genetics of schizophrenia and schizoid disease. *Science,* 1970, *167,* 249–256.

Hoffman, H. *Der Struwelpeter: Oder lustige Geschichten und drollige Bilder.* Leipzig, Insel.

Huessy, H. R. The adult hyperkinetic. *American Journal of Psychiatry,* 1974, *131,* 724–725.

Huessy, H. R., & Cohen, A. H. Hyperkinetic behaviors and learning disabilities followed over 7 years. *Pediatrics,* 1976, *57,* 4–10.

Kernberg, O. *Borderline conditions and pathological narcissism.* New York: Aronson, 1975.

Kohut, H. *The analysis of the self· A systematic approach to the psychoanalytic treatment of narcissistic personality disorders.* New York: International Universities Press, 1971.

Ludwig, A. M. Sensory overload and psychopathology. *Diseases of the Nervous System,* 1975, *36,* 357–360.

Mann, H. B., & Greenspan, S. I. The identification and treatment of MBD in adults. *Archives of General Psychiatry,* 1976, *133,* 1013–1017.

May, P., Wexler, M., Sackar, J., et al. Non-verbal techniques in the reestablishment of body image and self identity: A preliminary report. *Psychiatric Residents Report,* 1963, *16,* 68–82.

Mednick, S. A., & Schulsinger, F. Some premorbid characteristics related to breakdown in children with schizophrenic mothers. In D. Rosenthal & S. Kety (Eds.), *The transmission of schizophrenia.* New York: Pergamon, 1968.

Milkman, H., & Frosch, W. A. The drug of choice. *Journal of Psychedelic Drugs,* 1977, *9,* 11–24.

Mosher, L. R., & Feinsilver, D. Current studies on schizophrenia. *International Journal of Psychiatry,* 1973, *2,* 21–22.

Mosher, L. R., Pollin, W., & Stabenau, J. R. Identical twins discordant for schizophrenia. Neurologic findings. *Archives of General Psychiatry,* 1971, *24,* 422–430.

Orton, S. T. *Reading, writing and speech problems in children.* New York: Norton Press, 1937.

Quitkin, F., Rifkin, A., & Klein, D. Neurologic soft signs in schizophrenia and character disorders. *Archives of General Psychiatry,* 1976, *33,* 845–847.

Rochford, J. M., Detre, T., Tucker, G. J., et al. Neuropsychological impairments in functional psychiatric diseases. *Archives of General Psychiatry,* 1970, *22,* 114–119.

Sharp, V., & Bellak, L. Ego function assessment of the psychoanalytic process. *Psychoanalytic Quarterly,* 1978, *47,* 52–72.

Strauss, A. A., & Lehtinan, L. *Psychopathology and education of the brain-injured child,* Vol. 1. New York: Grune & Stratton, 1947.

Tucker, G., Campion, E., & Silberfarb, P. M. Sensorimotor functions and cognitive disturbances in psychiatric patients. *American Journal of Psychiatry,* 1975, *132,* 17–21.

Wender, P. H. *MBD in children.* New York: Wiley, 1971.

Wood, D., Reinherr, F., Wender, P., et al. Diagnosis and treatment of MBD in adults. *Archives of General Psychiatry,* 1976, *33,* 1453–1460.

CHAPTER TWENTY-FIVE

The Use of EFA in the Assessment of Borderline Pathology

LISA A. GOLDSMITH, EDWARD CHARLES, AND KENNETH FEINER

BACKGROUND LITERATURE: THE BORDERLINE CONCEPT

Issues of description and classification are rife in the literature on borderline pathology. Diagnostic difficulties were already crystallizing by 1955, when, in a panel on borderline patients, Greenson (in Rangell, 1955) indicated how troublesome it was to make classifications in an area that was only barely understood. Diagnostic positions at that time ranged to such a degree that there were those who said there was no such thing as "borderline," whereas others used the term to denote a transitional state between neurosis and psychosis, and yet others used the term to indicate a relatively stable, characterological clinical picture in which there are simultaneous indications of psychotic and neurotic as well as adaptive ego functioning.

Defined variously as a syndrome, a state, and a type of personality organization, the term *borderline* remains as varied in contemporary usage. Some authors (e.g., Kety, Rosenthal, Wender, & Schulsinger, 1968) subscribe to the notion that it is an attenuated form of schizophrenia, whereas others (e.g., Kernberg, 1975) speak of it as a broad, stable, and persistent level of personality organization, meant to apply to all who are neither psychotic nor neurotic (a normal range is curiously omitted) and to be conceptualized and dealt with on its own terms. Other groups of writers (e.g., Gunderson and Singer, 1975; Perry & Klerman, 1978; Spitzer, Endicott, & Gibbon, 1979) have chosen to stay at the level of descriptive analysis and the careful delineation of psychiatric signs and symptoms, applying the borderline designation to what is considered to be a discriminable syndrome.

The diversity in diagnostic schemata does not stop there; for instance, Klein (1977) ascribes to a conceptualization in which borderline constitutes an affective disorder that involves a hysteric–depressive state and is amenable to antidepressant medications. Stone (1979) uses the borderline designation as an adjective, meaning "adjacent" or "marginal" to the major psychotic conditions. Arguing not only against a conceptualization of a separate and distinct disorder but against the very issue of a diagnostic continuum, Dickes (1974) asserts that the pathological conditions subsumed under the disorder represent diverse and heterogeneous diagnostic entities with varying etiologies, courses, and outcomes. Specifically, Dickes asserts that the presence of both neurotic and psychotic symptoms does not necessarily point to a borderline state but may reflect multiple etiological factors influencing the person in a variety of ways. If a continuum exists at all, according to Dickes, it is in terms of a range of function and capacity, from the mild to the severe, and not in terms of some imagined continuum of disease entities.

In this varying literature we find a number of features to be noteworthy, and an attempt will be made here to bring them into some relief. First is the notion that the borderline rubric allows for ambiguity in large part because the disorder is as yet imperfectly understood. Since such a problem exists with almost every nosological entity, it is hardly unique to the borderline domain. It may in fact be premature, as Stone (1977) has suggested, to demand or expect a synthesis given the relatively recent history of systematic investigation.

Second is the compelling finding that, even in the face of such varying opinions as to the proper definition and even viability of the term, there seems to be significant agreement among clinicians in applying certain descriptive criteria to actual case material. From such diverse perspectives as those of Perry and Klerman (1980) and Spitzer, Endicott, and Gibbon (1979), to those of Abend, Porder, and Willick (1983) in their account of the findings of the Kris Study Group, there seems to be substantial agreement at the level of a phenomenological description of this group of patients. In fact, a consensus that appears to run like a thread through the literature—be it in the writings of Dickes, Kernberg, Abend et al., Gunderson and Singer, or others—is an acknowledgment that in these patients particular areas of ego functioning are severely impaired. Even in early descriptions, such as those of Stern (1938) and Knight (1953)—however the group was designated—ego functioning was characterized as uneven, unreliable, and, in Little's (1966) terms, "patchy." In other words, whatever the theoretical frameworks, clinicians seem to know who these patients are. As Giovacchini (1970) comments, when one describes the "emergency-taut atmosphere" that these patients create in their lives and so readily in their treatments, there is an immediate recollection of a case that fits such a description. Kernberg (1975) has articulated a configuration of poor ego integration that encompasses lowered anxiety tolerance, impulse control, and subliminatory capacity, in a setting of relatively preserved reality testing. Gunderson (1977) describes a clinical picture of intense negative affect, poor impulse control, and a proneness to intense clinging and to shallow relationships—features that he and his co-workers subsume under "disturbed ego functions." Regardless of the particular frame of reference, as Heimann (1966) comments, attention gravitates to impairments in ego functioning; for example, this group of patients is recognizable by their significant impairments in impulse control, integrative functions, certain areas of reality testing, and identity formation.

It is our intent in this paper to offer some discussion of such varying theoretical frameworks and to see how, within a context of psychoanalytic theory—and in particular by using the set of orienting concepts provided by psychoanalytic ego psychology—thinking about borderline phenomena may be clarified and some thorny diagnostic issues highlighted. Finally, it is our intent to show in a preliminary way how ego function assessment (EFA), as derived by Bellak, Hurvich, and Gediman (1973), might serve as one technique for articulating a final common pathway to the understanding of these patients—that is, how EFA might allow for description in terms of degrees and configurations of impairment in ego processes.

Major empirical studies of the borderline patient done from the descriptive orientation—such as those of Gunderson and Singer (1975), Perry and Klerman (1980), and Spitzer et al. (1979)—continue to emphasize the discriminability and stability of the syndrome, and they take such consistencies as indications for the clinical validity of the concept. As an instance, Gunderson and Singer (1975), in an effort to incorporate descriptive and psychodynamic considerations, adjudged that an initial step in demonstrating the validity of a discrete syndrome was to demonstrate its discriminability from other psychopathological groups with which diagnostic confusion often exists. They endeavored to do so on the basis of the list of readily recognizable clinical characteristics that they abstracted from a systematic review of the literature and incorporated into a semistructured clinical interview (Gunderson & Kolb, 1978). Five areas of functioning were delineated—social adaptation, impulse–action patterns, affects, psychotic symptoms, and interpersonal relations—and the authors did indeed find the areas to have value in differentiating borderline from both schizophrenic and neurotic patients. Of note is that it was the enduring and characteristic *patterns* (in this study primarily in the interpersonal and action-pattern spheres) that proved to have the greatest discriminatory value, and this in contrast to the isolated sign-and-symptom patterns so popularly relied on in the usual diagnostic systems. On the basis of their research, the authors took these discriminable patterns as providing evidence of a recognizable borderline personality disorder. At the same time, Kolb and Gunderson (1980) were clear in stating that although their efforts to operationalize the concept demonstrated interrater reliability and concurrent validity between clinical and research diagnoses, the issue of the borderline concept itself needed to be placed on a broader and firmer base.

Psychoanalytic Contributions

Although there is as yet no clear consensus at the level of descriptive classification, it seems to us that it is from the psychoanalytic study of such conditions—rooted as such studies are in the understanding of data in a context of structural, developmental, and dynamic considerations—that a clinical descriptive analysis can be given depth and coherence. It offers, in Pine's (1980) words, an "interior view" and complements the study of external manifestations. In addition it may help to provide some clarification of the diagnostic and nosological ambiguities so extant. In contrast to other current methodologies, psychoanalytic investigation puts greater emphasis on the study of character formation, on the organization and structural aspects of personality, and on a detailed assessment of ego processes. While in no way meant to coopt a clinical–descriptive point of view, the body of dynamic, genetic, and structural hypotheses can take us beyond the level of diagnostic labeling and facilitate our descriptive efforts. As Sugarman and Lerner (1980) have written, "The fact that the superficial adaptiveness of the borderline patient masks a chaotic inner world suggests the need for just that understanding of the underlying principles of personality organization that psychoanalytic theory provides" (pp. 15–16.) They further suggest that without such principles "the descriptive approach is limited to categorizing a puzzling and contradictory set of symptoms."

In a comparatively early paper in the area, Frosch (1964) noted how such varying identifying features may give the impression of multiple clinical syndromes or, on the other hand, of differing transitional states "on the way to or from psychosis." In Frosch's view, what justifies the unification into a common entity, and what gives order to what would otherwise seem a chaotic symptomatic and clinical picture, is that the clinical manifestations are an integral part of the character structure of these individuals. It is thus at the level of the crystallization of psychic structure that one begins to find a coherence and predictability in regard to adaptation and responses to stress. According to Frosch, we are dealing with a characterological phenomenon of a particular type and order.

Within certain psychoanalytic circles, the conceptualization developed, in Green's (1977) words, that "behind this descriptive rubric there in fact lies a unique concept," a concept to be considered in terms of variably impaired ego functions. The "borderline problem" thus came to be viewed from the standpoint of functions rather than of symptoms. In the context of psychoanalytic ego psychology, with the possibility of examining specific ego processes in addition to and beyond those serving defensive functions, Frosch (1964) chose as his principal frame of reference the "state and position" of the ego, and spoke of a particular and stable form of pathological ego structure that he designated as the "psychotic character."

It was Kernberg (1966) who took the major synthetic step and, drawing on numerous lines of thought, conceptualized borderline symptomatology as emerging from a unique personality organization. Moving beyond the descriptive analysis of borderline conditions within psychiatry (e.g., Zilboorg, 1941; Hoch & Polatin, 1949), and beyond those psychoanalytic analyses that essentially conceptualized such conditions as variants of psychotic illness (e.g., Knight, 1953), Kernberg postulated a stable form of pathological intrapsychic structural organization. Stern (1938), for instance, had designated a "border line group of neurotics" consisting of patients who fit neither psychotic nor neurotic categories but appeared to show a greater involvement of ego impairment and constellation of infantile traits than neuroses, making treatment more difficult and prognosis more grave than was typical in the treatment of neurotic patients. Stern concluded that within this group a "greater part of ego functioning" was implicated than had hitherto been considered. Deutsch (1942) seems to have been writing of a similar group of patients, whom she designated "as-if personalities." She considered this group of patients distinguishable from the neurotic by the extent of disordered object relationships, and from the psychotic, by reason of the maintenance of "relatively intact reality testing."

Knight's (1953) contributions were seminal in distinguishing a structural from a more descriptive point of view in regard to such patients and in emphasizing the importance of a differential versus a global assessment of areas of ego dysfunction. The fact that the "ego was laboring badly" in these "borderline schizophrenic" patients could give a new order of explanation to the chaotic and typically inconsistent symptom picture. Glover (1958) also noted that classificatory systems needed to include characteristic clusters of ego impairment in designating a group located diagnostically between the neuroses and the psychoses. He, as others, began to delimit particular areas of dysfunction beyond psychosexual considerations, writing of disturbances and instabilities of affect and drive expression, deficiencies in the structuralization of ego and superego components, a reduction of "reality valuation," an excessive reliance on projection in object relations, and a constitutionally low threshold of frustration. It was this configuration, this "multi-nuclear" aspect of the symptom constellation, that Glover considered most noteworthy and critical for diagnosis.

Controversies within Psychoanalysis

As previously noted, however, it was Kernberg (1966) who most firmly posited that we are dealing with a discrete, relatively stable, and internally consistent form of ego pathology—a level of pathology with implications that cannot be readily collapsed or subsumed under already established diagnostic categories. Implicit in his effort to reexamine the spectrum of borderline and character disorders from the point of view of structural derivatives was the argument that descriptive clarifications contain but "presumptive diagnostic elements." Drawing from the British object relations school and the structural theory of ego psychology, he postulated a unique form of personality organization—one to be differentiated from neurotic and psychotic levels of organization. He drew from Jacobson (1971) a conceptualization of the interplay of pathological internalized object relationships and the vicissitudes of ego and superego formation, and he shares her view that there are points nosologically where quantitative differences move into qualitative distinctions. Subsequently, and in no way precluding the impact of intrapsychic conflict, Jacobson (1971) stated that "the indistinct but convenient term 'borderline' epitomizes certain common features in the personality structure and the devised used by such patients in conflict solutions" (p. 285). In other words, Kernbrg's (1977) assertions as to a highly structured and fixed level of structural organization—the "borderline personality organization"—is a construct that is considered to mediate "between etiological features, on the one hand, and direct behavioral manifestations of illness, on the other." This organization of psychological functioning becomes the underlying matrix from which behavioral signs and symptoms emerge; in particular—and here one of Kernberg's more controversial conceptions is introduced—there is a structuralization of internalized object relationships that encompasses "hierarchically organized motivational sequences," and that crystallizes into a stable and pathological form of ego structure.

These patients manifest deficiencies in anxiety tolerance, impulse control, and sublimatory potential; they shift toward more primitive modes of thought, rely on specific primitive defensive operations, and, in symptoms of identity diffusion, manifest pathological internalized object relations. Although various overt manifestations will emerge, implying a broad array of determinants and different characterological styles, the common structural ego defects are ubiquitous, and the definitive diagnosis depends on this recurring pattern of ego pathology; it is the combination of the presence of identity diffusion, primitive defensive operations, and the maintenance of reality testing that clinically defines these conditions. As Smith (1980) writes in summarizing and supporting Kernberg's views, "borderline" is not a personality type but refers to a level of ego organization that can encompass several personality and characterological dispositions.

As for Kernberg's genetic hypotheses, mention previously was made of the nature of the structural matrix from which the overt symptomatology is assumed to emerge. From early in his writings Kernberg (1966) ascribed to a model of ego development in which splitting and synthesis are central mechanisms. He subsequently added to these conceptualizations, so that in terms of the defense of splitting—by which conflictual identifications based on aggression and affection are kept apart or alternatively activated—what was first considered a simple defect in integration is now seen to be a defensive formation arising in response to the pathological predominance of early aggressive conflicts, as well as being shaped by experiential and constitutional factors. In contrast to psychotics, whose self- and object representations remain undifferentiated, it is the active keeping apart of affectively polarized yet differentiated self- and object representations that so characterize borderlines. The lack of integration of these affectively determined constellations of self- and object images has its sequellae, according to Kernberg, in failures in ego integration, affective integration, and the establishment of object constancy; failures that Kernberg (1975) considers to be the major course for "nonpsychotic ego disturbances." Splitting and the organization of internal object relationships around splitting are presumed to be normal psychic phenomena in the infant and young child, where they are seen as precursors of mature tripartite structural organization. In the borderline, however, splitting is defensive, and the structural organization becomes fixated at this preoedipal level. While Kernberg (1977) places these considerations as to the prominence and sequellae of splitting on a dynamic base, he finds great value in focusing on structural and descriptive criteria, particularly at the level of diagnostic evaluation.

Arriving at a decidedly different position, Abend, Porder, and Willick (1983) summarize an extensive evaluation of the borderline concept that was done by the Kris Study Group—an evaluation that was derived from the psychoanalyses of a number of patients diagnosed as falling within the borderline rubric. As compared to other analysands with whom the study group had had experience, these patients, while considered "sicker" in many areas than the typical analysand, did not seem to necessitate conceptually the presumption that they were of a unique, sharply divisible group or require for their understanding the postulation of any distinct level of psychic organization. Although acknowledging that their clinical material derived from patients in office practice and was thus probably representative of the less severe end of the spectrum of disturbance, these observers felt their findings could be adequately encompassed by placing them within the framework of differences of degree of pathology rather than of kind. Further, those disturbances that were observed, such as disruptions in reality testing, over the course of analysis could be understood in terms of intrapsychic conflict, compromise formation, the role of unconscious fantasy, and other traditional psychoanalytic formulations; recourse to notions of particular mechanisms and fixations arising from or at the earliest phases of psychic development did not appear to this group to be required. Further, the concept of a splitting of self- and object images used by Kernberg to explain polarized conscious ego states was markedly challenged. Alterations in ego states were viewed as amenable to more parsimonious and accurate considerations as manifestations of such defenses as isolation, displacement, reaction formation, the use of one drive derivative to defend against another, and the like and were to be considered rather as the "tip of the iceberg," or, if you will, at the level of any other form of manifest content. The full range of defensive possibilities was observed in these patients, including—in contradistinction to the formulations of Kernberg—the repressive defenses. Where others have found recourse in a conceptualization of developmental defect and arrest of function, these authors relied instead on notions of varying aspects of ego regression in the face of conflict, with such elements then seen as impacting on the "general integration of the ego." What is called primitivity in these patients is but a reflection of disturbances of the full range of ego functions, according to these authors, who state: "The sicker a patient is, the more we see poor integration, poor ego organization, and breakdown of ego functions" (Abend et al., 1983, p. 171). Finally, acknowledging that the term *borderline* has achieved wide usage, they feel its continued utility can only be that of a reference to a broad, loose categorization as applied to severe levels of character pathology; distinctions drawn are quantitative ones, with no claim to a distinct diagnostic entity with characteristic defenses, conflicts, or developmental defects.

In considering that there are such varying points of view, even among those who share a psychoanalytic orientation, one is reminded of a refrain analogous to the defect-versus-conflict debate in the literature on psychosis (Arlow & Brenner, 1964; London, 1973), but now the effort is to come to terms with severe character pathology. The current debate is lively, with broad implications, and it is not limited to the writers just discussed. In support of the conflict position, Wohlberg (1973) asserted that rather than speaking of "ego weakness" or "ego defect" we should consider various forms of ego organization in a context of notions of conflict and defense. Holzman (1978) has noted that what unifies those patients referred to as borderline personalities is a characteristic inconsistency in reality contact. He believes, however, that what can be used as a basis for classification does not justify the assumption of a stable character constellation, disease entity, uniform etiology, or the like. In Holzman's view there has been a confounding of two lines in the search for diagnostic entities, one the search for symptoms of the descriptive psychiatric line and the other the search for "meaning in behavior" of the psychoanalytic line. There is marked heterogeneity within the range of clinical phenomena displayed by "borderlines," and Holzman suggests that what is so characteristic of these patients, inappropriately grouped under a common rubric, is the ease with which "control is loosened and organization impaired."

By contrast, many authors in addition to Kernberg have taken the position that there is an inner consistency to this group of patients, and a consistency that derives from a fundamental disturbance in ego functioning related to basic developmental defects. Grinker, Werble, and Drye (1968), in the first large scale study of ego function impairments in borderline patients, clearly stated that they were working within a theoretical framework that posited a structural defect in these patients deriving from early narcissistic and developmental trauma. In other words, they hypothesized that there are developmental deficiencies in the process of identification and in the formation of regulatory structures, on which a full array of defensive and adaptive behavior is overlaid. The core of the disturbance is to be found in the characterological peculiarities and "soft" thought disorder; it is not to be found "in symptomatic adaptive defenses, a mixture of which is found in all psychoses, neuroses, personality disorders and varieties of health, but in the basic ego defects in maturation and early development, expressed in ego dysfunctions" (Grinker et al., 1968, p. 97). Grinker et al. consider that despite the symptomatic variability, the syndrome itself is recognizable, giving rise to the adage "stable instability."

As Kanzer (1968) suggested in an effort to give some order to the functional ego disturbances observed in acting-out phenomena, the concept of ego distortions is hardly a new one, having its beginnings in Freud's (1924) writings on ego alterations, and many writers have associated deviations in ego development with serious character pathology. Chessick (1977), citing Gitelson's (1958) work on ego distortion, considers it well nigh impossible to approach an understanding of "borderline" patients without making use of the concept of narcissism and of the theoretical assumptions of psychoanalytic ego psychology. These patients represent, in many ways, according to Chessick, "the most subtle and complex malfunctions and maldevelopments of psychic structure of any patients that we deal with" (1977, p. 30). Blum (1972), in a similar vein, draws on what he interprets as Freud's formulations of a continuum of ego deficit. Blum holds that early deficits leading to structural impairments influence the way in which intrapsychic conflicts are dealt with, and he speaks of the "ego passivity" evidenced in the disturbed object relations, narcissistic features, intolerance of frustration, and lack of affect modulation in a certain group of patients. The propensity to regression itself has to be explained, and this propensity, along with other disturbed ego functions, Blum sees as characterizing the complex, unique borderline condition.

Similarly, Zetzel (1971) proposed that there is a distinction to be drawn between difficulties at the level of unresolved conflict and those that must be seen in the light of regressive changes that occur due to a vulnerability in the establishment of certain basic ego functions. She notes that failure in development may be "deceptively" expressed in the way of instinctual fantasy, but that it needs to be understood in terms of underlying structural and organizational weaknesses in the ego. According to Atkins (1975), in conjunction with such personality traits as ambivalence, aggressiveness, self-centeredness, empathetic failure, primitive superego manifestations, and pseudoadaptation of social roles, certain cases manifest fairly characteristic distortions in the autonomous functions of thought, cognition, and language, all of which speak, in his view, to an "integrative disjunction."

In all the literature cited there seems to be a convergence on the role of psychic structure formation, such that conflict and a variety of developmental and maturational factors are seen as coming to be, in the words of Gill (1954), "crystallized in structuralized, relatively enduring, relatively autonomous ego organizations" (p. 792). Modell (1963) indicates that when he uses the term *borderline* nosologically he is designating a structural and not a symptomatic diagnosis, encompassing notions of internalization processes, identity formation, self- and object differentiation, and the like; while for Masterson (1976) it is the structural considerations that knit the clinical contradictions together. Blanck and Blanck (1979) have stated that the era of ego psychology has forged a breakthrough in the attempt to understand borderline pathology. They have suggested that rather than simply conceptualizing borderline pathology as a failure of structuralization or the emergence of a too-rigid level of organization, what we are seeing is the "clinical expression of multifaceted complexities of development." Such complexities are not readily reducible either to a simple developmental arrest or to the vicissitudes of conflict and regression.

Loewald (1980), in his efforts to account for the vicissitudes of ego and superego formation, has postulated that it is useful to consider how defensive processes, by regression, make use of primitive psychic processes that "in their original state may better be viewed as subserving psychic organization and boundary setting, instead of being seen as defense mechanisms in the clinical sense of the term" (p. 175). Greenspan (1979) postulates a model that incorporates developmental-structural considerations so as to encompass dynamic and symptom-complex variables and reflect such basic disturbances as those of the formation of mental representations that impact, in turn, on the way stress and conflict are managed. Also taking a developmental-structural point of view is Robbins (1983). He espouses a two-model epigenetic hierarchy so as to encompass what he calls "primitive personality organization."

The phases of early psychic development articulated in the developmental psychoanalytic literature have been repeatedly invoked in the context of trying to define the borderline conditions. In no way presuming that the relationship between structure, phenomenology, and dynamics is equivalent in children and adults, many have suggested that the issues that are salient for early ego development—such as symbiosis, omnipotence, and immediate gratification—may be seen to dominate the clinical picture of borderline patients (Fries, Nelson, & Woolf, 1980).

Pine (1974) found it useful to specify common structural features underlying diverse "borderline" phenomena in children. He found failures in signal anxiety and reality testing and observed a "slippery connectedness to objects"—and these in contradistinction to the focal drive conflict to be found in the neurotic child. The borderline children seemed to lack the "basic stabilizers of functioning"; that is, they were without sufficient grounding in external reality and showed a dearth of patterned object relationships and reliable defenses. And yet, Pine's position, and one that we consider noteworthy, is that the delineation of critical features or the elucidation of a variety of syndromes in no way presupposes a search for a unitary concept of "the" borderline child. There need be no assumption of any single mechanism or developmental failure; rather, what emerges are certain structural commonalities in the aberrant development of ego functions and object relations. Pine speaks of "aspects of pathological phenomena" that are based in part on descriptive and in part on structural–developmental considerations; he does not speak in terms of entities. Just as we can strive for specification beyond the diagnostic term *neurosis,* so we can strive for specification within the borderline domain. *Borderline* is a concept that we, in line with Pine, choose to apply to a set of phenomena. And what it "really is" is just that—a concept.

Pine (1980) has written additionally on the topic of the borderline child and views the work by Knight (1953) and Redl (1951) as congenial to his own way of thinking. In this regard Pine cites Knight's emphasis on the existence of a range of ego pathology and a lack of any single etiological mechanism, and he notes Redl's (1951) adherence to the value of specifying and identifying particular ego disturbances in contrast to relying on such vagaries as "ego weakness" or "ego deficit." Meissner (1982–1983), too, has endeavored to map out syndromal possibilities within the domain, but his efforts have focused on adult patients. He has asserted, in line with Pine, that conditions within the "intermediate range of pathology" can be traced along several significant parameters, and this in preference to lumping them under a single descriptive heading.

Thus there appear to be continuing efforts to specify those areas of ego pathology that underlie diverse clinical and symptom pictures—to dimensionalize the concept of borderline—a position very congenial to our own. Also congenial with our position are those comments that draw attention to gaps in our existing knowledge. Sugarman and Lerner (1980), for example, have stated that although concepts derived from the study of early development may hold the promise of providing a wide explanatory scope, their precise applicability to such matters as the evolution of psychological structures, the modulation of affects, and the development of object relations still need to be spelled out.

Here, we would like to offer a few final statements on the theoretical debate so evident in today's literature. A major issue for us is whether one can take a firm stand at this point as to whether symptoms are restitutive or defensive. It is hardly the simplest of issues, and, as Wexler (1971) has pointed out in writing on psychosis, we may not be dealing with an either-or situation. Kernberg (1976) has himself stated that ego weakness in the sense of deficit reflects conflictually determined issues—deficit, in his view, encompasses defensive responses formed in the face of "intense and primitive object relations." Meissner (1978) has asserted that rather than offer simplistic conceptions of determinants to account for the multifaceted impairments found in borderline patients, one must consider the complexities of the factors involved in ego functioning at different levels of disturbance. Anna Freud (1974) articulated the need to regard the vicissitudes of both developmentally and conflictually based pathology. In addition to "abnormalities" caused by the incidence of trauma and conflict, one must also consider "defects in the personality structure itself caused by developmental irregularities and failures" (1974, p. 15). She spoke to the issue of how the temporal relations between pathological processes occur simultaneously and become "intertwined" in the clinical picture. The need to describe personality functioning in both structural and dynamic terms led her to conceptualize the notion of "lines of development" that could encompass the full array of maturational, adaptational, and conflictual variables.

In addressing the defect-defense as well as the preoedipal-oedipal debate, Frosch (1983) too suggests that one cannot consider such concepts as mutually exclusive. He writes: "defects may be borrowed in the service of defense . . . modes of defense are facilitated by defects or weaknesses already existing in the ego, which seem to be exploited in the service of defense" (1983, p. 410). Thus the very vulnerability to ego regression may need to be considered in terms of developmental traumata. Frosch considers psychic conflict, defenses, altered ego states, and defects in ego functions as all "very closely related." With the advent of the conceptual framework offered by psychoanalytic ego psychology, one has been able to begin to focus on processes that bespeak a continuous interplay of factors and operations and, as Frosch states, "it is only through a study of these processes that our understanding of clinical manifestations can be deepened" (1983, p. xii).

Psychoanalytic Ego Psychology—A Common Pathway

We recall that in his writing on the psychotic character Frosch (1964) chose as his frame of reference the state and position of the ego in regard to the external and internal environment. He spoke of adaptation established at different levels of organization, with evidences of regressive and progressive adaptations existing side by side. Particularly, it was in his efforts to delineate the exact nature of the reality disturbances in these patients—leading to a consideration of separate although interrelated aspects of the reality testing function—that significant diagnostic ramifications emerged. What we wish to emphasize here is that any effort to delineate the specific processes involved in any designated ego function—such as a disturbance with reality—can do much to illuminate the complex nature of the functions involved, be they autonomous, defensive, or admixtures thereof. A process-oriented approach need not preclude the kind of analysis that comes out of the psychoanalytic setting, in which one can attend to intrapsychic meaning, unconscious fantasy, and the like; it is a different slice of the pie, yet one that gives due respect to behavior in its multiple functions.

What we also find striking in the literature is that the differential assessment of regressed and distorted as well as intact ego processes is considered by most authors to be of fundamental importance in studying the "borderline" domain. Rangell (1955) asserted in one of the earliest symposia on borderline pathology that what is required for an improved nosology is the most careful evaluation of ego functions. Sadow (1969) proposed a diagnostic schema taking the role of the ego as an axis along which different pathologies could be considered and ordered. He believed that by "relating psychopathology intimately to differential ego capacities" sterile concepts of classification could be averted and means of comparison and cross-validation provided. Such an emphasis on ego processes, as Maenchen (1970) suggests, allows for a systematic way of observing the interrelationships among various currents in development.

It should be apparent by this point that we are in strong support of the position that a careful assessment of ego processes need not result in a prejudicial casting of the data into one or another conceptual framework, and that, moreover, we consider that there is heuristic value to be found in placing our clinical observations in what Grinker et al. (1968) call "appropriate frames." Further we believe that an approach that renders constructs empirically testable will be eminently useful in assessing the value of our constructs. It will be recalled that in the investigations reported by Abend et al. (1983) there were repeated attempts to delineate various ego functions—patient's object relations, defensive organization, intactness of reality testing, and the like. Thus even a group relying on a conflict model felt the need to dimensionalize their findings and found value in so doing.

Despite the absence of a theoretical consensus there does seem to be some unanimity in the literature as to the phenomenological coherence of "borderline" patients—that is, they are identifiable. Further, there seems to be a degree of consensus that assessment along the lines of variations in ego functioning can be, at least at this stage, of heuristic and theoretical value. It is our view that by refining our understanding of ego functions so as to enhance the descriptive clarity of our terms we might cut across issues of "entity," symptom picture, behavioral variability, discontinuity notions, and premature closure regarding etiology. It is our view that configurations and characteristic patterns may emerge from the assessment of an array of ego functions. Ego function assessment (EFA), as articulated by Bellak et al. (1973), has the potential to be useful in just this way. The EFA methodology attempts to render our clinical language less global and, further, what characteristic patterns do emerge may have a bearing on more differentiated hypotheses as to pathogenesis and etiology.

EFA allows for the assessment of the individual case; it does not preclude intergroup comparisons or presuppose the exclusivity of factors to any one diagnostic domain, nor does it presuppose an etiological commitment. As Bellak et al. (1973) reported, it was the configuration of ego function profiles that proved useful in distinguishing schizophrenic patients from neurotics and normals despite etiological heterogeneity. Relevant here is Schafer's

(1949, 1954) statement that it is in the constellation of "identifying characteristics," and in a full acknowledgment of overlap between and within diagnostic conceptualizations, that diagnostic clarification lies. We recall, too, Rapaport's (1950, 1954) observation that it is the patterning to be found in areas of strength and weakness that "allows for inferences concerning organization." As Glasner (1966) suggested, what proves to be so characteristic of the borderline patient is the "peculiar" amalgam and configuration of ego functions. Such a patterning is, as Horwitz (1977) suggests, not simply at the level of characterological dispositions, as these patients come in many "sizes and shapes . . . personality attitudes and behavioral dispositions." Where the commonality seems to lie is at the level of ego strength and weakness and organization.

AN APPROACH TO BORDERLINE PATHOLOGY USING EFA

In our preliminary study, we were interested in seeing whether we could observe patterns and configurations of ego processes within a small group of "borderline" patients. We chose to use EFA because, on the basis of observations made from manifest behavior, patient's self-observations, and clinical judgments, it would enable us to assess where patients stood on a range of ego functions rated along a continuum of adaptation. Kernberg and his colleagues (1981), working within their own particular framework, have also made efforts to utilize a semistructured interview format in assessing enduring structural features in borderline patients. Comparing their interview findings with data derived from other methods and scales, they asserted that the semi-structured interview format seemed to elicit a dimension of personality functioning different from what was available using the other methods studied.

As mentioned, Bellak et al. (1973) were able to utilize EFA in differentiating schizophrenic patients from neurotics and normals on the basis of patterns of ego function weaknesses and strengths, with results that attained a level of statistical reliability and discriminant validity. Subgroupings also emerged, as did individual differences. We hope that with replication and further study EFA will continue to help to define critical parameters and differentiate patterns useful to our understanding of the borderline domain. If recognizable patterns do emerge, we are not suggesting that the term *borderline* itself be substituted for precise descriptions. Rather the term might serve, as Leichtman and Shapiro (1980) have suggested, as a starting point for a satisfactory diagnostic portrait, alerting the diagnostician to possible impairments in ego functions.

In this spirit, and in light of the question as to whether the characteristics observed in borderline patients warrant a unified diagnostic consideration, we refer to Carpenter, Gunderson, and Strauss (1977) as to the advantages of a "mixed-model" approach in defining the borderline syndromes. They suggest a two-level ordering of the clinical data—a discrete and a continuous dimension. They would place considerations of disordered ego functioning and character development along a severity continuum but then would expect that, at certain segments of the continuum, characteristic signs and symptoms would arise to distinguish such patients from those in other diagnostic groups. Although we believe that such a typological effort might be premature, EFA profiling might prove useful in such a multiple-model endeavor.

EFA, emerging from a network of hypotheses within psychoanalytic ego psychology, affords quantifiable scores that are meant to facilitate and not to replace qualitative analysis. It must be remembered, too, that the clinical correlates of the obtained patterns are "identifying characteristics"—not labels, not entities, not typologies. To quote from Schafer (1949, 1954): "Research that proceeds by way of identifying personality characteristics rather than diagnoses as clinical criteria, individual variation as a focus of interest along with group trends . . . all this appears to hold great promise for personality investigation" (p. 211). It is our sense that EFA speaks to such needs.

Dahl (this volume) did in fact use EFA in a large investigation to assess the validity of the borderline category, comparing groups of hospitalized borderline, schizophrenic, affectively disordered, and neurotic patients. The borderline group did manifest significant differences in levels of ego functioning in comparison to the other diagnostic groups, its scores falling midway between neurotic and schizophrenic levels of functioning. While acknowledging certain methodological limitations in their study (e.g., judges were not "blind" to diagnosis, all patients were hospitalized, and there was no control for neuroleptic medication), they observed that EFA could be used reliably with a Norwegian population (pointing to EFA's cross-cultural potentialities), and lent support to a "dimensional" view of borderline psychopathology; that is, despite the variety of symptomatology, stable patterns of ego impairments were observed.

It was the purpose of our study to see where a group of outpatients, clinically diagnosed as borderline, would fall on specifiable dimensions of the EFA profile. Although Bellak et al. (1973) made no attempt to differentiate borderline patients in their original study, they made certain projections as to where such patients might fall on a continuum of adaptive ego functioning. Our study attempted to test the Bellak et al. projections by evaluating in depth four borderline patients randomly selected from a large psychiatric outpatient department. The patients were clinically diagnosed on the basis of intake interviews by two senior staff members with confirmation from two borderline assessment scales employing self-ratings (Sheehy, Goldsmith, & Charles, 1980; Conte, Plutchik, Karasu, & Jerrett, 1980). In addition, two neurotic outpatients were interviewed for preliminary comparison. Patients ranged in age from 19 to 48, and none were on medication. Our exclusionary criteria included drug habituation, alcoholism, organicity, or mental retardation (as assessed by a brief psychological test battery). The EFA interview schedule was slightly modified for our purposes; for example, not all subscales were included for the purposes of this preliminary analysis. The EFA interviews were conducted by one interviewer, and each interview was tape recorded in its entirety. Two raters, blind to diagnosis, then independently made their ratings from the tape recordings.

We hoped that our preliminary findings would suggest differences in configurations of impairment between our borderline and neurotic groups and that this would encourage further study. With regard to particular manifestations of impairment, we were interested in whether we might observe identifiable patterns in such areas as object relations, defensive functioning, reality testing, affect and impulse control, and subliminatory capacity.

Preliminary Findings

The establishment of interrater reliability for the diagnostic interview was a necessary first step before analyzing our results. The T-index, a chance-corrected statistic appropriate for ordinal level ratings, was used for this purpose. Three different analyses were conducted: the first to determine reliability when the criterion for agreement required identical ratings by the two judges, the second to establish the level of agreement when the raters could differ by one-half scale point, and the third to measure reliability when the raters could differ by no less than one scale point based on a seven-step scale.

Table 25.1. *Chance Corrected Interrater Agreement for Ego Function Ratings*

Subscale	Chi Square $(R2)$	Probability $(R2)$	T-Index $(R2)$
ARISE	9.511	.002**	1.00
Object Relations	5.067	.024*	.733
Reality Testing	.267	.012**	1.00
Judgment	9.511	.002*	1.00
Sense of Reality	9.511	.002**	1.00
Regulation and Control of Needs, Drives and Affects	9.511	.002**	1.00
Defensive Functioning	5.067	.024*	.733
Synthetic Functioning	9.511	.002**	1.00

Note: R2 = Differences among raters not greater than 1 scale point.
* $p < .01$
** $p < .05$

When the strictest criterion—that of identical ratings—was required, the analysis of the ratings shows a significant level of agreement for three ego functions—ARISE ($p < .001$), Object Relations ($p < .01$), and Judgment ($p < .001$). When a one-scale point difference between the raters was considered acceptable, the interrater reliability was significant for all ego function ratings except Reality Testing. Finally, Table 25.1 presents the chance-corrected interrater agreement when the two independent ratings had to be within 1.5 scale points of each other. Here the agreement was significant for all ego functions. This degree of reliability is substantial and compares favorably with that reported by Bellak et al. (1973) in their original study.

To determine whether there were differences between the borderline and neurotic subjects in the patterns of impairment in ego functioning, and as a comparison with the Bellak et al. projections, a mean profile for each group was formulated. Profiles were generated by computing a group mean rating for each ego function. Figure 25.1 presents the mean ego function ratings, as well as showing an overall mean, which was calculated by averaging the mean ratings for each group. An inspection of these measures shows that the overall mean for the borderline group ($\bar{x} = 6.64$) falls squarely within the projected range of 4–8, and the overall mean for neurotic subjects ($\bar{x} = 9.12$) also falls within the predicted range (6–10).

An examination of Figure 25.1, which depicts the ego function profiles of the two groups, allows a comparison of their patterns of impairment. Notably, for the neurotic group the ratings of all functions considered in the present pilot study, with the exception of Reality Testing, do fall within the predicted neurotic range.

Similarly, the pattern of scores for the borderline group was consistent with the predictions advanced by Bellak et al. (1973) for all functions except Judgment. Reality Testing, which fell within the expected range, was the next highest score. With regard to the particular configuration of ego functioning, it is noteworthy that the lowest scores were assigned to the functions of Object Relations and Defensive Functioning. Also in the lower range were Sense of Reality, ARISE, and Synthetic Functioning.

This preliminary investigation addressed two issues: first, whether overall ego function assessment ratings differentiate neurotic and borderline groups in terms of the range of ego functioning rated along a continuum of adaptation and, second, whether there are specific patterns of ego processes that are characteristic of each group and that further distinguish the two groups. In regard to the first issue, the results of this study support the notion of an ordering of diagnostic groups on a continuum of adaptive ego functioning. Thus the results suggest that the degree of ego impairments that characterizes patients diagnosed as borderline is more severe than the level of impairment for neurotic subjects.

As regards the profile of ego strengths and weaknesses within each group, the configuration of functions for the borderline group showed relative weak-

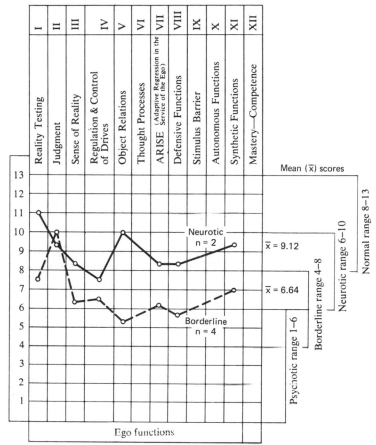

Figure 25.1. Profile of mean ego function ratings for borderline and neurotic groups.

nesses in all ego functions except for Judgment. In an attempt to make greater sense of these profiles, a preliminary inspection of the qualitative material was made. For this group, low scores on Object Relations seemed to reflect a tendency to display sadomasochistic relationships and extreme overreactions to separation and loss. The level of Object Relations for these subjects is exemplified by Ms. A., a 48-year-old woman with a past history of alcoholism. In the face of feeling "like an old rag"—left out and abandoned—she seemed to take recourse to violent attacks on others. She experienced her relationship with her husband as "a battleground" where each was constantly attempting to defeat the other. Such types of interactions were of a chronic and repetitive nature for Ms. A. and appeared fairly characteristic of this group as a whole.

In terms of defensive functioning the borderline patients seemed to rely on such defenses as denial, projection, and a schizoidlike withdrawal to stave off anxiety. Losses of impulse control were common, as were disruptions in the sense of reality.

It is noteworthy that all of the borderline subjects showed a relatively impaired sense of reality despite their ability to maintain the distinction between fantasy and reality. One subject described a history of episodic hypnagogic hallucinatory experiences and a feeling that she was "turning to stone." A 19-year-old male subject described painful feelings of depersonalization that emerged in the context of feelings of alienation from others. He stated, "I feel like I'm disintegrating . . . you know . . . fading away . . . as if I wasn't real." Another subject spoke of repeated, albeit episodic, states of feeling "blurry, light-headed, and dazed out."

In predicting what the ego profile for borderline subjects would look like, Bellak et al. (1973) suggested that Judgment and Reality Testing scores would be relatively elevated and Object Relations lowered in contrast to the profile for neurotics. In the present pilot study, the ego profile for the borderline group is strikingly consistent with Bellak et al.'s projections. One can conjecture that since these subjects performed relatively better on Judgment and Reality Testing than on the other dimensions, their social functioning seems on the surface less impaired than those areas of functioning that reflect other ego processes. Further, the ego profile for the neurotic subjects did reveal relatively higher levels of ego functioning than were observed for the borderlines in most areas, and, in particular, it was in the area of Object Relations that the greatest discrepancy in scores was evident; thus the findings were as predicted.

Although the findings are based on a relatively small sample, we are encouraged by them; they are promising signs that the study of specific constellations of ego processes may yield information useful to further dimensionalizing the area of "borderline" psychopathology. The EFA approach is one that may help to give systematic elucidation to the grouping that emerges at the level of clinical experience. Such studies as Dahl's (this volume) and our own are but a first step, a testing of the waters, and the need for broader sampling and cross-validation is obvious.

REFERENCES

Abend, S. M., Porder, M. S., & Willick, M. S. Borderline patients: Psychoanalytic perspectives. *Monographs of the Kris Study Group*, 1983, 7.

Atkins, S. Ego synthesis and cognition in a borderline case. *Psychoanalytic Quarterly*, 1975, *44*, 29–61.

Arlow, J., & Brenner, C. *Psychoanalytic concepts and the structural theory*. New York: International Universities Press, 1964.

Bellak, L., Hurvich, M., & Gediman, H. *Ego functions in schizophrenics, neurotics, and normals*. New York: Wiley, 1973.

Blanck, G., & Blanck, R. *Ego psychology II: Psychoanalytic developmental psychology.* New York: Columbia University Press, 1979.

Blum, H. P. Psychoanalytic understanding and psychotherapy of borderline regression. *International Journal of Psychoanalytic Psychotherapy,* 1972, *1,* 46–60.

Carpenter, W. T., Gunderson, J. G., & Strauss, J. S. Considerations of the borderline syndrome: A longitudinal comparative study of borderline and schizophrenic patients. In P. Hartocollis (Ed.), *Borderline personality disorders: The concept, the syndrome, the patient.* New York: International Universities Press, 1977.

Chessick, R. *Intensive psychotherapy of the borderline patient.* New York: Jason Aronson, 1977.

Conte, H. R., Plutchik, R., Karasu, T. B., & Jerrett, I. A self-report borderline scale: Discriminative validity and preliminary norms. *Journal of Nervous and Mental Disease,* 1980, *168*(1), 428–435.

Deutsch, H. Some forms of emotional disturbance and their relationship to schizophrenia. *Psychoanalytic Quarterly,* 1942, *11,* 301–321.

Dickes, R. The concepts of borderline states: An alternative proposal. *International Journal of Psychoanalytic Psychotherapy,* 1974, *3,* 1–27.

Freud, A. A psychoanalytic view of developmental psychopathology. *Journal of the Philadelphia Association for Psychoanalysis,* 1974, *1,* 7–17.

Freud, S. *Neurosis and psychosis.* Standard Edition (Vol. 19). London: Hogarth Press, 1961.

Fries, M. E., Nelson, M. C., & Woolf, P. J. Developmental and etiological factors in the treatment of character disorders with archaic ego function. *Psychoanalytic Review,* 1980, *67,* 337–352.

Frosch, J. The psychotic character: Clinical psychiatric considerations. *Psychiatric Quarterly,* 1964, *38,* 81–96.

Frosch, J. *The psychotic process.* New York: International Universities Press, 1983.

Gill, M. M. Psychoanalysis and exploratory psychotherapy. *Journal of the American Psychoanalytic Association,* 1954, *2,* 771–797.

Giovacchini, P. L. The need to be helped. *Archives of General Psychiatry,* 1970, *22,* 245–251.

Gitelson, M. On ego distortion. *International Journal of Psychoanalysis,* 1958, *39,* 245–257.

Glasner, S. Benign paralogical thinking. *Archives of General Psychiatry,* 1966, *14,* 94–99.

Glover, E. Ego distortion. *International Journal of Psychoanalysis,* 1958, *39,* 260–264.

Green, A. The borderline concept: A conceptual framework for the understanding of borderline patients: Suggested hypotheses. In P. Hartocollis (Ed.), *Borderline personality disorders: The concept, the syndrome, the patient.* New York: International Universities Press, 1977.

Greenspan, S. I. Intelligence and adaptation. *Psychological Issues,* 1979, *12*(3–4).

Grinker, R. R., Werble, B., & Drye, R. C. *Borderline syndrome: A behavioral study of ego functions.* New York: Basic Books, 1968.

Gunderson, J. G. Characteristics of borderlines. In P. Hartocollis (Ed.), *Borderline personality disorders: The concept, the syndrome, the patient.* New York: International Universities Press, 1977.

Gunderson, J. G., & Kolb, J. E. Discriminating features of borderline patients. *American Journal of Psychiatry,* 1978, *135*(7), 792–796.

Gunderson, J. G., & Singer, M. T. Defining borderline patients: An overview. *American Journal of Psychiatry,* 1975, *132*(1), 1–10.

Heimann, P. Comment on Dr. Kernberg's paper: Structural derivatives of object relationships. *International Journal of Psychoanalysis,* 1966, *47,* 254–260.

Hoch, P. H. & Polatin, P. Pseudoneurotic forms of schizophrenia. *Psychiatric Quarterly,* 1949, *23,* 248–276.

Holzman, P. S. What is a borderline patient? In S. Smith (Ed.), *The human mind revisited: Essays in honor of Karl A. Menninger.* New York: International Universities Press, 1978.

Horwitz, L. Group psychotherapy of the borderline patient. In P. Hartocollis (Ed.). *Borderline personality disorders: The concept, the syndrome, the patient.* New York: International Universities Press, 1977.

Jacobson, E. *Depression: Comparative studies of normal, neurotic, and psychotic conditions.* New York: International Universities Press, 1971.

Kanzer, M. Ego alteration and acting out. *International Journal of Psychoanalysis,* 1968, *49,* 431–435.

Kernberg, O. F. Structural derivatives of object relationships. *International Journal of Psychoanalysis,* 1966, *47,* 236–253.

Kernberg, O. F. *Borderline conditions and pathological narcissism.* New York: Jason Aronson, 1975.

Kernberg, O. F. Technical considerations in the treatment of borderline personality organization. *Journal of the American Psychoanalytic Association,* 1976, *24,* 795–829.

Kernberg, O. F. The structural diagnosis of borderline personality disorder. In P. Hartocollis (Ed.), *Borderline personality disorders: The concept, the syndrome, the patient.* New York: International Universities Press, 1977.

Kernberg, O. F., Goldstein, E. G., Carr, A. C., Hunt, H. F., Bauer, S. F., & Blumenthal, R. Diagnosing borderline personality: A pilot study using multiple diagnostic methods. *Journal of Nervous and Mental Disease,* 1981, *169,* 225–231.

Kety, S. S., Rosenthal, D., Wender, P. H., & Schulsinger, F. The types and prevalence of mental illness in the biological and adoptive families of adopted schizophrenics. In D. Rosenthal & S. S. Kety (Eds.), *The transmission of schizophrenia.* New York: Pergamon, 1968.

Klein, D. F. Psychopharmacological treatment and delineation of borderline disorders. In P. Hartocollis (Ed.), *Borderline personality disorders: The concept, the syndrome, the patient.* New York: International Universities Press, 1977.

Knight, R. P. Borderline states. *Bulletin of the Menninger Clinic,* 1953, *17,* 1–12.

Kolb, J. E., & Gunderson, J. G. Diagnosing borderline patients with a semistructured interview. *Archives of General Psychiatry,* 1980, *37,* 37–41.

Leichtman, M., & Shapiro, S. An introduction to the psychological assessment of borderline conditions in children: Borderline conditions and the test process. In J. Kwawer, H. D. Lerner, P. M. Lerner, & A. Sugarman (Eds.), *Borderline phenomena and the Rorschach test.* New York: International Universities Press, 1980.

Little, M. Transference in borderline states. *International Journal of Psychoanalysis,* 1966, *47,* 476–495.

Loewald, H. *Papers on psychoanalysis.* New Haven: Yale University Press, 1980.

London, N. J. An essay on psychoanalytic theory: Two theories of schizophrenia. *International Journal of Psychoanalysis,* 1973, *54,* 169–194.

Maenchen, A. On the technique of child analysis. *Psychoanalytic Study of the Child,* 1970, *25,* 175–208.

Masterson, J. F. *Psychotherapy of the borderline patient.* New York: Bruner Mazel, 1976.

Meissner, W. W. Theoretical assumptions of the concepts of borderline personality. *Journal of the American Psychoanalytic Association,* 1978, *26,* 559–598.

Meissner, W. W. Notes of the potential differentiation of borderline conditions. *International Journal of Psychoanalytic Psychotherapy,* 1982–1983, *9,* 3–49.

Modell, A. H. Primitive object relationships and the predisposition to schizophrenia. *International Journal of Psychoanalysis,* 1963, *44,* 282–292.

Perry, J. C., & Klerman, G. L. The borderline patient: A comparative analysis of four sets of diagnostic criteria. *Archives of General Psychiatry*, 1978, *35*, 141–150.

Perry, J. C., & Klerman, G. L. Clinical features of borderline personality disorder. *American Journal of Psychiatry*, 1980, *137*(2), 165–173.

Pine, F. On the concept "borderline" in children: A clinical essay. *Psychoanalytic Study of the Child*, 1974, *29*, 341–368.

Pine, F. On phase-characteristic pathology of the school age child: Disturbances of personality development and organization (borderline conditions) of learning, and of behavior. In S. I. Greenspan & G. H. Pollack (Eds.), *The course of life: Psychoanalytic contributions toward understanding personality development. Vol. II: Latency, adolescence, and youth.* National Institute of Mental Health, Washington, D.C., 1980.

Rangell, L. The borderline case. *Journal of the American Psychoanalytic Association*, 1955, *3*, 285–298.

Rapaport, D. The theoretical implications of diagnostic testing procedures. In R. P. Knight & C. R. Friedman (Eds.), *Psychoanalytic psychiatry and psychology.* New York: International Universities Press, 1954.

Redl, F. Ego disturbances. *American Journal of Orthopsychiatry*, 1951, *21*, 273–279.

Robbins, M. D. Towards a new model for the primitive personalities. *International Journal of Psychoanalysis*, 1983, *64*, 127–148.

Sadow, L. Ego axis in psychopathology. *Archives of General Psychiatry*, 1969, *21*, 15–24.

Schafer, R. Psychological tests in clinical research. In R. P. Knight & C. R. Friedman (Eds.), *Psychoanalytic psychiatry and psychology.* New York: International Universities Press, 1954.

Sheehy, M., Goldsmith, L. A., & Charles, E. A comparative study of borderline patients in a psychiatric outpatient clinic. *American Journal of Psychiatry*, 1980, *137*(11), 1374–1379.

Smith, K. Object relations concepts as applied to the borderline level of ego functioning. In J. Kwawer, H. D. Lerner, P. M. Lerner, & A. Sugarman (Eds.), *Borderline phenomena and the Rorschach test.* New York: International Universities Press, 1980.

Spitzer, R. L., Endicott, J., & Gibbon, M. Crossing the border into borderline personality and borderline schizophrenia: The development of criteria. *Archives of General Psychiatry*, 1979, *36*, 17–24.

Stern, A. Psychoanalytic investigation of and therapy in the border line group of neurotics. *Psychoanalytic Quarterly*, 1938, *7*, 467–489.

Stone, M. H. Psychodiagnosis and psychoanalytic psychotherapy. *Journal of the American Academy of Psychoanalysis*, 1979, *7*, 79–100.

Sugarman, A., & Lerner, H. D. Reflections on the current state of the borderline concept. In J. Kwawer, H. D. Lerner, P. M. Lerner, & A. Sugarman (Eds.), *Borderline phenomena and the Rorschach test.* New York: International Universities Press, 1980.

Wexler, M. Schizophrenia: Conflict and deficiency. *Psychoanalytic Quarterly*, 1971, *40*, 82–99.

Wohlberg, A. R. *The borderline patient.* New York: Intercontinental Medical Book Corporation, 1973.

Zetzel, E. R. A developmental approach to the borderline patient. *American Journal of Psychiatry*, 1971, *127*(7), 43–47.

Zilboorg, G. Ambulatory schizophrenia. *Psychiatry*, 1941, *4*, 149–155.

CHAPTER TWENTY-SIX

The Capacity for Adaptive Regression and Humor and Its Relation to Suicide Lethality

LISA A. GOLDSMITH

Two major propositions are investigated in the present chapter. First, that there are stylistic aspects to the way suicidal people think and, second, that creative resources, such as the saving grace of humor, are not available to them during states of suicidal stress.

To date, the research literature has taken note of features of cognitive functioning and ego adaptation that are characteristic of suicidal individuals despite their array of dynamic conflicts. Hartmann and Loewenstein (1962) suggested that the decisive factor in suicide, given a depressive context, was to be observed in the pathology of the ego. Empirical research has frequently characterized the thoughts and cognitive controls of suicidal patients as rigid and inflexible (Farberow, 1965; Levinson and Neuringer, 1971). A loss of

Portions of this chapter are reprinted from L. A. Goldsmith, Adaptive regression, humor, and suicide. *Journal of Consulting and Clinical Psychology,* 1979, *47,* 628–630. Copyright 1979 by the American Psychological Association. Reprinted by permission of the publisher.

perspective, a paucity of alternatives, and an overall cognitive rigidity have been observed repeatedly in these patients—captured in Farber's (1968) allusion to the "no exit" character of the suicide. The relationship between perceptual styles and suicidal behavior was noted also by Shevrin (1971) in summarizing the cognitive-style research of Gardner and Voth. It has been hypothesized in the clinical literature that a potential outcome of such cognitive and perceptual inflexibility under stress is pathological regression, where, in its extreme, tension tolerance and reality judgment may give way to primitive action (Sappenfield, 1954). Such pathological regression is considered one of the major factors underlying suicidal behavior.

Although regressive behavior has typically been portrayed in maladaptive terms, that is, as the "antithesis of conduct adapted to reality" (Hartmann, 1964, p. 13), in the context of an effort to account for creative processes and humor, Kris (1952) introduced the concept "regression in the service of the ego" (RISE) to psychoanalytic ego psychology. Kris pointed to certain adaptive uses of regression and elaborated the ways in which regressive processes facilitate the mastery of stresses and new situations and provide an alternative to pathological regression and psychological disorganization. In fact, RISE, as conceptualized by Kris, has subsequently become one criterion for differentiating adaptive from pathological activity. When the regressive process is under the aegis of the ego, not only is tension relieved, not only is there a staving off of a sterile constriction and impoverishment of ego functions, but pleasure is attained from the very mastery of regression and the acceptance of infantile modes of thought. There is an active process of taking "intellectual liberties," and it is a process starkly differentiated from the terrifying, passive experience of being overwhelmed by affect and tension. Significant relationships have consistently been reported in the literature between RISE and measures of creativity, humor, and cognitive flexibility (Derman, 1968; Wild, 1965; Fitzgerald, 1966; Feirstein, 1967; and O'Connell, 1964).

There appears to be a parallel that can be drawn between those very factors delineated as crucial dimensions in suicide (e.g., issues relating to regression, degree of rigidity, management of depression, capacity to master stresses), and those factors often ascribed to one function of RISE—the humor process. Menninger, in fact, spoke of the "saving graces of wit and humor" (1938, p. 376) in the battle of man against self-destruction. Freud identified humor as "one of the highest psychic functions devised by man to evade the compulsion to suffer" (1928, p. 3). Interestingly, Freud's chief example of the elevating quality of humor pertained to the reactions to one's imminent death. In gallows humor the protagonist does not decompensate under pressure but rather responds with a certain lofty perspective to inescapable circumstances. Grotjahn (1958) and Reich (1949) stated that in both comedy and melancholia there is an attempt to deny and prevent the pain of loss and abandonment through regressive means. It is, however, in humor that there is a process of active, adaptive conquering of conflict as the ego controls the regressive resolution, allows for a sublimated expression of impulses, permits a temporary denial of reality, and thus restores psychological equilibrium (Kramer, 1958; Schafer, 1960). The brief and episodic regression that in humor is experienced without guilt may virtually forestall pathological regression, preserve the sovereignty of the ego, and simply give the humorist the strength to face reality. Kris's (1952) work is of such value because it emphasizes the ego factors that make the regression in humor creative.

The adaptive aspects of the process of transforming passive helplessness into active mastery were noted by Rapaport (1967) to lie at the very core of structure formation. Creative processes in general, and humor in particular, are characterized by such mastery, and may thus be recognized to both reflect and effect permanent transformations of the ego. This permanence, as noted by Kris (1952), is in contrast to the transitory gains to be had from wit and hypomania. Schafer (1958) gives the construct RISE the status of a psychic structure with a "tool or means character" that is not contingent on each new occasion of stimulation but is triggered in the face of current internal or external pressures. He delineated a set of overlapping factors as crucial precursors of RISE, such as a flexibility of defenses and controls and the presence of well-developed affect signals, noting that a relative incapacity for adaptive regression was found to occur where there was the least tolerance for and most rigid defense against conscious fantasy and feeling. Pine and Holt (1960), using operationally defined scores in their study of creativity and adaptive regression, also suggest that modes of dealing with primary process can become generalized as broad cognitive controls reflected in many areas of thinking.

The ascription of structural properties to capacities that regulate shifts in levels of psychic functioning is the rather unique contribution of psychoanalytic ego psychology. With the concept of RISE it now becomes possible to assess modes of expression and control of primary process material underlying diverse dynamics. Bellak, Hurvich, and Gediman (1973) in fact included Adaptive Regression in the Service of the Ego (ARISE) in their ego function assessment model. That these capacities for RISE are significantly impoverished in the suicidal individual has been suggested in the literature. Kris (1952) stated that those to whom the comic is unknown lack precisely the flexibility and ego strength that allow for an active conquering of conflict. Such inflexibility has been ascribed both to humorless people and to the suicidal individual.

In light of such formulations it seems to follow that the capacity to use humor would be impoverished in suicidal people. As opposed to the whole subclass of depressive conditions, the seriously suicidal individual is likely to suffer a degree of inflexibility that precludes recourse to humor and paves the way for regression to primitive action. Spiegel et al. (1969) studied the thematic content of favorite jokes of suicide attempters and found the suicidal subjects to express significantly more jokes with self-punishing themes than did their nonsuicidal controls. The focus of Spiegel's study was on manifest content, however, with no mention of possible structural and stylistic differences between the two groups. The literature reveals virtually no reference to a formal relationship between RISE and humor in the suicidal individual, and it was to fill that gap that the present study was conducted—with the theoretical formulation of RISE providing the unifying construct and Bellak et al.'s definition of ARISE providing its operational base.

The present study explored the relationship between capacity for adaptive regression and degree of suicide lethality or potentiality (at times often referred to as "suicide severity"). It was predicted that when certain adaptive functions of the ego are deficient and the context is a depressive one, the potential for rigidity and acting out is increased. Thus, a consistent relationship was predicted between the capacity for adaptive regression and the behavioral manifestations of its impoverishment. Specifically, the central hypothesis was that measures of adaptive regression would bear an inverse relationship to degree of suicidal risk. Humor, as one manifestation of RISE, and one distinguished from hostile wit and resignation, was expected to stand in an inverse relationship to suicide severity and in a positive relationship to measures of ego strength. A final hypothesis—predicated on the construct of adaptive style as a relatively stable structure—was that various measures of adaptive regression would be positively related.

METHOD

In conjunction with a previous study conducted at the Bronx Municipal Hospital Center (Goldsmith, 1979), 31 female inpatients between the ages of 18 and 35 years who had been consecutively admitted to the psychiatric service over a period of six months were selected for study. All the subjects had a minimum of a high school education and diagnoses typical of patients on the service. Approximately 82% of the sample presented with some past or present history of suicidal ideation and/or behavior. Approximately 3% of the subjects sampled were excluded from the study because they were disoriented, organic, or uncommunicative on initial intake.

A series of tests was administered to all subjects: The Whittemore Suicide Potentiality Rating Schedule served as the measure of suicide severity, and the D scale of the Minnesota Multiphasic Personality Inventory (MMPI) was used additionally to assess degree of depression. The 68-item Barron Ego Strength Scale (ES) was chosen to assess relatively stable integrative and adaptive capacities of the ego.

Bellak, Hurvich, and Gediman's (1973) interview guide for the clinical assessment of ego functions explicitly measures degree of "adaptive regression on the service of the ego" (ARISE). ARISE, as previously mentioned, is defined as the capacity of the ego to make appropriate shifts in levels of psychological functioning, thereby permitting the emergence and integration of new and creative configurations (e.g., "Can you let go and think strange and 'nutty' thoughts without being upset or frightened?" "What is one of the most creative things you've ever done?" "The most spontaneous thing?").

The O'Connell (1964) Story Test was used to measure appreciation of wit and humor. This test consists of 18 jokes with three alternative punch-line endings for each joke, representing, respectively, resignation wit, hostile wit, and humor. Humor is designated as the most mature and hostile wit as the least mature selection. Subjects' humor-choice scores were derived from their preferred punch-line endings. Favorite jokes were also elicited and sorted according to the morbidity of joke content (e.g., themes of death, self-destruction, damage, downfall, and the macabre), as well as according to degree of humorousness. Scores on all but the MMPI scales were derived from independent judges' ratings; interrater agreement, as measured by Pearson Product-Moment Correlations, ranged from .72 for the lethality scale to .97 on the ARISE interview.

RESULTS

To test the hypothesis of an inverse relationship between adaptive regression and suicide lethality, each subject's score on the lethality scale was correlated both with the ARISE score and with choice scores on the Story Test. Correlational analysis revealed a significant inverse relationship between lethality and the ARISE score ($r = -.52$, $p < .01$). The correlation between lethality and humor-choice scores, although in the expected negative direction, did not reach statistical significance ($r = -.27$, $p < .10$). A point-biserial correlation coefficient was derived for morbid–nonmorbid jokes and lethality scores, with an obtained r value of .65 ($p < .001$). Thus, suicide lethality was significantly and positively associated with jokes judged to be of morbid thematic content. (One severely suicidal woman offered the following favorite joke: "Hitler told the Jews he had good and bad news for them. For the good news, he said, 'Half of you are going north and half south. And now for the bad news—the top halves of you will be going north and the bottom halves, south.'" Such an example is typical of the category of high morbidity of joke content.) Correlations between lethality scores and the second dimension, humorousness, were not significant.

Further statistical analysis, in the form of partial correlation, was employed to remove the potential effects of the depression factor; no significant trends were observed, and thus it was unlikely that any of the obtained results could be reduced to an underlying relationship with depression, as assessed on the rating scale. In line with predictions, ego strength as measured by Barron's scale was positively associated with appreciation of humor ($r = .35$, $p < .05$) and was negatively associated with suicide potentiality ($r = -.46$, $p < .01$). Finally, the humor score on the Story Test was positively correlated with the ARISE score ($r = .50$, $p < .01$), in contrast to the hostile wit and resignation scores on the Story Test, which were consistently associated with the ARISE score in a low and negative direction. Correlations between humor as measured on the Story Test and the humorousness dimension of the Favorite Joke were also statistically significant [Eta coefficient = $.55$ ($F = 5.71$; $p < .01$)].

DISCUSSION

In considering the findings, it seems likely that those measures that yielded significant results (i.e., Bellak et al.'s ARISE interview and the Favorite Joke technique) were more sensitive to individual differences in cognitive organization, shifts in defensive control, and stylistic patterns of coping than were the other measures. The Story Test, from which the humor-choice score was derived, merely elicits a discrete response, with no allowance for an evaluation of differential adaptive and defensive resources. Kris (1952), Zwerling (1955), and others have emphasized that complex structural and personality factors—ego strength in particular—are needed to understand humor. Indeed, when correlating the adaptive capacity for humor with ego flexibility, consistent positive trends were observed in this study between those two dimensions. Furthermore, the introduction of the concept of RISE and the use of instruments that were derived from or could be related to that concept made it possible to assess and interpret fairly predictable styles of functioning, observable in a variety of contexts. Although one must consider the restricted nature of the sample studied, a wide array of diagnostic groupings were in fact represented. On the other hand, it should be noted that Herron (1962) and Frank (1967) have both indicated that no single measure, be it Barron's scale or others, appears completely adequate as a measure of ego strength. It is generally agreed that ego strength is a somewhat vaguely defined construct; yet it is principally with the continued delineation of the behavioral and structural correlates of the construct that its precision will improve.

The findings are reminiscent of Kris's (1962) emphasis on the double-edge character of humor and RISE: It is only when the ego is strong enough to master anxiety and master shifts in functioning that regression can be used in the service of the ego. It would follow that the rigidity observed in our high-lethal group not only might have precluded a recourse to RISE but would have made such recourse psychologically dangerous. When there is morbidity of humor, pathological expression of hostile wit, and severe suicide risk, crucial controls and modulations of the ego are unlikely to be adequate to the task of creative regression. That ego strength, a relatively stable attribute of the person, was inversely related to suicide lethality may indicate a chronic state of marginally immobilized ego functions in the more serious suicidal person. Thus, Zwerling's statement that we laugh at what makes us anxious may be only partially correct. People laugh at what makes them anxious if they have the ego strength to do so.

To see if any qualitative distinctions could be made that might enrich the quantative findings, a content analysis of the individual ARISE interviews was made. Although the uniqueness of each personality was evident in style and verbalization, three major groups could be recognized in the data. The majority of subjects in the sample fell within the mid-range of suicide lethality. Within this mid-group ($N = 16$) there seemed to be a predominance of subjects manifesting features of a hysterical-like cognition, in that suicidal ideation seemed itself to serve a defensive function—almost as an analogue of repression. Recurrent suicidal thoughts and lethal ruminations seemed to ward off other thought content for these women, and even when conscious fantasy and other forms of ideation were actively elicited, suicidal material and action propensities seemed to replace thought and fantasy expression.

The interplay between suicidal thoughts and conscious fantasy can be observed in the following excerpts from the ARISE protocol material of Miss J., a young woman who fell within this mid-range of lethality.

I: Are your daydreams ever put to any use?
S: Yes—tried to kill myself. When I think of anything—try to kill myself.
I: What about your dreams?
S: I don't dream—I don't fantasize.
I: If you have a serious problem to solve how do you go about solving it?
S: Try to kill myself.
I: Do you ever let your thoughts wander and then, later, organize them and come up with a good solution?
S: Nothing, except killing myself.
I: What is the most spontaneous thing you've ever done?
S: It's the same answer—trying to kill myself.

Each and every time inner ideation was elicited, suicidal material and action propensities seemed to replace thought and mitigate against fantasy expression. Excerpts from the interview material of another woman within this group further illustrate such repressive functions of action and suicidal ideation:

I: Do you enjoy letting your hair down and just giving into fanciful feelings?
S: No, because when I think what I want to think it's usually bad and I end up doing things.
i: Have you ever come up with an answer to a problem in a dream?

S: Yes—but all the wrong ones. I tried to commit suicide. There's solutions to every problem—no?

I: Are you ever able to think strange and nutty thoughts without being upset or frightened?

S: Thoughts or actions? Mostly actions—I do crazy things like try to kill myself.

One insight into what these defensive actions and thoughts may forestall was gleaned from the characteristic favorite joke material of this group. Evident in the group as a whole were a preponderance of starkly sexual and hysterical jokes with recurrent themes of oral sexuality, promiscuity, prostitution fantasies, and homosexual wishes reflected in the content. One such example of a favorite joke from a woman in this mid-range group was the following: "Oh, none come to mind—oh, I know one, but it's not a clean joke. This girl went to see her doctor—she's complaining that she's so tired she doesn't know what to do. This girl was a prostitute to begin with and she went to the doctor and told him about her problems. He told her the only advice he could give her was to stay out of bed for two weeks." It is possible that suicidal ideation prevents the acting out of certain forbidden sexual fantasies.

It is interesting that Shneidman (1967) posited that very frequently fantasies of suicide are disguised sexual perversions, where defenses and the prospect of death itself have become libidinized. He also stated that one motive for suicide may be to avert the possibility of yielding to forbidden impulses. Richman (1968), in his survey of jokes dealing with suicide and death themes, observed a major covert relationship between sex and death, where the opposite of death was not life but sex, especially forbidden or illicit sex. Whether repressive forces are in the service of libidinal or other drive derivatives, what can be suggested is that such tremendous defensive expenditures do not foster the active participation in primary process activity that would lead to ARISE. In fact, this mid-group was typified by subjects who appeared empty, limited, isolated, and stimulus-bound, with no particular primary process talent or evidence of its development. The paucity of primary process activity and the pervasive avoidance of fantasy and ideation characteristic of this group is reflected in the following excerpts from one woman's protocol:

I: Do you daydream?

S: No—as a child I sometimes did—but no, not really.

I: Tell me something about what you do with your dreams?

S: I haven't had dreams in so long—seldom dream. Just go to sleep and wake up the next morning.

I: Are you ever able to let go and think strange and "nutty" thoughts without being upset or frightened?

S: Very seldom do I think of awful thoughts—can't think of any.

I: What is one of the most creative things you've ever done?

S: Creative? In what line of work? In high school we used to make our own patterns.

In sum, what this repressor group of women appear to display is a reliance on hysterical-like defenses and sporadic acting out, which, in part, avoid and militate against access to their inner life. It is not surprising that such marked repressive efforts and such rigid and stereotyped attempts to simplify the world and block out change would not lead to the "flexibility of repression" that would be observed in adaptive regression and humor.

Typical of a second group ($N = 6$) were those women whose defenses against regression and psychotic primitivization of thought were markedly tenuous. The distinctions between thought and action and between ideas and reality were marginal in these people; primitive fantasies were on the verge of erupting, resulting in fear and guardedness against any primary process material. Temporary and well-regulated regression was virtually impossible for such subjects. As this group was only marginally represented in the sample, it is premature to relate their responses directly to suicide lethality. However, the devastating effects that vulnerability to severe ego regression and impaired capacity for affect modulation have on the accessibility for ARISE seem evident in the following excerpt:

I: Tell me something about what you do with your dreams?

S: Sometimes my dreams come real and I believe in them and that's what brings me into the hospital. I dreamed I killed my parents in one of my dreams and I believed it so strongly I believed it. (?) No, I don't believe it now, though I have flashbacks about it. One other time I was in the hospital I dreamt my psychiatrist jumped out a window and committed suicide and I was broken up about it because I love him.

Another woman who displayed reactions characteristic of this group gave the following response:

I: Have you had the experience of the thoughts and feelings of a dream continuing when you woke up?

S: Yes—I wake up and I'm wide awake—but I can't move—I'm paralyzed and I still feel the dream going on even when I'm awake—I want to scream.

The temporary and well-regulated regressions observable in ARISE are virtually impossible for such patients. There is little in the way of the freedom of moving back and forth between levels of organization with the assurance of later establishing equilibrium.

Finally, there was a group of subjects ($N = 4$) characterized by a previous reliance on ideational and obsessive-like defenses and a once impressive capacity for ARISE. Neither primarily hysterical nor repressive modes seemed dominant in this group. Rather, there appeared to be a breakdown and a relatively acute and insidious change in a once developed capacity to accept and utilize primary process derivatives. While no precise quantitative statements can be made, it is of note that all those women who manifested a decompensation of obsessive and ideational modes of defense were in the high-lethality ranges of the study sample. One woman who scored within this high-lethality range offered the following material:

I: Tell me something about what you do with your dreams?

S: I remember my dreams—one was so incredibly beautiful. I dreamt it about a year ago—last winter. I dreamt about an orange red rose growing out of the snow—tried to draw it so many times, to get the color, the feeling—so beautiful.

I: Have you ever had the experience of when there is a problem to solve of just letting your thoughts go and then later coming up with a good solution?

S: Now I can't—I get crazy—when I have a real problem I just hang on it—it won't get out of my head.

The one woman in the sample who did eventually kill herself, Mrs. M., was included in this cluster of subjects. Some of the ARISE protocol material from Mrs. M. follows:

I: What do you do when you're alone and have nothing to do?

S: I usually pace the floors. I don't do much of anything any more except to think of ways to kill myself. Sometimes I try to live in a fantasy world where things are always right. But now the only answer I can come up with is death.

I: Are you ever able to let go and think strange and "nutty" thoughts without being upset or frightened?

S: Yah—I could do that—when I took the razor blades I had a strange and nutty thought.

I: Do you ever find that things you do with a playful attitude can later be put to serious purpose?

S: Used to—a lot—would explore things, liked to see what things are made of—why is it that way? But no more.

A major disruption seems to have occurred at some point in this woman's life, and neither obsessive, ideational routes nor recourse to psychosis have allayed suicidal material. She is not characterized by the repressive devices that prevailed in the first group, nor does she, like subjects in the second group, find some diminution or alleviation of tension through psychotic means. It is ironic that it was a joke of "going downhill" that Mrs. M. chose to tell as her favorite. "What is black and white—and black and white—and black and white? A nun rolling down a hill! I'm not a very good joke teller."

In an effort to understand this last group of subjects one could speculate that a decompensation of a previous capacity for ARISE, combined with active suicidal propensities, is perhaps more ominous than a chronic incapacity for ARISE. Such a formulation might account for what seems to be a discordant incidence of suicide in groups of impressively gifted, creative, and humorous people—for example, the suicides of Lenny Bruce and Sylvia Plath. When access to inner life and emotional nuance are no longer under the mastery of the ego, the sense of devastation and loss may be suffered more markedly by those who have known the rewards of such access than by those who have not. Again, formulations regarding the double-edged character of creative regression are relevant.

The preceding qualitative impressions seem to fall into line with a model introduced by Goldberger (1961) in a study of experimentally induced perceptual isolation. Goldberger found that adaptive versus maladaptive reactions to the isolation were associated with "characterological differences" in the capacity to tolerate primitive modes of thought. He formalized such differences along a continuum of modes of handling primary process, ranging from uncontrolled, ego-alien breakthroughs of primary process elements into consciousness, through complete repression of primary process, to the controlled, modulated use of primary process material in the service of the ego. Goldberger's first mode does seem to encompass the functioning of those subjects described in the present sample as threatened and overwhelmed by primitive material. His mid-group seems to parallel the first group of hysterical repressors who, perhaps because of a heavy expenditure of repressive forces, allowed little primary process material into consciousness. Possibly, those low on the range of suicide lethality and high on ego strength and ARISE would approach Goldberger's final mode. Goldberger (1961) explicitly proposed that his concept of differences in ego structure that allow for the "freedom to abandon secondary process operations temporarily" (p. 301) is comparable to Kris's concept of RISE. It is also noteworthy that such clusterings could be independently observed with Bellak et al.'s ARISE interview.

Schafer (1968) similarly distinguished along a continuum of a readiness to suspend and restore "reflective self-representations." He referred to a capacity that enables a person to disappear for a moment as "the thinker" and momentarily experience his thoughts as though they were concrete realities. He conceptualized this shift as one to primary process ideation, likening it to a regression in the service of the ego that invariably entails a temporary disappearance of reflective self-representations. The three groups Schafer describes—the rigid, the flexible, and the fluid—again bear a resemblance to the clusters derived from the qualitative interview material of the present study. It is interesting, however, that neither Goldberger's nor Schafer's model explicitly encompasses the last group herein described—namely, those who once could but can no longer exercise ARISE. It would be worthwhile in a future study to observe what happens to the "flexibles" when they decompensate. For example, is there a propensity for them to become "fluid"?

So far findings have been discussed within a theoretical framework, but there are practical implications as well. For one, the delineation of stylistic and fairly stable modes of ego adaptation and regulation in depressive clinical syndromes may generate not only systematic analysis but also specific predictions of subsequent life-threatening behaviors. Farberow (1950) has repeatedly cautioned suicide researchers against interpreting data following a suicide attempt as representing the psychological state prior to the action. In the present study structural resources of the ego that allow for tension reduction in times of stress were examined. It is hoped that by specifying such characteristic styles of functioning, temporal and other sampling difficulties might be reduced.

In addition, the findings suggest the usefulness of incorporating humor assessment and other ARISE measures into diagnostic batteries particularly in such clinical settings as psychiatric facilities and suicide prevention centers. For example, self-generated humor productions of "lethal" content might be added as indicators of suicidal risk, and differences in overall capacities for ARISE and humor might help distinguish between various types of depression. In concluding, however, it must be cautioned that broader sampling is needed to articulate the applicability of the concept RISE, as well as to determine those other tension-reducing behaviors that, used in conjunction with ARISE, promote adaptation. Finally, while RISE has been discussed principally in terms of structural propositions, this is not to underestimate the developmental and object relations implications of the construct. Kernberg (1970), for example, had suggested that the capacity for RISE involves as a critical dimension, the "reactivation of past internal object relationships in times of stress or loss of external support, or of loneliness" (p. 82). It is no surprise that the literature on suicidality consistently reports a history of unresolved object disruptions in the clinical histories of suicidal individuals, as well as an incidence of object loss itself as a most frequent acute precipitant of suicidal crises (Dorpat et al., 1965).

SUMMARY

With the advent of psychoanalytic ego psychology attention has been focused on the adaptive aspects of ego functioning—structural elements that serve not only defensive purposes but modulate tension in times of stress.

Within this framework, Kris's (1952) concept of regression in the service of the ego heralded the notion that the regressive process could itself be in the service of adaptation and enrichment of the ego; he included humor within his domain of regressive processes serving adaptation.

The present study explored the relationship between humor, as a manifestation of the capacity for adaptive regression, and suicide lethality, as a manifestation of a pathological regressive process. Subjects were assessed on Bellak et al.'s clinical rating scale of "adaptative regressive in the service of the ego" (ARISE), humor measures derived from O'Connell's Story Test, the Favorite Joke technique, and a suicide potentiality rating scale. Suicidality and humor were also correlated with measures of ego strength and depression. Results largely confirmed a hypothesized significant negative relationship between suicidality and both adaptive regression and ego strength, as well as a positive relationship between ego strength and humor and between different measures of adaptive regression. The finding of a relationship between the capacity for humor and the capacity to deal with depressive affect and ideation were interpreted in line with those formulations of psychoanalytic ego psychology that posit a relationship between adaptive forms of regression and psychic structure formation. Implications for the use of ARISE and humor measures in diagnostic and prognostic assessment were also discussed.

REFERENCES

Bellak, L., Hurvich, M., & Gediman, H. K. *Ego functions in schizophrenics, neurotics, and normals*. New York: Wiley, 1973.

Derman, B. I. Adaptive versus pathological regression in relation to psychological adjustment. *Dissertation Abstracts*, 1968, *28* (11-B), 4574–4755.

Dorpat, L. L., Jackson, J. J., & Ripley, H. S. Broken homes and attempted and completed suicide. *Archives of General Psychiatry*, 1965, *12*(2), 213–216.

Farber, M. *Theory of suicide*. New York: Funk & Wagnalls, 1968.

Farberow, N. L. Personality patterns of suicide mental hospital patients. *Genetic Psychology Monographs*, 1950, *42*, 3–79.

Farberow, N. L. Summary. In N. L. Farberow & E. S. Schneidman (Eds.), *The cry for help*. New York: McGraw-Hill, 1965, pp. 290–324.

Feirstein, A. Personality correlates of tolerance for unrealistic experiences. *Journal of Consulting Psychology*, 1967, *31*, 387–395.

Fitzgerald, E. T. Measurement of openness to experience: A study of regression in the service of the ego. *Journal of Personality and Social Psychology*, 1966, *4*, 655–663.

Frank, G. H. A review of research with measures of ego strength derived from the MMPI and the Rorschach. *Journal of General Psychology*, 1967, *77*, 183–206.

Freud, S. Humor. *International Journal of Psychoanalysis*, 1928, *9*, 1–6.

Goldberger, L. Reactions to perceptual isolation and Rorschach manifestations of primary process. *Journal of Projective Techniques*, 1961, *25*, 287–302.

Goldsmith, L. Adaptive regression, humor, and suicide. *Journal of Consulting and Clinical Psychology*, 1979, *47*, 628–630.

Grotjahn, M. *Beyond laughter*. New York: McGraw-Hill, 1958.

Hartmann, H. *Essays on ego psychology*. New York: International Universities Press, 1964.

Hartmann, H., & Loewenstein, R. Notes on the superego. *Psychoanalytic Study of the Child*, 1962, *17*, 42–18.

Herron, W. G. The assessment of ego strength. *Journal of Psychological Studies*, 1962, *13*, 173–203.

Kernberg, O. G. Treatment of narcissistic personalities. *Journal of the American Psychoanalytic Association*, 1970, *18*, 51–85.

Kramer, P. Note on one of the preoedipal roots of the superego. *Journal of the American Psychoanalytic Association*, 1958, *6*, 38–46.

Kris, E. *Psychoanalytic explorations in art*. New York: International Universities Press, 1952, pp. 173–239.

Levinson, M., & Neuringer, C. Problem-solving behavior in suicidal adolescents. *Journal of Consulting and Clinical Psychology*, 1971, *37*(3), 433–436.

Menninger, K. *Man against himself*. New York: Harcourt, Brace, 1938.

O'Connell, W. E. Resignation, humor and wit. *Psychoanalytic Review*, 1964, *51*, 49–56.

Pine, F., & Holt, R. R. Creativity and primary process. *Journal of Abnormal and Social Psychology*, 1960, *61*, 370–379.

Rapaport, D. O. *Collected papers of David Rapaport*. M. M. Gill (Ed.). New York: Basic Books, 1967.

Reich, A. The structure of the grotesque-comic sublimation. *Bulletin of the Menninger Clinic*, 1949, *13*, 160–171.

Richman, J. *Suicide, homicide, death and jokes: A study of social and psychological attitudes*. Paper presented at the Annual Meeting of the American Association of Suicidology, 1968.

Sappenfield, B. *Personality dynamics: An integrative psychology of adjustment*. New York: Knopf, 1954.

Schafer, R. Regression in the service of the ego: The relevance of a psychoanalytic concept for personality assessment. In G. Lindzey (Ed.), *Assessment of human motives*. New York: Holt, Rinehart and Winston, 1958, pp. 119–148.

Schafer, R. The loving and beloved superego in Freud's structural theory. *Psychoanalytic Study of the Child*, 1960, *16*, 163–188.

Schafer, R. *Aspects of internalization*. New York: International Universities Press, 1968.

Shevrin, H. Recent perspectives on treatment and diagnoses. *Bulletin of the Menninger Clinic*, 1971, *35*, 461–478.

Shneidman, E. S. *Essays in self destruction*. New York: Science House, 1967.

Spiegel, D., Keith-Spiegel, P., Abrahama, J., & Kranitz, L. Humor and suicide: Favorite jokes of suicidal patients. *Journal of Consulting and Clinical Psychology*, 1969, *33*(4), 504–505.

Wild, C. Creativity and adaptive regression. *Journal of Personality and Social Psychology*, 1965, *2*(2), 161–169.

Zwerling, I. The favorite joke in diagnostic and therapeutic interviewing. *Psychoanalytic Quarterly*, 1955, *24*, 104–114.

PART FOUR

EFA Research in Personality and Development

CHAPTER TWENTY-SEVEN

Symbolization, Fantasy, and Adaptive Regression as Developmental Tasks of the Latency Period

GERARD J. DONNELLAN

Evidence from a variety of disciplines supports the conclusion that the latency period is a time when children expand cognitive skills and mature in the use of adaptive ego functions. Psychoanalytic theory has traditionally portrayed the latency period as a time of calm and truce, of lessening sexual and aggressive drives. This view of the latency period, from 5½ to 12 years, was first proposed by Freud (1905) and later elaborated on by Bornstein (1951).

Freud's contributions first shed light on this stage of development, a stage that hitherto had received little attention. His work raised many questions, especially concerning what factors were involved in the developmental changes of latency. The present study, exploring some of these factors, focused on two ego functions, *symbolization* and *adaptive regression in the service of the ego,* as these were manifested in the stories of a 7½-year-old boy.

The literature touching on the latency period derives from a variety of sources. Developmental psychology, cognitive theories, psychoanalytic research, and models that utilize a combination of these all contribute some information concerning latency.

Developmental psychology offers evidence to indicate that the time between $5\frac{1}{2}$ and 12 is a time for an ongoing series of achievements, especially in the area of mastery of cognitive skills (Kagan and Moss, 1962; Elkind, 1973). Longitudinal research suggests that the mastery of cognitive skills also relates to the more encompassing mastery of control mechanisms—mechanisms for cognitive control as well as impulse control. Cognitively, the child learns to deploy attention efficiently, which facilitates the educational process (Pendleton, 1973); the child also learns ways to delay and redirect the discharge of impulses, thereby developing a broader range of outlets for his or her drives.

Other models of development, which stress ego functioning, offer frameworks for ordering the knowledge derived from developmental research. The psychoanalytic model, with its emphasis on the vicissitudes of ego growth, appears to be the most comprehensive. One branch of the psychoanalytic model focuses on the varied functions of the ego. In this framework the ego is conceptualized as a network of interrelated functions. These functions, such as motility, perception, reality testing, defensive functioning, and adaptive regression, all have a developmental course leading to increased differentiation of the ego (Hartmann, 1958, 1964).

Much of the psychoanalytic research has focused on the early stages of development before latency. Recent formulations derived from this research suggest that ego development proceeds at a predictable, steady pace and is directly related to the quality and intensity of the child's early object relations (Mahler, Pine, & Bergman, 1975). This proposition derived from early development may be applied to latency; latency is also a time of increased differentiation and growth of the ego. The present research examined specific aspects of this proposition and did so by expanding the use of the ego function assessment model of Bellak et al. (1973) to include this period of development.

The literature on fantasy and play is also suggestive of developmental changes during latency. The literature supports three possible alternatives for the relation between play and fantasy: play and fantasy are one and the same process during infancy; fantasy is regarded as the single prior process, leading gradually to motor expression in play; or play is regarded as the single prior process, leading to schematization, and thereby, fantasy formation (Piaget, 1945, 1962).

Each alternative is possible. The most convincing evidence indicates that play and fantasy are linked and that they have separate sequences of development that parallel each other (Klinger, 1971). Latency children spend much of their free time in play that involves fantasy. The research literature suggests that fantasy and play both serve functions during latency: Both can allow for the expression and discharge of impulses in a less direct mode and both are considered to be associated with the ego functions of symbolization and adaptive regression in the service of the ego. Achieving impulse discharge in less direct modes is an important milestone in latency, since most children live in societies that do not condone direct, unmodulated expression of impulses, especially sexual and aggressive impulses.

It is with the work of Sarnoff (1971, 1976) that latency receives comprehensive treatment. Sarnoff's model, which served as the basis for this study, maintains that latency encompasses a number of cognitive organizing periods; this view provides a clear outline of the functional changes of the ego during latency.

The core of Sarnoff's theory is designated as the "structure of latency." In this construct, he describes the configuration of defenses in the latency child that allow for the expression of impulses through fantasy. Fantasy becomes an important outlet for the discharge of drives during latency. In prelatency, wishes are expressed more directly, and in adolescence real substitute objects can be sought. The developing latency-age child begins to use play and fantasy as a less direct means of discharge. With maturation, other sublimatory channels in addition to play and fantasy are utilized. This process, as delineated by Sarnoff, takes place in specified cognitive organizing periods. It is but a short step to the view that eventually support from developmental and cognitive researchers, psychoanalytic investigators and biological scientists will fill out a comprehensive model of development during this period.

AIMS OF THE STUDY

Symbolization and adaptive regression were chosen for study because recent work reveals their fundamental significance during latency (Sarnoff, 1976).

Symbolization refers to the psychoanalytic concept of symbol formation. Jones (1916, 1948) assumes that psychoanalytic symbols are formed through the work of repression; a position that asserts that the association between a symbol and its referent is broken. Symbols may arise from various intrapsychic conflicts. As the child matures he begins to gain distance from conflicts and develops cognitive skills that allow him to deploy his attention in nonconflictual areas. The child's ability to use symbols and symbolic communication (e.g., language) permits him to devote his energies to school, play, friends, and parents. The unfolding of symbolic capacities in this manner seems to be one of the aims and results of the latency period.

Adaptive regression in the service of the ego refers to the ability to "let go" of cognitive and perceptual acuity and relax controls. The term was introduced by Kris (1952) to describe a transient state of loss of ego autonomy. Often the term, used with reference to creativity, implies a controlled regression that enables the person to create new syntheses not available in other forms of thought.

As used in this study, adaptive regression signifies the relaxation of controls, thus permitting the child to tell a playful, fanciful story. Bellak et al. (1973) suggest that the term encompasses two ideas: (1) that of regression to an earlier level of functioning and (2) that of the regression being used in the service of adaptation. These two components are necessary if the child is to tell an enjoyable "make-believe" story.

One subject was chosen for study for a number of reasons. Other single-subject [$N = 1$] researchers have demonstrated the utility of such research for opening up unexplored areas for study (Hersen & Barlow, 1976). As discussed elsewhere (Donnellan, 1978), $N = 1$ research affords the researcher the opportunity of focusing on one person in depth. Finally, this type of research, by its design, lends itself to studies on the process of change in psychotherapy.

THE BOY

Ben was 7½ years old at the time he was brought by his parents to the child guidance clinic for evaluation and treatment. He was restless and fighting in school; he was enuretic at night and soiled during the day. The oldest of two adopted children, both he and his sister, 2 years his junior, were both adopted a few days after birth.

Besides the precipitating stress of Ben's disruptive behavior at school Ben's father had a change of work assignment almost 2 years previously. Transferred to another city, hundreds of miles away, he commuted home on weekends.

When Ben began therapy he was introduced to the "mutual storytelling technique" (Gardner, 1971). Ben made up a story during each session, followed by a similar story told by the therapist. The aim of the therapist's story was to interpret the child's story and clarify his concerns. The storytelling became part of the regular routine of the therapy. All stories were recorded. Ben was seen weekly for 8 months.

As to the hypotheses of the study, it was proposed that, as Ben progressed through treatment, he would show a significant improvement in the use of symbolization and adaptive regression as measured by particular scales to be described. The CAT (Children's Apperception Test) and other psychological tests were administered before and after treatment to establish a baseline from which to compare the stories during treatment.

Two scales were used for the rating of Ben's stories. One, the ARISE (Adaptive Regression in the Service of the Ego) scale, was modified from the work of Bellak et al. (1973); the other, the SYM scale (Symbolization) was designed for the study. The scales were dimensionalized along a five-point continuum, ranging from maladaptive to adaptive (see the appendix to this chapter for rating scales).

The maladaptive end of the ARISE scale (stop 1) describes the child's story thus: Regressions are very prominent and primitive; the story seems "wild" and confused, chaotic and disrupted; the child is totally carried away by the story; characters appear and disappear. The child, then, is not in control of the regression, nor is the regression adaptive. This is in contrast to stop 5, where the regressions are described as controlled and pleasurable.

This maladaptive–adaptive continuum applies to the SYM scale as well. At the lower end there is minimal or no symbolization: The fantasy appears fragile; drives appear close to the surface; language may be concrete and idiosyncratic. This contrasts sharply with stop 5, where the fantasy is complex and dramatic, the symbols are true "psychoanalytic symbols," and thus "masked" very well and the child shows distance from drives. The stories at this level are highly symbolic, but not necessarily transparent in their meaning.

A group of three raters was trained in the use of the scales. They rated Ben's CAT stories (16) and treatment stories (26) on both scales. Written transcripts, as well as recordings, were used for the ratings.

The specific hypotheses as they relate to the stories told before, during, and at the end of psychotherapy included the following predictions: (1) a positive change in Ben's use of symbolization and adaptive regression on stories told in response to the CAT; (2) positive changes for the same variables on the treatment stories; and (3) overall improvement in the use of adaptive regression and symbolization.

RESULTS AND DISCUSSION

The ratings were analyzed by the split-middle method of trend estimation described by Kazdin (1976). This statistical technique was developed specifically for $N = 1$ designs as a means of describing change over time. The results of the analysis of the data indicated substantial support for the prediction of an improvement in capacities reflected in the two measures over the course of treatment. Although there was no significant change in performance on the CAT before and after treatment, ARISE and SYM increased at stable rates during treatment, with ARISE showing the most improvement. The prediction of an overall positive change in the use of ARISE and SYM was also substantially supported. Treatment did seem to have an effect, especially on ARISE. The results for SYM are less well defined.

These findings permit some exploration and discussion of the factors involved in the process of change observed in Ben during treatment.

Treatment was divided into two phases prompted by a vacation break and due to the fact that, shortly after the break, Ben asked about termination. He was told that he would be seen until the summer and then treatment would end because the therapist was leaving the clinic. As a consequence, even though, like most 8-year-olds, Ben did not comprehend the concept of "3 months," he still felt angry, rejected, and confused.

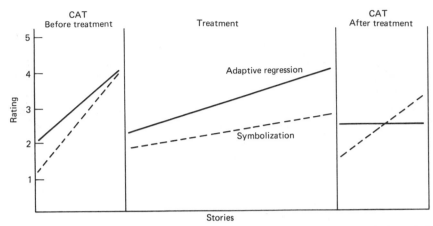

Figure 27.1 Slopes of stories rated for adaptive regression and symbolization before, during, and after treatment.

Ben's stories before the vacation break reflect his positive feelings toward the therapist and the beginning of a sense of comfort in the treatment. One story illustrates a recurring theme:

> Okay. One day there was a . . . duck! A yellow duck and he swam in the pond. One day hunters came and shot his mother. Then he was all alone. Then one day he found a boy duck. They swam and swam. Then they both got married that same night. The end.

After the therapist gave his story Ben gave this lesson: "Sometimes you can be happy with other people." The lesson and the story are indicative of Ben's concerns about separation and his pleasure in forming attachments, as indicated in his relationship to the therapist. The story also reflects his ambivalent feelings about close relationships—a theme that pervades many of his stories in treatment.

Ben told the following story in a session following the 2-week hiatus in treatment:

> Let's get the show on the road. "The New Manager." Once there used to be a manager of the A's named Charlie Findlay. One day he retired. A new guy came in. His name was Ben. He said, "Okay, guys, let's get the show on the road. Let's go down to Los Angeles and play those Angels." The Angels got . . . 10 home runs. It was 10 to nothing. Three outs and the A's were up. All the A's men got home runs. The A's won the game. The end. The lesson is . . . sometimes you can be outsmarted.

Many of the stories told during this period reflected themes related to the news of termination and spoke to a sense of not getting enough or of being outsmarted. However, with the interpretation and discussion of this material, subsequent stories began to show a clear move toward the adaptive end of the scales. Toward the end of the treatment the tone of the sessions became more structured and almost ritualistic. Ben would tell his story at the beginning of the session, sometimes reluctantly, and then would engage the therapist in a competitive activity such as baseball. He would show real pleasure in his victory. At the end of many sessions Ben would play "Ghosts": He would turn off the lights of the playroom and therapist and child would then take turns throwing a ball at each other. Ben particularly enjoyed the game and would save it for the end of the session. The game is significant in that it appears related to separation from the therapist and to an identification with the therapist as the ambivalently loved object.

Some Implications

Sarnoff's (1976) characterization of the latency child as a "physiologically impotent dwarf-warrior" is an apt description of the child's incapacity to express sexual and aggressive drives fully with real objects in the external world. He must find substitutes, as he cannot afford to lose his parents. Thus, the playful, aggressive games observed at the end of the treatment sessions could be interpreted as an attempt at restitution and reunion with the father. Albeit overdetermined, turning off the light and allowing himself to be in the same room as the feared–loved object appeared as an attempt at working through his ambivalence.

Similarly, baseball became symbolic of Ben's wish to vie with the father. Over a number of sessions the character of the game changed, becoming more of a mutually shared experience and less of a repetition of beating the "father." This change in the sessions is related to the marked increase in the ratings for symbolization during the second phase of treatment. The assumption that symbolization provides for the redirection of impulses is supported by this finding. The therapist's interpretations may have served as a wedge between fantasy and action; they provided the child with a "cognitive handle"—inhibiting the move toward action and fostering expression through other modes.

Almost all the stories told by Ben reflected his internal conflicts. As he achieved some distance from these conflicts through repression and symbolization, his stories revealed that distance. He appeared more comfortable with fantasy and more in control of his actions. Furthermore, the observed repetition of fantasy themes seemed significant in the working through and mastery of the conflicts. The capacity to move in and out of fantasy also made Ben appear less bound by the fantasy and more in control of his activity. The achievement of mastery through fantasy indicates a crucial difference between the latency child and prelatency child.

Termination and the Role of the Father

Ben's history reveals no significant pathology prior to entering kindergarten. Noteworthy in the family situation was the father's intermittent absence for over a 2-year period. The parents accepted living in different cities and this separation undoubtedly exacerbated Ben's problems on entering kindergarten.

These factors must be considered in terms of what terminating therapy meant to Ben. He had no control over it; it was the therapist's decision. Thus, there may be a parallel between the lack of control Ben felt both in regard to the separations from the father and the termination of treatment.

The resolution of oedipal issues as they appeared in Ben's play and stories seemed to be facilitated by a better command of language and an increased ability to express wishes through the linguistic mode. This enhanced behavioral control and linguistic capacity seemed to reflect an increased utilization of symbolization.

The emergence of latency, initiated by the resolution of the oedipal conflict, is reflected by the behavioral indices of the child's ever-increasing capacity to differentiate fantasy from reality. This cognitive change fosters further psychological shifts: a further disengagement from oedipal themes, a growing interest in school, an interest in social relations with peers, and the wish to grow up and be in control of oneself. Conflicts and prohibitions are increasingly internalized and by late latency are expressed in less direct modes and more symbolic and verbal modes.

These psychological changes in early latency are likely to be fostered in situations where the boy (in this case) has emotional access to both male and female parental figures. The early relationship of parents and child seems to encourage the development of a coherent sexual identity and the establishment of control mechanisms. The absence of Ben's father came at a crucial time in his development. With the father absent from the home most of the time Ben did not have the opportunity to "bounce up against" him—literally and figuratively. Ideally, the father at this time allows the boy to test his own strengths in opposition to the father.

The task in early latency is one of establishing new boundaries of the self in relation to parents and others. Cognitive and emotional changes allow the child to gain some distance from the intensity of conflicts. It appears that in Ben's case this process was interrupted by the father's absence. At such a normally unstable time the pull is to regress to preoedipal levels. It will be recalled that during this period Ben began bed-wetting, soiling his pants, fighting, and developing reading difficulties. The father's absence came at a crucial time in Ben's development and took its toll in Ben's stormy entrance into latency.

To turn to the issue of termination, it is evident that separation and loss were central issues in Ben's development. A fortunate aspect of the termination was that it occurred *after* the return of the father to the home. Father and son were already beginning to establish a stable relationship at this time, and so Ben's loss of the therapist was softened by a revitalized relationship with his father.

Ekstein (1977) suggests that child therapy is coming to a close when the symptoms are resolved and the child can now deal with the normal developmental tasks for his age. These tasks, of course, are not removed by treatment, but the child's willingness to confront them is an indicator that treatment has done its work. In Ben's case, fostering the structure of latency was the aim of therapy. That some measure of success was achieved is evidenced by the result of this study.

SUMMARY

Through the study of the psychotherapy of a latency-age boy, it was observed that the thematic material elicited throughout the course of treatment revealed a widening of mastery and control mechanisms through the use of symbols. Specifically, the two ego functions chosen for study, adaptive regression and symbolization, were hypothesized to be involved in the processes of fantasy, storytelling, and play. As demonstrated by the course of treatment, the ascendance of more adaptive ego functioning in the areas under investigation seemed critical in helping Ben to plant his feet firmly in latency.

Since single-subject ($N = 1$) research is a rather recent development, the methodologies and statistics appropriate to such research are still evolving. This study of Ben and his stories suggests that such research is possible and can address underlying structural and ego-adaptive capacities of the child. Clearly, more systematic studies on a broad range of subjects are indicated and would continue to provide further validation of the scales used in the present study.

REFERENCES

Bellak, L., Hurvich, M., & Gediman, H. *Ego functions in schizophrenics, neurotics, and normals.* New York: Wiley, 1973.

Bornstein, B. On latency. *Psychoanalytic Study of the Child,* 1951, *6,* 279–285.

Donnellan, G. Single-subject research and psychoanalytic theory. *Bulletin of the Menninger Clinic,* 1978, *42,* 352–357.

Ekstein, R. Termination in child psychotherapy. Presentation at Children's Hospital, San Francisco, February 1977.

Elkind, D. *Children and adolescents.* New York: Oxford University Press, 1970.

Freud, S. The interpretation of dreams (standard ed., Vols. 4, 5). London: Hogarth Press, 1900; 1953.

Freud, S. *Three essays on the theory of sexuality* (standard ed., Vol. 7). London: Hogarth Press, 1905; 1953, pp. 135–243.

Freud, S. *Creative writers and daydreaming* (standard ed., Vol. 9). London: Hogarth Press, 1908; 1959, pp. 141–153.

Gardner, R. A. *Therapeutic communication with children: The mutual storytelling technique.* New York: Science House, 1971.

Hartmann, H. *Ego psychology and the problem of adaptation.* New York: International Universities Press, 1958.

Hartmann, H. *Essays on ego psychology*. New York: International Universities Press, 1964.

Hersen, M., & Barlow, D. *Single-case experimental designs: Strategies for studying behavior change*. New York: Pergamon, 1976.

Jones, E. The theory of symbolism. *Papers on psychoanalysis*. Baltimore: Williams & Wilkins, 1916; 1948.

Kagan, J., & Moss, H. A. *Birth to maturity: The Fels study of psychological development*. New York: Wiley, 1962.

Kazdin, A. E. Statistical analyses for single-case experimental designs. In M. Hersen & D. Barlow, *Single-case experimental designs: Strategies for studying behavior change*. New York: Pergamon, 1976, pp. 265–313.

Klinger, E. *Structure and functions of fantasy*. New York: Wiley.

Kris, E. *Psychoanalytic explorations in art*. New York: International Universities Press, 1952.

Mahler, M. S., Pine, F., & Bergman, A. *The psychological birth of the human infant*. New York: Basic Books, 1975.

Meers, D. A diagnostic profile of psychopathology in a latency child. *Psychoanalytic Study of the Child*, 1966, *21*, 483–526.

Pendelton, R. Maturity of object relations and the process of attention. *Dissertation Abstracts International*, 1973, *73–14*, 169.

Peskin, H. Pubertal onset and ego functioning. *Journal of Abnormal Psychology*, 1967, *72(1)*, 1–15.

Piaget, J. *Play, dreams, and imitation in childhood*. New York: Norton, 1945; 1962.

Sarnoff, C. Ego structure in latency. *Psychoanalytic Quarterly*, 1971, *40*, 387–414.

Sarnoff, D. *Latency*. New York: Aronson, 1976.

Shapiro, T., & Perry, R. Latency revisited: The age 7 plus or minus 1. *Psychoanalytic Study of the Child*, 1976, *31*, 79–105.

Williams, M. Problems of technique during latency. *Psychoanalytic Study of the Child*, 1972, *27*, 598–617.

APPENDIX: RATING SCALES OF CHILDREN'S STORIES

Adaptive Regression in the Service of the Ego (*ARISE*)

Scale: 1 . . . 2 . . . 3 . . . 4 . . . 5

Stop:

1. Regressions very prominent and primitive.
   Disrupts adaptive behavior severely.
   Story seems "wild," confused, and chaotic.
   Appears that child is "carried away" by story and is totally confused.
   Characters appear and disappear; the clarity and "point" of the story are lost.

2. Regressions still observed, but not as primitive or chaotic.
   Story has moments of clarity.

Or
>   Virtual absence of regressive phenomena.
>   Inability to loosen controls.
>   (CAT) Story is concrete; child describes the card.
>   Inability to be playful or humorous.

Or
>   Child may enjoy playfulness but does not recover from it.

3. Child enjoys primitive regression and playfulness.
    Regressions somewhat controlled, or may be difficult to achieve.

4. Fairly high enjoyment but may regain control prematurely.
    Shows fair amount of control in "letting go" and reemerging.
    Tends to be humorous, playful, "silly."

5. Regressions controlled and child shows maximal enjoyment of them.
    A creative story—may be "fantastic" but enjoyable and not over-
       whelming.
    Images are vivid and engrossing.
    High level of spontaneity.

Psychoanalytic Symbolization Scale

Scale: 1 . . . 2 . . . 3 . . . 4 . . . 5

Stop:

1. Symbolization minimal or absent; no fantasy.
    Symbolic process easy to understand—symbols represent primitive
       drives, fantasies, impulses.
    Fantasy appears simple and very fragile.
    Child keeps fantasy very short and seems to be distancing self from it—
       tries not to be involved in it.
    Related to fragility: drives close to surface; child may lose fantasy and
       act out impulse.
    Language minimal for expression of concrete desires.
       Greater reliance on metaphor than on symbol.
       Speech may be idiosyncratic.

2. Presence of symbols intermittent. Fantasy present.
    Beginning of masking in fantasy. Symbols bear direct resemblance to
       that symbolized. Symbols transparent.
    Fantasy seems fragile.
    Fantasy tends to be short; child distant but manages some involvement
       with it.

Drives and conflicts close to surface; child may stop fantasy, refuse to continue.

Child uncomfortable with use of symbols. May have difficulty finding correct words. May perseverate and resort to neologisms.

3. Use of symbolization more regular and consistent in fantasy.

Masking function seen in child's ability to sustain fantasy.

Symbols less directly connected to that symbolized.

Symbols transparent.

Fantasy less fragile, more structured; more complex.

Child shows interest and energy in the fantasy. Distances occasionally as anxiety increases.

Link broken between drives and symbols. Child shows no interest in meaning of symbols. Child may still stop prematurely.

Language understandable; child facile in its use. May occasionally resort to "baby talk."

4. Whole fantasy rich in symbols.

Masking function very adequate. Symbols not transparent.

Inference necessary to make connection between symbol and that symbolized.

Fantasy resilient; shows complex structure. Child interested in telling story.

Very little distancing from story.

Child shows greater distance from drives underlying symbols.

Occasional slips of tongue.

Child comfortable in using language as symbolic communication.

5. Maximal use of symbolization.

Symbols more difficult to understand—masks very well.

Fantasy is complex, intricate, and engrossing to child.

Child deeply involved in fantasy. May give different voices to characters; has flair for the dramatic.

Child consistently distanced from drives; symbols keep child in control.

Child very comfortable in expressing self symbolically.

Apparent that language is true sublimatory channel.

— *CHAPTER TWENTY-EIGHT* ————————

Ego Functioning Patterns Among Families of Schizophrenic and Neurotic Patients

AUGUSTINE MEIER, WILLIAM BARRY, AND MICHELINE BOIVIN

PROBLEM

The purpose of the study was to compare ego functioning patterns in families with an adult schizophrenic male with members of families with an adult schizophrenic female on adaptive levels of ego functioning. Two groups, one composed of members of families with a neurotic male offspring and the other composed of members of families with a neurotic female offspring, were used as controls. This study investigated psychopathology, membership, and sex differences with respect to ego functioning as defined and measured by Bellak and associates (1973).

The early family studies of schizophrenia focused on the parent–patient, patient–sibling, and husband–wife relationships with the purpose of shedding light on the etiology of schizophrenia and the factors that contribute to one sibling becoming symptomatic (Alanen, 1958, 1966; Lidz, 1957a, 1957b,

1963). Parents of schizophrenics manifested more serious marital problems than control groups and were found to be more severely disturbed.

A neglected area in family studies has been the investigation of parental competencies (ego functions) or incompetencies in dealing with inner and outer reality and in relating to their offspring. It is commonly accepted by researchers adhering to a psychodynamic model that healthy ego (function) development is, in part, related to the provision of nurturant and reality-oriented childhood experiences by the parents, particularly the mother or her substitute (Bellak et al., 1973; Lidz, 1973; Mahler, 1968, 1974, 1975; Spitz, 1958). Schizophrenia can also be characterized by disturbances in ego functioning brought on, in part, by ego deficits found in the mother (Alanen, 1966; Bellak et al., 1973; Hartmann, 1965; Lidz, 1973). Yet past research has not specifically investigated the relationship between the schizophrenic patient's ego capacities and those of his or her parents. Moreover, the severity of ego deficits in emotionally disturbed persons has been found to be positively related to the degree of their psychopathology (Bellak et al., 1973; Bellak and Hurvich, 1969; Hartmann, 1950; Witkin et al., 1962).

Clinical and empirical observations suggest the following relationships: (1) The severity of ego deficits is positively related to the degree of psycho-pathology (Bellak et al., 1973); (2) the parents and siblings of schizophrenic patients show greater emotional disturbance than the parents and siblings of neurotic patients (Alanen, 1966, 1971; Pollack, 1969); and (3) the type of behavioral patterns observed between fathers and mothers of male schizophrenics differs from that observed between fathers and mothers of female schizophrenics (Fleck et al., 1963; Lidz et al., 1957b). These considerations led the authors to hypothesize that differences in ego functioning would be observed among members of families with a schizophrenic and neurotic patient.

The major hypotheses of this study, based on psychodynamic theory and the results from family investigations, are:

1. There is a significant relationship between the group mean scores on the dependent variables (ego functions) when the combined sample is divided according to the psychiatric status (psychopathology) and sex of the patient and family membership (member).

2. There is a significant relationship between the group mean scores on the dependent variables when the families with a schizophrenic patient and neurotic patient, taken separately, are divided according to member and sex.

3. There is a significant relationship between the group mean scores on the dependent variables when the patients, siblings, fathers and mothers, taken separately, are divided according to psychopathology and sex.

4. There is a significant relationship between the group mean scores on the dependent variables when the families with a male patient and the

families with a female patient, taken separately, are divided according to psychopathology and member.

In summary, ego functioning patterns among families of schizophrenic and neurotic patients are hypothesized to be related to three independent variables, namely, the psychiatric status of the patient, the patient's sex, and family membership.

SAMPLE

The subjects for the study and the criteria for their inclusion were:

1. Eight schizophrenic males, eight schizophrenic females, seven neurotic males, and eight neurotic females who:
    a. Were 18–30 years of age at date of admission
    b. Were consecutively admitted to the inpatient, day-care, or outpatient programs of the Royal Ottawa Hospital (a psychiatric hospital that admits about 80% of all psychiatric patients in the region)
    c. Were diagnosed as definite schizophrenic and definite neurotic (anxiety, obsessive–compulsive neurosis, hysteria) by psychiatrists using the criteria of Spitzer and associates (1975)
    d. Did not have a secondary diagnosis of chronic brain syndrome, alcoholism, drug dependence, or mental retardation. The neurotics were also required not to meet the secondary diagnoses of homosexuality and antisocial behavior
    e. Had living biological parents who were both Caucasian and spoke English
    f. Had at least one same-sexed, full sibling of 16 years or older, and in the case of the neurotic patients only, could not have a schizophrenic diagnosis
2. The biological parents of the schizophrenic and neurotic patients
3. The patient's same-sexed full sibling who was 16 years of age or older at the time of the patient's admission

The combined sample consisted of 124 subjects (31 intact families), divided equally for family membership. Patients were admitted to the study between December 1, 1976, and August 30, 1978.

INSTRUMENTS

The manual for Rating Ego Functions from a Clinical Interview (MANUAL) as devised by Bellak et al. (1973) was the principal tool used in the present study. The MANUAL provides descriptive criteria on the basis of which material from clinical interviews can be rated as to the adaptive level of 12 ego functions and their component factors.

In line with Bellak et al. (1973), each of the 12 ego functions and their component factors can be globally rated as to the lowest, highest, current, and characteristic level of functioning. *Lowest* and *highest* ordinarily apply to functioning during a reasonable time period (at least 2 months). *Current* refers to the adaptive level of ego functioning at the time of the interview. The characteristic level is constituted by the frequency, intensity, and pervasiveness of any phenomena rated and is inferred from a subject's current, lowest, and highest levels of functioning.

Bellak and associates (1973) studied the predictive validity of the MANUAL by investigating its ability to discriminate between three groups differing as to degree of psychopathology. For their study the authors used 50 schizophrenics, 25 neurotics, and 25 normals as subjects. The one-way analysis of variance of the three group means for each ego function (except mastery–competence which was not included in the study) produced F ratios that were highly significant, and all mean differences were in the predicted direction. The Duncan Multiple Range Test showed that the differences between the group means of the schizophrenics and neurotics, and between those of neurotics and normals for each of the ego functions, were significant beyond the .001 level. The authors interpreted their findings as supporting the predictive validity of the MANUAL as a technique to rate ego functions from interview material.

The reliability of the MANUAL has been determined by two techniques, namely, interrater reliability and the extent of disagreement in scale points among raters. Based on the 100 cases used in their study, Bellak and associates (1973) obtained a mean interrater correlation coefficient of .77 with a range of .61 and .88 for the 11 ego functions. Bellak and associates also calculated the extent of disagreement among raters in scale points, which they then converted into percentages. Using the raters' scores for the 100 cases of their study, the authors obtained a total agreement between two judges on 24% of the ratings, 60% were within one scale point, 84% within two scale points, and 94% within three scale points. The authors interpreted these results as reflecting a substantial degree of agreement among the raters, more than is suggested by the reliability coefficients.

Bellak and associates (1973) investigated, as well, the interrelationship of the ego functions by performing a principal-components factor analysis with varimax rotation on the matrix of intercorrelations. The matrix of intercorrelations was computed using one rater's scores for the 11 ego functions obtained from the schizophrenic group because they showed the least intercorrelation, and presumably, the least halo and response effects. In all, four factors were extracted. The Synthetic, Autonomous, and Defensive functions loaded heavily on Factor 1; Judgment, Sense of Reality, and Reality

Testing loaded on Factor 2; Regulation and Control, and Object Relations loaded on Factor 3; and Thought Process and ARISE loaded on Factor 4. Stimulus Barrier did not load heavily on any of the factors and thus was considered as the fifth factor. The results of the factor analysis indicates a relative degree of dependency among groups of scales and suggests that the 11 ego functions are reducible to five factors.

PROCEDURE

Selection of the Sample

The subjects were selected by a hospital psychiatrist according to the criteria described earlier. A psychiatrist interviewed all 18–30-year-old males and females in the sample with an initial hospital diagnosis of schizophrenia or neurosis. The patients, who according to the judgment of the psychiatrist met the preceding criteria indicated, were admitted, together with their biological parents and one same-sexed full sibling, as potential subjects for the study.

The sample for the present study was drawn from the accumulating pool of potential subjects and was group-matched for socioeconomic status (Blishen et al., 1976), for age, and individually for sex. The schizophrenic females were used as the reference group for all matching and were, consequently, the first selected. Age was matched within 5 years and socioeconomic level within one class of the female schizophrenic. The father's occupation when the patient was 16 years of age was used to determine the socioeconomic status of all patients (McRoberts, 1975)

A two-factor (psychopathology × sex), fixed-effects analysis of variance was conducted separately on the social status mean scores of the patients, and on the mean age scores of the patients, siblings, fathers, and mothers. The ANOVA failed to produce significant social status and age differences between compared groups, thus confirming that the patients were group-matched for social status and age and that the siblings, fathers, and mothers were group-matched for age as well.

Conducting Clinical Interviews

Once family units (consisting of the patient, his or her biological parents, and one same-sexed full sibling) qualified for the study, the psychiatrist explained to them the purpose and nature of the study and solicited their participation. The researcher was not informed as to who were patients and siblings and who were the parents of the schizophrenic and neurotic patients until all coding and interviewing were completed. These eligible patients, their biological parents, and their same-sexed siblings were interviewed individually according to the questionnaire.

Rating Adaptive Levels of Ego Functioning

The ego functions were rated by five advanced undergraduate and doctoral students (designated as A, B, C, D, and E) enrolled in the psychology program at the University of Ottawa.

Prior to the study proper, the raters participated in a specially designed 20-hour training program, where they became thoroughly familiar with the MANUAL and independently scored five tape-recorded practice protocols. After scoring each of the taped practice protocols, scores for each ego function were compared and discrepancies discussed. Practice sessions continued until the level of agreement (percentage of agreement within two scale points) paralleled that reported by Bellak and associates (1973).

The five raters were grouped into seven pairs, namely, AB, AC, AE, BD, BE, CD, and DE. Each pair independently rated the interviews of one block of "four families" (16 subjects) except for raters AC, who rated the interviews of two blocks of "four" families (32 subjects). Each block of "four families" consisted of the following subjects: one male schizophrenic and his biological parents and same-sexed sibling, one female schizophrenic and her biological parents and same-sexed sibling, one male neurotic and his biological parents and same-sexed sibling, and one female neurotic and her biological parents and one same-sexed sibling.

Computation of Scores

Two raters independently evaluated each subject on the 12 ego functions according to his or her highest, lowest, and characteristic level of functioning. Thus, each subject received two ratings for each of the three levels of functioning for each of the 12 ego functions. To compute one score for each level of functioning for each of the 12 ego functions, the researcher averaged the two rater's scores. This procedure was followed in the calculations of all scores for the three levels of functioning and for each of the 12 ego functions. These scores were used for all statistical calculations that involved group comparisons.

Formation of Testing Groups

To test the hypotheses, the sample was divided into 16 groups using family membership and the psychiatric status and sex of the patient as a basis. These groups can be thought of as Patient, Sibling, Father, and Mother groups divided according to the psychiatric status and sex of the patient. The number of subjects varied from seven to eight per group.

TECHNIQUES OF ANALYSIS

Computation of Interrater Reliability

Interrater reliability was computed by the use of two techniques, namely, the Pearson Product Moment Coefficient of Correlation r and the calculation of disagreements among raters in terms of scale points.

The Pearson r's were corrected by the Spearman–Brown formula (Guilford, 1965, p. 458) because of the small number of subjects assessed by each rater. The Spearman–Brown corrected correlations for the seven pairs of raters for each of the 12 ego functions are presented in Table 28.1. The correlations were computed using the ratings for the characteristic level of ego functioning. The table shows that the means for the paired raters across the 12 ego functions range from .55–.85, and the means for the 12 ego functions across raters range from .55 to .83. The mean correlation is .74. The correlations obtained in this study are somewhat lower than those obtained by Bellak and associates (1973). In the latter study, the corrected correlations ranged from .61 to .88, with a mean of .77. Nevertheless, the magnitude of the correlations in both the Bellak and the present study ranges from moderate to high.

The second method used to evaluate interrater reliability consisted of calculating the extent of disagreement among raters in terms of scale points. For example, if rater A assigned a value of 6 for Reality Testing, and rater B assigned a value of 5 for the same ego function, the extent of disagreement between the two raters would be one scale point. Bellak and associates (1973) employed this technique in calculating interrater reliability in their study and stated that this method reflected a greater degree of agreement than was suggested by correlation coefficients (pp. 303–304).

The mean disagreements on a 13-point scale for each pair of raters on the 12 ego functions for the combined sample are presented in Table 28.2. The mean disagreements for each ego function across the seven pairs of raters and the mean disagreements for each pair of raters across the 12 ego functions are presented as well. For these calculations the ratings for the characteristic level were used so that the findings could be evaluated in view of Bellak and associates' results.

Table 28.2 shows that the mean disagreements for the seven pairs of raters across the 12 ego functions range from 1.00 to 1.40 scale points and that the mean disagreements for the 12 ego functions across the seven pairs of raters range from .89 to 1.65 scale points. The mean disagreement is 1.23 scale points.

Bellak and associates did not report mean disagreements among the raters for each ego function for the combined sample. However, using their data for the schizophrenic, neurotic, and normal groups, mean disagreements can be computed (Bellak et al., 1973, p. 303). The results of these computations

Table 28.1.   Correlation Coefficient Corrected by the Spearman–Brown Formula for the Seven Pairs of Raters for Each of the 12 Ego Functions

Ego Function	Raters							
	AB	AC	AE	BD	BE	CD	DE	Mean
I. Reality Testing	.54	.68	.87	.91	.90	.89	.95	.82
II. Judgment	.82	.73	.63	.63	.84	.92	.94	.79
III. Sense of Reality	.67	.83	.82	.78	.87	.95	.92	.83
IV. Regulation and Control of Drives	.80	.62	.62	.43	.83	.79	.85	.71
V. Object Relations	.26	.73	.80	.57	.85	.70	.82	.68
VI. Thought Process	.79	.65	.67	.18	.88	.82	.94	.70
VII. ARISE	.48	.28	.51	.86	.57	.67	.48	.55
VIII. Defensive Functioning	.48	.71	.75	.52	.83	.55	.90	.68
IX. Stimulus Barrier	.57	.75	.85	.31	.67	.91	.77	.69
X. Autonomous Functioning	.45	.82	.92	.66	.92	.81	.93	.79
XI. Synthetic Functioning	.38	.84	.65	.66	.84	.84	.92	.73
XII. Mastery–Competence	.41	.84	.84	.84	.88	.76	.81	.77
Mean	.55	.71	.74	.74	.82	.80	.85	.74
Range	.26–.82	.28–.84	.51–.92	.18–.91	.57–.90	.55–.95	.48–.95	.55–.83

Table 28.2 Mean Disagreements on a 13-Point Scale for Each Pair of Raters on the 12 Ego Functions for the Combined Sample

				Raters						
Ego Function	AB (N = 11)	AC (N = 31)	AE (N = 14)	BD (N = 16)	BE (N = 17)	CD (N = 16)	DE (N = 12)	Range	Mean (N = 112)	Bellak Mean
I. Reality Testing	1.82	1.96	.71	.82	1.00	1.00	.92	.82–1.96	1.18	1.48
II. Judgment	1.10	1.46	1.07	1.26	1.05	1.00	.83	.83–1.46	1.11	1.54
III. Sense of Reality	1.36	1.30	1.07	1.12	.82	.62	1.08	.62–1.36	1.05	1.41
IV. Regulation and Control of Drives	1.00	1.46	1.36	1.12	1.52	1.06	1.50	1.00–1.52	1.05	1.29
V. Object Relations	1.46	1.12	1.14	1.62	1.64	1.44	2.33	1.23–2.33	1.54	1.33
VI. Thought Process	.46	1.48	1.00	1.38	.94	.62	1.00	.46–1.48	.98	1.33
VII. ARISE	1.64	2.00	1.71	1.06	1.88	1.42	1.83	1.06–2.00	1.65	1.60
VIII. Defensive Functioning	1.64	1.10	1.36	1.38	1.11	1.26	1.50	1.11–1.64	1.34	1.21
IX. Stimulus Barrier	1.46	.96	1.50	1.56	1.52	.56	1.42	.56–1.56	1.28	1.61
X. Autonomous Functioning	1.54	.90	.50	1.18	.59	1.12	1.17	.50–1.54	1.00	1.34
XI. Synthetic Functioning	.90	1.36	1.07	1.12	1.18	.76	1.50	.76–1.50	1.13	1.60
XII. Mastery–Competence	1.28	1.10	2.00	1.50	1.35	1.12	1.67	1.10–2.00	1.43	—
Range	.46 to 1.82	.90 to 1.96	.50 to 2.00	.82 to 1.62	.59 to 1.88	.62 to 1.44	.93 to 2.33	.46 to 2.33	.98 to 1.65	1.21 to 1.60
Means	1.24	1.33	1.21	1.26	1.22	1.00	1.40		1.23	1.43

are presented in Table 28.2, under Bellak. The mean disagreements among raters in Bellak's study range from 1.21 to 1.60, with a mean of 1.43. The results of the present study are in general comparable to those of Bellak.

The extent of agreement and disagreement was also calculated in terms of percentages. These data are presented in Table 28.3. The table shows that there was total agreement between the two raters on 26% of the ratings, 65% were within one scale point, 87% were within two scale points, and 95% were within three scale points. The results are very similar to those obtained by Bellak and associates, whose percentages of agreement for the same scale points were, respectively, 24, 60, 84, and 94.

The extent of interrater agreement was also computed by the use of the Lawlis-Lu chi square and a T index (Tinsley and Weiss, 1975, p. 367). The chi squares and the T values obtained by the application of the Tinsley and Weiss procedure to rater agreement within two scale points indicated that all chi squares were significant beyond the .001 level, and that the T values, ranging from .80 to .85 indicated both high and positive agreement among raters. (The chi squares for the seven pairs of raters were: 10.13, 36.50, 15.20, 18.84, 16.27, and 11.83, all of which were significant at the .005 level or better. The corresponding T values were: .72, .80, .78, .81, .72, .90, and .74, all of which indicate both high and positive agreement.)

The results of the analysis of interrater reliability indicate that there is substantial agreement among raters even though the magnitude of the correlation coefficients ranges from moderate to high. The interrater reliability

Table 28.3. Percentages of Agreement for Zero to Six Scale Points Differences Obtained by the Combined Pairs of Raters (N = 117)

	Ego Function	Scale Point Difference						
		0	1	2	3	4	5	6
I.	Reality Testing	33	38	15	7	5	1	1
II.	Judgment	27	46	16	7	4	0	0
III.	Sense of Reality	33	36	25	6	1	0	0
IV.	Regulation and Control of Drives	21	43	21	10	4	0	0
V.	Object Relations	21	31	21	20	15	0	0
VI.	Thought Processes	35	36	18	5	4	0	2
VII.	ARISE	14	38	23	14	9	3	1
VIII.	Defensive Functioning	25	36	26	13	1	0	0
IX.	Stimulus Barrier	24	44	21	9	3	0	0
X.	Autonomous Functioning	32	41	25	2	0	0	0
XI.	Synthetic Functioning	26	42	25	7	1	0	0
XII.	Mastery–Competence	17	44	25	8	6	0	0
Mean percentage		26	39	22	8	4	.21	.33
Cumulative percentage		26	65	87	95	99	99	100

data obtained in this study are similar to those obtained by Bellak and associates in their study.

Analysis of Differences Among Group Mean Ego Function Scores

Intercorrelations among the 12 ego functions for each of the three levels were computed separately. The obtained intercorrelations matrices were factor analyzed using a principal components factor analysis followed by a varimax rotation. The derived factor scores were analyzed from group differences using a two-factor, fixed-effects analysis of variance.

The intercorrelations among the 12 ego functions for characteristic (CH), low (LO), and high (HI) levels are presented in Table 28.4. The mean correlations for CH, LO, and HI levels are, respectively, .67, .69, and .64, and their ranges are, respectively, .12–.88, .24–.83, and .16–.88. The mean correlation coefficients obtained in this study are somewhat higher than those obtained by Bellak and associates (1973). Their correlation coefficients ranged from .45 to .57 (pp. 313–314).

The data in Table 28.4 show that the lowest coefficients were obtained when the ego function ARISE was compared to the other 11 ego functions. These coefficients range from .09 to .44 across the three levels of functioning. All other comparisons produced coefficients that range from .47 to .88 across the three levels of functioning.

The intercorrelation matrices for each level of functioning taken separately were factor-analyzed using a principal components factor analysis followed by a varimax rotation. The results of these analyses are summarized in Table 28.5. The loadings on the extracted factors for the three levels of functioning are presented in the same table.

The results of these analyses show that for the CH level, only one extracted factor had an eigenvalue that exceeded 1.00. This factor with an eigenvalue of 8.71 accounted for 72.6% of the variance. All 12 ego functions, except ARISE, loaded heavily on the factor. Similar results were obtained for the LO level of functioning, where the first factor, with an eigenvalue of 8.55, accounted for 71.3% of the variance. Again, all ego functions except ARISE loaded heavily on the factor.

A factor analysis of the HI level of functioning produced two factors with eigenvalues greater than 1. The first factor had an eigenvalue of 8.36 and accounted for 69.7% of the variance, and the second factor had an eigenvalue of 1.02, which accounted for 8.5% of the variance. All ego functions, except ARISE, loaded heavily on the first factor, whereas ARISE alone loaded heavily on the second factor.

On the basis of the factor analysis, the 12 ego functions can be reduced to two factors (one factor and one item) for each level of functioning. The first factor, which comprises 11 of the 12 ego functions, is labeled Composite Function (C); the second factor comprises the scores from the ego function

Table 28.4. Correlation Coefficients Between Ego Functions for the Three Levels of Functioning

Ego Function	RT	JU	SR	RD	OR	TP	AR	DF	SB	AF	SF	MC
Reality Testing (RT)	—	.77	.79	.73	.75	.78	.33	.73	.54	.77	.74	.70
	—	.88	.83	.79	.73	.66	.23	.71	.60	.79	.75	.67
Judgment (JU)	.87	—	.80	.75	.76	.70	.37	.73	.64	.78	.79	.79
		—	.86	.82	.74	.71	.24	.76	.63	.75	.78	.80
Sense of Reality (SR)	.87	.88	—	.78	.80	.76	.33	.73	.64	.81	.78	.74
			—	.79	.76	.66	.16	.74	.68	.81	.80	.75
Regulation and Control of Drives (RD)	.78	.79	.83	—	.79	.67	.40	.82	.65	.75	.72	.70
				—	.77	.64	.34	.79	.61	.74	.81	.70
Object Relations (OR)	.76	.75	.82	.77	—	.65	.44	.79	.69	.74	.75	.69
					—	.55	.26	.80	.69	.70	.73	.76
Thought Processes (TP)	.79	.75	.76	.68	.65	—	.36	.67	.47	.74	.75	.67
						—	.33	.60	.47	.62	.66	.55
Adaptive Regression in the Service of the Ego (AR)	.29	.26	.24	.37	.33	.39	—	.50	.24	.28	.43	.40
							—	.34	.09	.14	.26	.24
Defensive Functioning (DF)	.77	.76	.80	.81	.82	.66	.36	—	.70	.75	.77	.76
								—	.73	.73	.77	.78
Stimulus Barrier (SB)	.61	.62	.68	.64	.68	.51	.12	.74	—	.64	.62	.57
									—	.65	.59	.63
Autonomous Functioning (AF)	.79	.72	.85	.73	.72	.71	.15	.74	.65	—	.83	.83
										—	.82	.76
Synthetic Functioning (SF)	.79	.82	.86	.75	.73	.76	.30	.78	.59	.84	—	.81
											—	.79
Mastery–Competence (MC)	.76	.78	.83	.71	.77	.70	.32	.79	.60	.81	.82	—

Notes: (1). Top half of the table along the diagonal presents the interscale correlation coefficients for the low and high level of functioning. The upper number represents the coefficient for the low level of functioning, whereas the lower level number represents the high level of functioning. (2). Lower half of table along the diagonal represents the interscale correlation coefficients for the characteristic level of functioning.

Table 28.5. Factor Loadings for the 12 Ego Functions on the Extracted Factors for the Three Levels

Ego Function	Level of Functioning: Characteristics,[a] Factor 1	Low,[a] Factor 1	High: Factor 1	High: Factor 2
Reality Testing	.90	.85	.87	−.04
Judgment	.90	.87	.90	−.00
Sense of Reality	.94	.90	.91	−.15
Regulation and Control of Drives	.87	.86	.89	.11
Object Relations	.86	.87	.85	−.01
Thought Processes	.80	.80	.72	.14
ARISE	.33	.43	.30	.71
Defensive Functioning	.88	.88	.87	.07
Stimulus Barrier	.71	.71	.73	−.17
Autonomous Functioning	.87	.89	.87	−.16
Synthetic Functioning	.90	.89	.89	.00
Mastery–Competence	.88	.84	.83	−.03

[a] Number of iterations terminated after the first because the second eigenvalue was less than 1.

ARISE and is labeled ARISE (7). The three levels of the Composite Function are labeled Composite High (CHI), Composite Low (CLO), and Composite Characteristic (CCH); the three levels of ARISE are labeled ARISE high (HI7), ARISE low (LO7), and ARISE characteristic (CH7).

Intercorrelations among the three levels (LO, HI, CH) for the two functions (Composite and ARISE) taken separately were computed. The correlation coefficients for CLO versus CHI, CLO versus CCH, and CHI versus CCH were, respectively, .92, .95, and .95; and for LO7 versus HI7, LO7 versus CH7, and HI7 versus CH7 they were, respectively, .54, .79 and .82. The results show that the scores for the three levels of functioning are highly intercorrelated.

A principal components factor analysis was carried out on the correlation matrix obtained from the scores on the three levels of functioning for the two functions taken separately. The factor loadings for the three levels of the two ego functions are presented in Table 28.6. The table shows that only one factor can be extracted from each of the Composite Function and ARISE. In the case of the Composite Function, the eigenvalue for Factor 1 is 2.54 and accounts for 98.3% of the variance; for ARISE, the eigenvalue for Factor 1 is 2.76 and accounts for 92.0% of the variance.

The results from the factor analysis suggest that only two factors can be extracted from the 12 ego functions across the three levels. One factor,

Table 28.6.   Factor Loadings for Composite and ARISE on the Three Levels of Functioning [a]

Ego Function	Level of Functioning	Factor Loadings
Composite	Low	.97
	High	.99
	Characteristic	.99
ARISE	Low	.91
	High	.91
	Characteristic	.99

[a] Number of iterations terminated after the first because the second eigenvalue was less than 1.

which will be called Global Ego Function (GEF), comprises the combined scores of 11 ego functions from the three levels, and the second factor, which will be called Adaptive Regression in Service of the Ego (ARISE), comprises the combined scores from ARISE for the three levels of functioning.

In the present research, member, psychopathology, and sex differences (the three independent variables) on GEF and ARISE were the two factors studied as dependent variables, using a three-factor and a two-factor analysis of variance. GEF and ARISE were analyzed separately. The univariate and multivariate analysis of variance computer program designed by Finn (1976) was used for all univariate analysis.

Whenever significant differences were found in the analysis of variance, the Duncan Multiple Range Test was used as a post hoc procedure (Kirk, 1968). The Duncan method, used by Bellak and associates in their study, was chosen because the assumption of equal sample size could be met and because it is a powerful test when all pairs of experimental groups are compared. For the present study, group differences at the .05 level or less were interpreted as being significant.

RESULTS

The results from the analysis of the data are presented under four major classifications in accordance with the four sets of hypotheses tested. The data were analyzed by the use of either a two-factor or a three-factor, fixed-effects analysis of variance.

To test the hypothesis that a relationship exists between the two dependent variables when the combined sample is divided according to psychopathology, member, and sex, means (M) and standard deviations (SD) were

Table 28.7.   Means and Standard Deviations Obtained on GEF Scores for the Combined Sample Divided According to Psychopathology, Family Membership, and Sex

Pathology and Sex of Patient	Family Membership							
	Patients		Siblings		Fathers		Mothers	
	M	SD	*M*	SD	*M*	SD	*M*	SD
Schizophrenic male	230.56	41.03	282.75	20.32	316.25	19.52	293.50	29.46
Schizophrenic female	223.44	35.60	268.06	74.27	320.50	29.04	291.25	40.29
Mean	227.00	37.00	275.41	53.14	318.38	24.00	292.38	34.11
Neurotic male	270.57	45.55	279.50	28.68	297.29	22.60	301.14	23.47
Neurotic female	234.75	24.45	284.69	33.80	308.75	16.74	318.75	11.88
Mean	251.47	39.12	282.27	30.52	303.40	19.85	310.53	19.73
Mean across psychopathology and sex	238.84	39.55	278.73	43.11	311.13	23.01	301.16	29.13

computed for each of the groups for GEF and ARISE. These data are presented in Tables 28.7 and 28.8, respectively. Means and standard deviations for each member group across psychopathologies are given as well.

With respect to main effects, significant differences between members within families were observed on both the GEF and ARISE group means ($F = 26.07$, $p < .0001$; $F = 3.63$, $p < .015$; respectively), but no significant psychopathology and sex differences were found, nor were there significant interactions among the independent variables. Hypothesis 1, therefore, was rejected in part.

The means, differences between means, and levels of significance for post hoc comparisons on GEF and ARISE, for the sample divided according to member, are presented in Table 28.9, rows 1 and 6, respectively, The Duncan Multiple Range Test was used for all post hoc comparisons.

In the post hoc comparisons, the mean GEF scores of the fathers and mothers differed significantly from the mean GEF scores of the patients ($p < .01$) and siblings ($p < .01$), with the mean scores of the fathers and mothers significantly higher than the means of both groups. The mean GEF scores of the siblings differed significantly ($p < .05$) from the mean GEF scores of the patients, with the latter having the lower score. The mean GEF scores of the fathers and mothers, however, did not differ significantly from each other.

In the post hoc comparisons of ARISE group means, the mean score of the patients differed significantly from the mean score of the siblings ($p <$

Table 28.8.   Means and Standard Deviations Obtained on ARISE Scores for the Combined Sample Divided According to Psychopathology, Family Membership, and Sex

Pathology and Sex of Patient	Family Membership							
	Patients		Siblings		Fathers		Mothers	
	M	SD	*M*	SD	*M*	SD	*M*	SD
Schizophrenic male	22.75	3.27	24.63	3.84	24.13	4.95	22.13	2.80
Schizophrenic female	22.00	2.37	25.63	5.33	22.63	4.18	24.94	3.71
Mean	22.38	2.79	25.13	4.52	22.38	4.49	25.53	3.49
Neurotic male	22.00	2.52	23.79	2.63	23.21	3.19	25.07	2.32
Neurotic female	23.19	3.91	26.75	3.39	23.44	5.20	27.00	2.56
Mean	22.63	3.28	25.37	3.32	23.33	4.23	26.10	2.56
Mean across psychopathology	22.50	2.99	25.24	3.92	23.35	4.29	24.77	3.30

.01) and the mothers ($p < .05$). The mean ARISE scores of all other comparisons did not differ significantly from each other. The siblings obtained the highest mean score on ARISE, whereas the patients obtained the lowest ARISE score.

Summarizing the results, member was found to correlate with mean GEF and ARISE scores; psychopathology and sex, however, did not relate to the scores on the two dependent variables. Moreover, the findings on GEF and ARISE were not similar.

The second hypothesis, that there is a relationship between the group mean scores for the two dependent variables when the families with a schizophrenic patient are divided according to member and sex, was tested by performing a two-factor analysis of variance on the GEF and ARISE group means (Tables 28.7 and 28.8). Significant differences were found on GEF mean scores for member ($F = 15.06$; $p < .0001$), but no significant differences were found on mean ARISE scores. The means, differences between the means, and the levels of significance for post hoc comparisons on GEF are presented in Table 28.9, row 2.

In the post hoc comparisons, the mean GEF scores for fathers, mothers, and siblings differed significantly ($p < .01$) from the mean GEF scores of the patients. The mean GEF scores of the fathers also differed significantly ($p < .05$) from the mean score of the siblings. All other comparisons did not yield significant differences. However, the differences between the fathers' and mothers' mean GEF scores just failed to reach significance.

On the basis of previous research concerning the family studies of schizo-

Table 28.9. *Comparison of Mean Scores Obtained by Member Groups, Using the Duncan Multiple Range Test*

Row	Dependent Variable	Sample Size	Comparative Groups[a]					
			Fa-Mo	Fa-Sib	Fa-Pat	Mo-Sib	Mo-Pat	Sib-Pat
1	GEF	Combined	9.97[b]	32.40**	72.29**	22.43**	62.32**	39.89**
2	GEF	Schizophrenic	26.00*	42.97**	91.38***	16.97	65.38***	48.41***
3	GEF	Neurotic	-7.13	21.13**	51.93***	28.26**	59.06***	30.80***
4	GEF	Male patients	10.33	26.17*	56.17***	15.84	47.84***	32.00***
5	GEF	Female patients	9.63	37.85**	85.54**	28.22**	75.91***	47.69***
6	ARISE	Combined	-1.42	-1.89	.85	-.47	2.27*	2.74**
7	ARISE	Neurotic	-2.77*	-2.04	.70	.73	3.47*	2.74*
8	ARISE	Female patients	-2.94*	-3.16*	.44	-.22	3.38*	3.60*

Note: * Level of significance is .05 or less, ** level of significance is .01 or less.

[a] Fa—fathers; Mo—mothers; Sib—siblings; Pat—patients.

[b] Values represent differences between the means. The mean of the second in the pair is always subtracted from the first listed.

phrenia, the fathers were expected to differ from the mothers on mean GEF scores. To test this hypothesis, the mean GEF scores of the fathers and mothers were reanalyzed using a two-factor analysis of variance. The results of this analysis showed significant differences ($F = 5.82$; $p < .023$) among member groups with the fathers scoring higher. No other significant differences were found.

In summary, member was found to be related to GEF scores, but not to ARISE scores. Sex related to neither GEF nor ARISE scores. The results of the analysis of mean GEF scores showed that the fathers scored significantly higher than all other members and that the mothers and siblings, who did not differ significantly from each other, also scored significantly higher than the patients.

A two-factor analysis of variance was used to test the second part of the second hypothesis, that is, that there is a relationship between the group mean scores for the two dependent variables when the families with a neurotic patient are divided according to member and sex. Significant differences were found among members' mean scores on both GEF ($F = 13.22$; $p < .001$) and ARISE ($F = 3.39$; $p < .025$), but no significant sex differences were found. In view of these findings, hypothesis 2 was partially rejected.

The differences between means and the levels of significance for post hoc comparisons on GEF and ARISE are presented in Table 28.9, rows 3 and 7, respectively. In the post hoc comparisons, the mean GEF scores of the mothers and fathers differed significantly from the mean GEF scores of the siblings ($p < .01$ and $p < .05$, respectively, for mothers and fathers) and of the patients ($p < .01$). The mean GEF scores of the siblings also differed significantly from the mean scores of the patients ($p < .01$). All other comparisons failed to yield significant differences. The mothers obtained the highest mean GEF score and the patients obtained the lowest score.

To test the hypothesis that there is a relationship between the group mean scores on the two dependent variables when the patients' siblings, fathers, or mothers are divided according to psychopathology and sex, a two-factor analysis of variance was carried out on the GEF (Table 28.7) and ARISE mean scores (Table 28.8) for each member group taken separately. The means on GEF showed no significant differences for main effects and no psychopathology–sex interaction. The means on ARISE revealed significant psychopathology ($F = 6.01$; $p < .021$) and sex ($F = 5.18$; $p < .03$) differences only for the combined mother groups, but not for any of the other groups. There was no significant psychopathology–sex interaction on ARISE. On the basis of these results, the only hypothesis in this group to be rejected had to do with the relationship between pathology and sex with the two dependent variables for the mother group.

When the means on ARISE are compared, the mean for the mothers of neurotics ($M = 26.04$) is significantly higher than that for the mothers of schizophrenics ($M = 23.53$), and the group mean of mothers of females ($M = 25.97$) is significantly higher than that for the mothers of males ($M = 23.50$). The mothers of male schizophrenics obtained the lowest mean score ($M =$

22.13) on ARISE, whereas the mothers of neurotics obtained the highest mean score ($M = 27.00$) on the same function.

Additionally, the hypothesis that states that there are no significant psychopathology and member differences on GEF and ARISE mean scores for the combined families with a male patient was tested by separate two-factor analysis of variance. The means on GEF showed significant differences among member groups ($F = 10.66$; $p < .001$), but no significant psychopathology difference was found, nor was there a significant psychopathology–member interaction. The analysis of the mean scores on ARISE yielded no significant main effects, nor was there a significant psychopathology–member interaction.

The differences between means and the levels of significance for post hoc comparisons on GEF are presented in Table 28.9, row 4. In the post hoc comparisons the mean GEF score of fathers was significantly higher than the mean scores for both the siblings and the patients; this score did not differ significantly from that of the mothers. The mean scores on GEF for both the mothers and siblings differed significantly from that of the patients. All other member comparisons yielded no significant differences.

To test the latter hypothesis with regard to families with a female patient rather than with a male patient, a two-factor analysis of variance was carried out on the GEF and ARISE mean scores for the families with a female patient divided according to psychopathology and member. Significant member differences were found on the mean scores for both GEF ($F = 16.54$; $p < .001$) and ARISE ($F = 3.66$; $p < .018$), but no significant psychopathology differences or significant psychopathology–member interactions were found on the two dependent variables.

The differences between the means, the levels of significance for the comparisons on GEF and for ARISE are summarized in Table 28.9, rows 5 and 8, respectively.

In the post hoc comparisons, the mean GEF scores of the fathers, mothers, and siblings differed significantly ($p < .01$) from the mean GEF scores of the patients. The mean GEF scores of the fathers and mothers also differed significantly ($p < .05$) from that of the siblings. All other comparisons yielded no significant differences.

In the post hoc comparisons of ARISE scores, the siblings and mothers scored significantly higher ($p < .05$) than both the father and patient groups. All other comparisons yielded no significant differences.

In summary, member alone was found to be related to both GEF and ARISE mean scores. The post hoc findings on GEF for the families with a female patient are very similar to the post hoc findings for families with a male patient. However, the findings on ARISE for the two samples are not similar.

To summarize, the present study yielded the following findings:

1. Family membership related significantly with GEF but the orderings for member differed for the two psychopathological groups.

2. Differences in the psychiatric status of the patient were significantly related to ARISE for the mother groups, but not for any other group member.
3. There was a significant relationship between family membership and ARISE for the combined sample, for families with a neurotic patient, and for families with a female patient.
4. Differences in the sex of the patient were significantly related to ARISE for the mother but not for any other group.

DISCUSSION

The results of the present study must be interpreted in view of three limiting conditions. First, the findings are generalizable to intact families of schizophrenic patients who have at least one full sibling of the same sex. Second, the neurotic patients who served as a comparison group represented the more serious end of the neurotic spectrum. Therefore, the findings might have been different if a more representative sample of neurotics was utilized. Last, the families studied in this project are predominantly from the higher socioeconomic strata.

The findings will be discussed in accordance with the three independent variables: psychopathological status of patient, member, and sex differences.

Psychopathological Differences

Among the various intergroup comparisons a single psychopathological difference was observed. This difference appeared on the ARISE scores, where the mothers of the neurotics scored significantly higher than the mothers of the schizophrenics. The ego function ARISE has been defined as the ability to shift perspectives, which allows for the emergence of new configurations and creative adaptations (Bellak et al., 1973). It is also associated with the mother's capacity to be attuned to the needs of the infant—a function considered essential for the child's ego development (Mahler, 1974; Mahler & Furer, 1968).

The finding that the mothers of schizophrenics scored lower than the mothers of neurotics on ARISE is consistent with empirical data. The mothers of schizophrenics, when compared to mothers of controls, were found to be impervious to the needs and demands of the child (Lee, 1975), lacking in empathy (Alanen, 1958; Fleck et al., 1963; Lidz et al., 1965), more concerned with the satisfaction of their own needs rather than with those of the child (Stabenau & Pollen, 1965; Summers & Walsh, 1977), emotionally cold and impoverished (Alanen, 1958), and symbiotically protective toward their children (Wolman, 1965).

The finding on ARISE provides evidence in support of propositions concerning ego development and the psychodynamic theory of schizophrenia interpreted in light of ego disturbances. According to this orientation the ego is believed to evolve within a context of object relationships, particularly within the context of a mother–child symbiotic relationship (Jacobson, 1964; Mahler, 1968, 1974; Spitz, 1965). It is conjectured that the capacity for ARISE equips the prospective mother for participation with the neonate in the affective interchanges that are important for his or her ongoing development (Spitz, 1965). Bellak (1958) states that inadequate mothering, which includes an inflexibility, a lack of emotional availability and rapport, and an incapacity to regress in service of the ego (ARISE), is associated with the etiology of schizophrenia.

In brief, the finding is consistent with published empirical data and with a psychodynamic interpretation of schizophrenia. However, the precise manner in which a mother's low score on ARISE relates to a neonate's ego deficiencies requires further empirical investigation.

There were no significant psychopathological differences observed on GEF. This finding conflicts with the implication of empirical data, indicating that the family members of schizophrenics are, in general, more emotionally disturbed than the family members of controls. The implication is that the former are expected to manifest greater ego deficiencies than the latter.

On the other hand, the failure on the part of the three groups—patients, fathers, and mothers—to reach a level of significance should be cautiously interpreted because the failure might be a function of the size of the sample utilized, of the severity of the emotional disturbance of the control patients, and/or of the patient's social status. In comparison with Bellak's and associates' study (1973), the neurotic patients of the present study were more seriously disturbed. Last, a power test indicated that one could be confident in the results only by increasing the sample size to 65 subjects per group.

Bellak and associates (1973) were able to differentiate a sample of schizophrenics significantly from a sample of neurotics on each of the 12 ego functions by the use of a one-way analysis of variance. To determine more precisely the comparability between the results of the present and the Bellak et al. study, the mean scores of the patients (divided according to psychopathology) for each of the 12 ego functions were subjected to a two-way (psychopathology by sex) analysis of the variance. The results indicated that the schizophrenics scored significantly lower than the neurotics on five ego functions, namely: Reality Testing, Sense of Reality of the World and of the Self, Object Relations, Thought Processes, and Mastery–Competence. On the remaining seven ego functions, the mean scores of the schizophrenics were lower than those of the neurotics. The results of the two studies are not identical, but comparable and reflect similar trends.

The failure to differentiate the two sibling groups on ARISE and GEF scores was unexpected and is not consistent with the results from empirical studies. Alanen (1966), for example, observed that 8% of the siblings of schizophrenic patients were schizophrenic themselves, while none of the siblings of neurotic patients were schizophrenic. He also noted that, when compared to the siblings of neurotics, a greater percentage of siblings of schizophrenics were more disturbed than simple neuroses. The difference in the two findings might be related to the nature of the sample. In his study, Alanen used all available siblings, whereas in the present study the siblings selected were those of the same sex as the patient and nearest to him or her in age. It is still debated whether siblings nearest in age and of the same sex as the patients are more disturbed than siblings of the opposite sex and more distant in age. If the response to the preceding debate is positive, then the siblings used in the present and in the Alanen studies are not comparable and, this difference might then account for the inconsistencies observed between the two studies. Further investigations are required to clarify this issue.

In summary, the only psychopathological difference observed was on ARISE, where the mothers of schizophrenics scored lower than the mothers of neurotics.

Member Differences

When member differences on GEF are examined, a pattern becomes apparent. The fathers and mothers, who do not differ significantly from each other, except in the case of families with a schizophrenic patient, scored higher than the sibling; the siblings, in turn, scored higher than the patients. This finding is consistent with the implications of Alanen's (1966) finding. He noted that the extent of psychopathology among the siblings of schizophrenics and neurotics was greater than that among the combined parents of the same patients, but less than that among the patients themselves.

Of particular significance is the finding that the fathers of schizophrenic patients scored higher on GEF than did the mothers. This is not true for the fathers and mothers of neurotics, where no differences were observed. These findings can also be compared to those of Alanen (1966), where he found that 3% of the fathers and 10% of the mothers of schizophrenics were schizophrenic themselves. None of the fathers or mothers of neurotics were schizophrenic. Moreover, among the families of schizophrenics a greater percentage of the mothers than of the fathers was psychotic (30 and 23%, respectively).

An interesting pattern emerges when the mean GEF scores of the parents divided according to member and psychopathology are considered. The fathers of schizophrenics obtained the highest mean score, the mothers of schizophrenics the lowest, and the mothers of neurotics scored higher than the fathers of neurotics.

The fact that the mothers and fathers of schizophrenics represented the two extremes on a continuum of GEF mean scores has theoretical implications. It suggests that the mother's ego capacities play a most vital role in the development of the child's ego and can do so despite the ego capacities of the father. This is supported by the fact that the fathers of neurotics tend to be more deficient in terms of ego functioning than the fathers of schizophrenics, yet it is the child of the latter that is more seriously disturbed.

Member differences were observed on ARISE as well, but only within the families of the combined sample and within the families of neurotic patients. No member differences were found on ARISE within the families of schizophrenic patients. In the case of the combined sample, the fathers, mothers, and siblings scored higher than the patients but did not differ from each other. In the case of the families of neurotics, the mothers and siblings scored higher on ARISE than the patients, but the mothers alone scored higher than the fathers. Earlier it was observed that the mothers of neurotics scored higher on ARISE than the mothers of schizophrenics. Now it is seen that they also score higher than the fathers of neurotics. It may very well be that the child who becomes a neurotic is kept from more serious psychopathology in part because of the more adequate grounding in ego development given to him by his mother than that given to the child reared by a mother who is deficient in ARISE. It would be interesting to know what happens to families where the father compensates for the mother's deficiency in ARISE. Nevertheless, the preceding findings and deductions give support to the theories concerning ego development and its role in the etiology of schizophrenia.

Sex Differences

When the sample was divided according to the sex of the patient, very similar GEF patterns emerged for the two groups. In the case of female patients, the fathers and mothers, who did not differ significantly from each other, performed better than the siblings, while the siblings performed better than the patients. In the case of male patients, the only divergence from the preceding pattern was that the mothers did not differ from the siblings while the fathers showed the same pattern as in the case of female patients. Thus, the mothers of male patients were found to be more deficient in their level of adaptive ego functioning than the fathers.

It is interesting to note that the GEF pattern for the families with a female patient is identical both to that observed for the combined families of schizophrenic and neurotic patients and to that observed for the combined families of neurotics divided according to member. In the case of male patients, the family GEF pattern is similar to that observed for the families of schizophrenics divided according to member.

The GEF findings, in general, are consistent with empirical data, particularly with those of Alanen (1966), who observed that the siblings of both neurotics and schizophrenics demonstrated less personality disorders than the patients, but greater disorders than the parents of the patients. Also consistent with the empirical data is the observation that mothers of male patients demonstrate less adaptation in terms of ego capacities when compared to their husbands. That is, mothers of male patients have been found to be more disturbed emotionally than the mothers of female patients (Alanen, 1966; Lidz et al., 1965).

In the case of ARISE, member differences were observed for families with a female patient but not for families with a male patient. Both the mothers and siblings performed better on ARISE than the fathers and patients. The difference on ARISE scores in the case of female patients is accounted for by the elevated scores by the group of mothers and by the group of siblings, and not by a lower score of the patients, since the mean ARISE scores for the four groups of patients are similar.

In a second analysis investigating the relationship of the sex of the patient to GEF and ARISE scores, each of the four member groups was divided according to the sex of the patient. Only one significant difference was observed and that was for the mothers on ARISE. The mothers of females performed significantly better than the mothers of males on ARISE. Earlier it was noted that the mothers of neurotics obtained higher ARISE mean scores than the mothers of schizophrenics. It seems that this difference is in large part due to the neurotic mothers' higher ARISE mean score and to the lower mean score of mothers of male schizophrenics.

The findings on ARISE indicate that the mothers can be differentiated not only on the basis of the patient's psychiatric status but also on the basis of the patient's sex. These findings are in accord with those of Alanen (1966), Lidz and associates (1965), and Sathyvathi (1974). Lidz and co-workers (1965) observed the mothers of male schizophrenics to be more disturbed than those of female schizophrenics.

In summary, the results of this study on the families of schizophrenic patients provide data that are in part consistent with contemporary psychodynamic theory and with previous findings. The finding that mothers of schizophrenics scored lower on ARISE is consistent with previous findings and with contemporary psychodynamic theory, which emphasizes the importance of the maternal role in the evolution and structuring of the neonate's ego. The fact that family members differed significantly on GEF, with the parents scoring the highest and the patients the lowest, is also consistent with previous findings, which suggest a positive relationship between the level of ego functioning and the status of psychiatric health. There are, however, some obvious inconsistencies between the findings of the present study and those of previous investigations. Whereas previous studies found the fathers of schizophrenics to be more disturbed in every respect than fathers of neurotics, the present study failed to provide evidence to confirm this generalization. The present study failed, as well, to provide evidence differentiating the schizophrenics and their siblings and mothers from the neurotic patients and their siblings and mothers, respectively, on GEF. This observation is inconsistent with previous findings and fails to support Lidz's theory, which postulates that family pathology is more severe in families of schizophrenics and is, as well, related to the patient's illness. The failure to differentiate the two families on GEF scores should, however, be cautiously interpreted, given the level of significance ($p < .07$).

ACKNOWLEDGMENTS

The authors wish to express their appreciation to David R. Offord, M.D., and to James G. Mullin, M.D., psychiatrists, formerly at the Royal Ottawa Hospital, Ottawa, Canada, for their collaboration in every phase of the project. Without their generous assistance this project would not have been possible.

Gratitude is expressed to Paul O'Grady, Ph.D., and to Maureen Slatterly-Durely, Ph.D., professors at the University of St. Paul, Ottawa, Canada, for their critical comments and suggestions of earlier versions of this paper.

REFERENCES

Alanen, Y. O. The mothers of schizophrenic patients, *Acta Psychiatrica Neurologia Scandinavica*, 1958, *33* (Supplement 124), 5–361.

Alanen, Y. O. The family in the pathogenesis of schizophrenia and neurotic disorders. *Acta Psychiatrica Neurologia Scandinavica*, 1966, *42*, Supplement 189), 654.

Bellak, L. The schizophrenic syndrome: A further elaboration of the unified theory of schizophrenia. In L. Bellak (Ed.), *Schizophrenia: A review of the syndrome*. New York: Logos Press, 1958.

Bellak, L., & Hurvich, M. A systematic study of ego functions. *Journal of Nervous and Mental Disease*, 1969, *148*(6), 569–585.

Bellak, L., Hurvich, M., & Gediman, M. K. *Ego functions in schizophrenics, neurotics, and normals*. New York: Wiley, 1973.

Blaker, R. M. Psychopathology and familial communication. In Michael Brenner (Ed.), *The structure of action*. Oxford: Basel Blackwell, 1980, pp. 211–263.

Blishen, B. R., & McRoberts, H. A. A revised socioeconomic index for occupations in Canada. *The Canadian Review of Sociology and Anthropology*, 1976, *13*, 71–79.

Finn, J. D. *Multivariance: Univariate and multivariate analysis of variance, covariance, and regression—A Fortran IV program*. New York: National Educational Resources, 1976, p. 134.

Fleck, S., Lidz, T., & Cornelison, A. Comparison of parent–child relationships of male and female schizophrenic patients. *Archives of General Psychiatry*, 1963, *8*, 1–7.

Guilford, J. P. *Fundamental statistics in psychology and education*. Toronto: McGraw-Hill, 1965, p. 605.

Hartmann, H. Comments on the psychoanalytic theory of the ego (1950). In Heinz Hartmann, (Ed.), *Essays on ego psychology: Selected problems in psychoanalytic theory*. New York: International Universities Press, 1964, pp. 113–141.

Hartmann, H. (Ed.) *Essays on ego psychology: Selected problems in psychoanalytic theory*. New York: International Universities Press, 1965.

Jacobson, E. *The self and the object world*. New York: International Universities Press, 1964, p. 225.

Kirk, R. E. *Experimental design: Procedures for the behavioral sciences.* Belmont, Calif.: Brooks/Cole, 1968.

Lee, A. R. Levels of imperviousness in the schizophrenic's family. *Psychiatry: Journal for the Study of Interpersonal Processes,* 1975, *38,* 124–131.

Lidz, T. *The origin and treatment of schizophrenic disorders.* New York: Basic Books, 1973.

Lidz, T., Cornelison, A., Fleck, S., & Terry, D. Intrafamilial environment of the schizophrenic patient: I. The fathers. *Psychiatry,* 1957a, *20,* 329–342.

Lidz, T., Cornelison, A., Fleck, S., & Terry, D. The intrafamilial environment of the schizophrenic patient: II. Marital schism and marital skew. *American Journal of Psychiatry,* 1957b, *114,* 241–248.

Lidz, T., Fleck, S., Alanen, Y. O., Cornelison, A. R. Schizophrenic patients and their siblings. *Psychiatry,* 1965, *26,* 1–18.

Mahler, M. S. Symbiosis and individuation: The psychological birth of the human infant. *The Psychanalytic Study of the Child,* 1974, *29,* 89–106.

Mahler, M. S., & Furer, M. *On human symbiosis and the vicissitudes of individuation.* New York: International Universities, 1968.

Mahler, M. S., Pine, F., & Bergman, A. *The psychological birth of the human infant.* New York: Basic Books, 1975.

McRoberts, H. A. *Social stratification in Canada: A preliminary analysis.* Unpublished doctoral dissertation, Ottawa, Ontario, Carleton University, 1975.

Meehl, P. E. Schizotaxia, schizotypy, schizophrenia. *American Psychologist,* 1962, *18,* 827–838.

Pollack, M., Woerner, M., Goldberg, P., Klein, D. F., & Oaks, G. Siblings of schizophrenic and non-schizophrenic psychiatric patients. *Archives of General Psychiatry,* 1969, *20,* 652–658.

Sathyvathi, K. Perception of parents by schizophrenics: A consideration of instrumentality-expressivity roles. *Psychiatry,* 1974, *37,* 261–266.

Spitz, R. *The first year of life: A psychoanalytic study of normal and deviant development of object relations.* New York: International Universities Press, 1965.

Spitzer, R. L., Endicott, J., & Robins, E. *Research diagnostic criteria.* New York: New York State Psychiatric Institute, Biometrics Research, 1975, pp. 1–34.

Stabeneau, J. R., & Pollin, W. Comparative life history differences of families of schizophrenics, delinquents, and normals. *American Journal of Psychiatry,* 1968, *124,* 1526–1534.

Summers, F., & Walsh, F. The nature of the symbiotic bond between mother and schizophrenic. *American Journal of Orthopsychiatry,* 1977, *47,* 484–494.

Tinsley, H. E. A., & Weiss, D. J. Interrater reliability and agreement of subjective judgements. *Journal of Counseling Psychology,* 1975, *22*(4), 358–376.

Wild, C., Singer, M., Rosman, B., Ricci, J., & Lidz, T. Measuring disordered styles of thinking: Using the object sorting test on parents of schizophrenic patients. *Archives of General Psychiatry,* 1965, *13,* 471–476.

Witkin, H. A., Dyk, R., Faterson, H., Goodenough, D., & Karp, S. *Psychological differentiation.* New York: Wiley, 1962, p. 418.

Wolman, B. B. Family dynamics and schizophrenia. *Journal of Health and Human Behavior,* 1965, *6,* 163–169.

CHAPTER TWENTY-NINE

Stimulus Barrier Functioning and Patterns of Arousal in Schizophrenics and Normal Controls

RICHARD L. RUBENS AND
LEAH BLUMBERG LAPIDUS

Stimulus barrier functioning (e.g., Gediman, 1971; Bellak et al., 1973) is a complex area of processes concerned with the regulation and modulation of the individual's relationship to arousal from internal as well as external origins of stimulation. Maladaptive arousal patterns have been inextricably linked with schizophrenic processes (e.g., Lapidus & Schmolling, 1975; Rubens & Lapidus, 1978).

STIMULUS BARRIER AND AROUSAL

In recent years, increased interest in the specific adaptive functions of the ego has led many clinicians and dynamically oriented theorists such as Beres

We are grateful to the American Psychological Association for permission to use this material, which was previously published as "Schizophrenia Patterns of Arousal and Stimulus Barrier Functioning," *Journal of Abnormal Psychology*, 1978, 87(2), 199–211. Copyright 1978 by the American Psychological Association.

(1956); Engel (1962); Gediman (1971); and Bellak, Hurvich, and Gediman (1973) to undertake examinations of the role of arousal in schizophrenia. In particular, the concept of stimulus barrier—long relegated to the laboratories of the psychophysiologists—has begun to be explored by psychodynamically oriented clinicians and researchers in relation to its implications in schizophrenic dysfunctions.

Gediman (1971) has traced the evolution of the concept of stimulus barrier from its genesis in the writings of Freud (1892/1961, 1920/1961, and 1940/1961) as a passive screen for filtering potentially dangerous stimuli through the work of Bellak (1963) and Wallerstein (1967), in which the stimulus barrier was viewed as an active mechanism functioning to provide the organism with an optional level of stimulation, not merely a reactive process to protect against a destructive excess of stimulation. This concept of stimulus barrier is incorporated into the work of Bellak et al. (1973), which quantifies the adaptiveness of an individual's functioning in this area.

The present study integrates two contrasting approaches that are designed to measure an individual's reactivity to his or her environment. The first involves a psychophysiological experiment designed to obtain information about the autonomic patterns of the participant's orienting responses to simple stimuli as reflected in the GSR pattern he or she exhibits. The second approach consists of a structured psychological interview designed to assess the adaptive and coping characteristics, as well as the level of sensory thresholds, that constitute an individual's stimulus barrier, when the stimulus barrier is viewed as an adaptive ego function. The GSR data and the ratings of stimulus barrier functioning were compared to examine the relationship between these two approaches. The study was also designed to explore the nature of the maladaptive arousal patterns in schizophrenic conditions. The existence of the overresponder–underresponder differentiation found by Gruzelier (1973) was retested, and its stability over time for individual schizophrenics was systematically examined. The present research was further designed to ascertain whether an individual schizophrenic remains in a single pattern or moves back and forth between the two patterns characteristic of schizophrenics in general.

In addition, an exploration was undertaken of the relationships between the overresponder–underresponder differentiation and the participant's anxiety, mood, and behavior as both subjectively reported and clinically observed.

METHOD

Subjects

The two experimental groups each consisted of 20 schizophrenic patients, selected at random by staff at the facilities involved. The outpatient group was composed of subjects drawn from the outpatient departments of a community mental health center in New Jersey. These patients had no more than 1 year of total accumulated psychiatric hospitalization (with a mean length of hospitalization of 4.1 months), they had never been hospitalized consecutively for more than 6 months, and they had not been hospitalized within the 3 months prior to the testing. The inpatient group was drawn from the chronic wards of a New Jersey state psychiatric hospital. These patients were currently institutionalized, with their present hospitalization beginning at least 4 years prior to testing. They had an average of 142.6 months of accumulated psychiatric hospitalization.

All of the subjects were adult males. All patients included in the experimental samples were independently diagnosed as schizophrenic by the senior staff clinicians. When a patient's records suggested that there was a question of organic brain impairment, chronic alcoholism, or drug addiction, he was excluded from the study. None of these schizophrenics had been lobotomized or had received electroconvulsive therapy or insulin coma treatments. Subdiagnoses were obtained from the patients' charts. Patients with schizoaffective disorders were not included in the samples. All patients included in the sample had no change in medication between the first and second testing sessions, and those patients receiving psychotropic medications other than antipsychotic medication, tricyclic antidepressants, or anti-Parkinsonian agents were excluded from this research.

The control group consisted of 20 normals with no psychiatric history. They were drawn from the professional and nonprofessional male employees of two New York religious institutions and included clergymen, teachers, administrators, guards, janitors, telephone operators, and so forth. They were selected after the experimental groups had been formed, and an attempt was made to match them to the experimental groups with respect to age.

Materials and Procedures

The participants were administered the following procedures in order in an initial session and follow-up repeat measurement 6 weeks later.

1. The subject was asked to fill out the Beck Depression Inventory, Short Form (Beck et al., 1961).
2. Electrodes were attached to the volar surface of the distal phalanges of the first and second fingers of the right hand. An adhesive insulating tape ring with a hole 1 cm in diameter was then applied to the area to expose only a standardized area for electrode contact.
3. The stimulus barrier assessment interview was then administered. This interview is Section 9 of the 12-part interview for the clinical assessment of ego functions developed by Bellak et al. (1973). Bellak operationally defined *stimulus barrier functioning* as a measure of ego strength in regulating and responding to internal and external stimulation. The stimulus barrier assessment is composed of 14 areas of

inquiry into the subject's sensory thresholds and adaptive and coping mechanisms for dealing with stimulation. In each area specific questions are provided, and the type and extent of probing or prompting for further information are delineated. The lower the score the less able the individual to tolerate and cope with stimulation.

4. Headphones were placed over the subject's ears and attached to an audio signal generator. The audio signal generator was designed and built by the Speech Research Laboratory of Teachers College, Columbia University.

5. Skin conductance was measured by a Lafayette Instrument Company GSR Amplifier (Model 7601 TP), operating in a DC mode. GSR characteristics were recorded directly on a Lafayette Instrument Company Polygraph (Model 7603-1A SP).

   After allowing the subject's skin conductance level to stabilize (in a period that ranged from 2 to 5 minutes), the habituation sequence was begun. It consisted of fifteen 1000-Hz, 1-second tones at an intensity of 75 dB SPL (American National Standards Institute, 1969). The tones were presented binaurally at preset intervals ranging between 24 and 60 seconds. The pattern and length of the intervals in the sequence were identical for each subject. The pattern was established prior to the beginning of the study, using computer-produced random numbers (within a predetermined range of 20–60 seconds).

6. The subject's hearing was screened using the audio signal generator. A single tone (1000 Hz, 1 second) at an intensity of 18 dB SPL (re: ANSI, 1969) was presented monaurally to each of the subject's ears, first right and then left. The subject was asked to indicate when he heard a tone. Any subject unable to detect the tone in both ears was excluded from the study.

7. The Structured Clinical Interview (SCI; Burdock & Hardesty, 1969) was administered to each participant. The SCI is a psychological research technique for the assessment of levels of psychopathology in 10 different dimensions of functioning listed by Burdock and Hardesty.

8. Finally, the Taylor Manifest Anxiety Scale (TMAS; 1953) was administered.

Full details of the procedures and demographic data are presented in Rubens and Lapidus (1978).

RESULTS

Overresponder–Underresponder GSR Patterns of Schizophrenics

A normal subject in reaction to a novel stimulus that is repeatedly presented will exhibit a series of orienting reactions followed by a process of habituation through which the response to the particular stimulus will be extinguished. It was predicted that schizophrenics would not exhibit this normal pattern of orienting responses and subsequent habituation but rather would exhibit either of two maladaptive GSR response patterns. One of these maladaptive patterns was termed the *overresponder mode* and was operationally defined as a pattern to which orienting responses were initially exhibited but in which habituation to criterion (viz., the absence of orienting responses to three consecutive stimuli) failed to occur within the 15 trials of the tone sequence. The second maladaptive response pattern was termed the *underresponder mode* and was operationally defined as a pattern in which either no orienting response was exhibited or only an isolated first-trial response occurred, without any further orienting activity.

The resulting GSR data are presented in Table 29.1. Because these data did not meet the criteria of normal distribution, Kruskal–Wallis nonparametric analyses of variance were employed. To control for the possibility of an inflation in the rate of Type I errors, an $\alpha + .01$ was utilized in the analysis of these data.

Response Frequency.   Of the 40 schizophrenics in the study, approximately half (18 during the first session and 19 during the second) manifested the overresponder pattern. The other group (22 during the first session and 21 during the second) were underresponders. Of the outpatients, approximately 75% of the underresponders exhibited an isolated Trial 1 response, whereas the remainder exhibited no orienting response at all. Less than half of the inpatient underresponders exhibited even an isolated Trial 1 response.

The comparison of the response frequencies of the overresponder, underresponder, and control groups indicated that the effect of response pattern was significant at the $p < .001$ level. The graphic representation of these data in Figure 29.1 supports the predicted division of schizophrenics into two GSR patterns, different both from each and from the normal pattern. A sharp contrast exists between the habituation pattern of the controls (all of whom initially exhibited three to eight orienting responses followed by habituation to criterion) and the patterns of the schizophrenics, all of whom exhibited either an overresponder pattern (with a range of response frequencies of 11–15) or an underresponder pattern (with response frequencies of either 0 or 1).

Skin Conductance Level.   In every case, the effect of response pattern on skin conductance level was found to be highly significant. Inspection of the data showed that this was in the direction of overresponders having higher skin conductance levels than controls and underresponders having lower levels.

Spontaneous Fluctuations.   There was a highly significant effect of response pattern on the number of spontaneous fluctuations, with the overre-

Table 29.1. Effects of Response Pattern on GSR Measures and Bellak Stimulus Barrier Ratings

Variable	Outpatients Over-responders M	SD	Outpatients Under-responders M	SD	Inpatients Over-responders M	SD	Inpatients Under-responders M	SD	Controls M	SD	Comparison of Outpatient Groups and Controls	Comparison of Inpatient Groups and Controls
	First Session											
	(n = 11)		(n = 9)		(n = 7)		(n = 13)		(n = 20)			
Frequency	13.64	1.36	.78	.44	14.14	1.22	.46	.52	3.80	1.06	$H(2) = 32.89$**	$H(2) = 32.60$**
Skin conductance level[a]	12.66	3.99	5.03	1.50	12.30	4.05	4.16	2.27	7.75	2.03	$H(2) = 21.18$**	$H(2) = 20.47$**
Spontaneous fluctuations	23.36	9.53	1.56	1.24	20.86	5.15	1.62	1.80	5.45	1.60	$H(2) = 31.96$**	$H(2) = 28.87$**
Amplitude[a]	.92	.72	—	—	.51	.21	—	—	.49	.20	$H(1) = 2.47$	$H(1) = .06$
Latency[b]	1.73	.44	—	—	2.09	.43	—	—	1.90	.39	$H(1) = 1.52$	$H(1) = .88$
Recovery time[b]	5.15	2.12	—	—	2.14	.73	—	—	5.12	2.19	$H(1) = .14$	$H(1) = 11.20$**
Bellak stimulus barrier rating	4.55	1.23	6.89	1.17	3.57	1.72	6.23	1.69	8.95	1.43	$F(2, 37) = 41.22$**	$F(2, 37) = 33.62$**
	Second Session											
	(n = 11)		(n = 9)		(n = 8)		(n = 12)		(n = 20)			
Frequency	14.36	1.03	.67	.50	13.50	1.31	.33	.49	4.15	1.50	$H(2) = 32.89$**	$H(2) = 32.78$**
Skin conductance level[a]	13.66	3.66	5.15	1.90	12.50	3.52	3.56	1.52	7.64	1.87	$H(2) = 24.28$**	$H(2) = 26.03$**
Spontaneous fluctuations	28.45	12.07	2.22	1.64	19.12	6.66	1.67	1.75	5.50	1.64	$H(2) = 30.33$**	$H(2) = 30.43$**
Amplitude[a]	1.05	.80	—	—	.46	.19	—	—	.47	.24	$H(1) = 6.55$*	$H(1) = .00$
Latency[b]	1.95	.81	—	—	2.05	.37	—	—	1.92	.42	$H(1) = .07$	$H(1) = .47$
Recovery time[b]	4.11	1.79	—	—	2.62	1.36	—	—	4.96	1.92	$H(1) = 1.24$	$H(1) = 7.82$*
Bellak stimulus barrier rating	4.36	1.12	6.78	.83	3.75	1.28	6.58	1.44	9.10	1.52	$F(2, 37) = 48.44$**	$F(2, 37) = 40.62$**

Note: * $p < .01.$, ** $p < .001.$ [a] in μmhos.   [b] in secs.

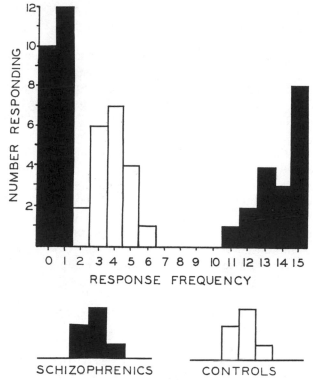

Figure 29.1. Distribution of response frequencies for schizophrenics and controls (first session).

sponder groups exhibiting a higher incidence of spontaneous fluctuations than the control group and the underresponder groups exhibiting a lower incidence.

Response Characteristics.   Response characteristics (viz., amplitude, latency, and recovery time) were compared only for the overresponder and control groups because the underresponders either did not exhibit any response at all or they exhibited only an isolated initial response. For the second session, as predicted, the outpatient overresponders had a significantly higher response amplitude than the controls. The corresponding comparison for the first session, although failing to reach a significant level of difference, approached significance in the predicted direction. The inpatients were not significantly different from the controls in either session. No significant differences were found between the latency times of overresponders and controls. Significantly faster recovery times were found in the inpatient overresponders than in the control group, but no significant difference was found between the outpatient overresponders and the controls.

Relationship Between the Overresponder–Underresponder Differentiation and Stimulus Barrier Ratings

In the analysis of variance performed on the Bellak stimulus barrier rating data, response pattern was found to be highly significant. Examination of these findings indicated differences in the predicted direction of lowest Bellak ratings (indicative of most pathological stimulus barrier functioning) for the overresponder schizophrenics, less pathological ratings for the underresponder schizophrenics, and highest ratings for the controls.

The Bellak stimulus barrier ratings were also highly correlated with the overresponder–underresponder differentiation. In the multiple regression analyses performed on the non-GSR variables, with the overresponder–underresponder dichotomy as the dependent variable, the Bellak scale was uniformly the best predictor of group membership (with simple correlations significant at the $p < .001$ level, $r = .62–.78$). Moreover, the Bellak score accounted for more than half of the total variance in every regression equation, except for the first session of the inpatient group. [Complete results of these analyses are presented in Rubens (1976).]

Relative Instability of the Overresponder–Underresponder Differentiation Over Time

Eight of the outpatient schizophrenics changed from one of the maladaptive arousal patterns in the first session to the other maladaptive pattern in the second: four of the first session overresponders exhibited underresponder patterns during the second session, and four of the first session underresponders became second session overresponders. Three of the inpatient schizophrenics shifted patterns, with two first session underresponders becoming overresponders during the second session and one first session overresponder becoming an underresponder. None of the controls exhibited anything other than a normal habituation pattern (viz., exhibiting three to eight orienting responses before habituating to criterion) during either of the two sessions.

As predicted, there was a significantly higher proportion of schizophrenics than normals who changed: outpatients, $z = 3.16$, $p < .001$, one-tailed; inpatients, $z = 1.80$, $p < 0.041$, one-tailed [computed by the test of difference between two proportions (Bruning & Kintz, 1968)].

Additional Relationships

As predicted, the existence of two dichotomous patterns of responsivity resulted in their division into two groups, overresponders and underresponders. The predicted existence of certain schizophrenics who changed from one schizophrenic GSR pattern to the other was also demonstrated. Thus, the samples were further subdivided into dichotomous groups by change status: (1) changers, who exhibited one schizophrenic GSR pattern during the first session and the other schizophrenic pattern at the time of the second session; and (2) nonchangers, who exhibited the same GSR pattern during both sessions.

In order to examine how these groups compared on the other measures obtained during this study, a two-way analysis of variance was computed for change status and response pattern. All the previously utilized variables were reanalyzed according to these divisions, with the exception of those demographic variables whose level of measurement did not permit such a procedure and the GSR variables concerned with response characteristics (for which such an analysis would have resulted in comparisons involving characteristics that were not present in underresponders). Employing the multivariate analysis of variance (MANOVA) program (Applebaum, 1974), the interaction effects were examined, and where they proved to be significant, an analysis of simple effects was performed. The effects of change status and response pattern were then examined, also using the MANOVA program. Full data and the results of these analyses are presented in Rubens and Lapidus (1978).

Interaction Effects.   Where the interaction between response pattern and change status was significant in the outpatient sample, the analysis of simple effects indicated the following:

1. For the skin conductance level, changers showed lower levels than nonchangers in the overresponder pattern, $F(1,36) = 19.80, p < .001$, whereas the difference was not significant in the underresponder pattern, $F(1,36) = 3.10$, ns (see Figure 29.2). It is of interest to note that the skin conductance levels associated with the response patterns of changers were less extreme than those of the nonchangers.
2. For the TMAS, changers had higher levels of anxiety than nonchangers in the underresponder phase, $F(1,36) = 11.72, p < .002$, but not in the overresponder phase, $F(1,36) = .09$, ns. The scores for changers of both patterns were approximately equal to the overresponder scores of nonchangers.
3. For the SCI Perceptual Dysfunction Scale, changers were rated more pathological on this measure than nonchangers in the overresponder pattern, $F(1,36) = 9.97, p < .003$, but not in the underresponder pattern, $F(1,36) = .13$, ns.
4. For the SCI Physical Complaints Scale, changers voiced more complaints than nonchangers in the overresponder pattern, $F(1,36) = 4.80, p < .033$, but not in the underresponder pattern, $F(1,36) = 1.17$, ns.

In the inpatient sample, a significant interaction effect was present only in the case of skin conductance level, similar to that found in the outpatient

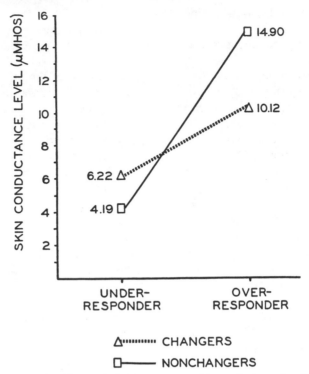

Figure 29.2. The simple effects of change status on skin conductance level for the two response patterns (outpatient sample).

sample: The levels associated with the response patterns of changers were less extreme than those of nonchangers.

The Effects of Response Pattern.   In the outpatient sample, the effect of response pattern was highly significant in the case of the Fear–Worry Scale of the SCI, with overresponders rated more pathological than underresponders. The effect of response pattern was not significant in the inpatient sample for the TMAS or any of the SCI scales.

In neither the inpatient nor the outpatient sample were any significant effects of response pattern found to hold for the Beck Depression Inventory, medication, length or number of psychiatric hospitalizations, or age. A separate analysis of demographic variables (viz., education, occupation, marital status, or subdiagnostic category of schizophrenia) by response pattern yielded no significant differences.

The Effects of Change Status.   In the outpatient sample, it was found that changers were rated as more pathological than nonchangers on the Anger–Hostility, Incongruous Ideation, and Self-depreciation scales of the SCI. On the SCI Incongruous Behavior Scale, nonchangers were rated more pathological than changers. Nonchangers also showed significantly greater accumulated psychiatric hospitalization time. The only significant effect of change status in the inpatient sample was that changers had more physical complaints (SCI Scale 8) than nonchangers.

In every instance, changers, while in their underresponding phase, exhibited isolated Trial 1 responses. Although there were nonchanger underresponders who also exhibited this particular phenomenon (six in all, equally distributed between the inpatient and outpatient samples), it was striking that each of the 11 changers invariably manifested this special subpattern of underresponsivity. [A fuller presentation of these exploratory relationships is given in Rubens (1976).]

DISCUSSION

The findings of the present study support those of Gruzelier (1973) in that all schizophrenics were found to exhibit one of two abnormal arousal patterns, overresponder and underresponder, each of which was distinct from the arousal patterns of the nonschizophrenic subjects.

It is important to note the similarities of these findings regardless of whether the phenomenon was examined in terms of psychophysiological arousal, as suggested by Gruzelier (1973), or in terms of adaptive ego function of stimulus barrier, following the work for Bellak et al. (1973). Although the nonschizophrenics were midway between the two schizophrenic groups in terms of the GSR measures and at the opposite extreme from them in terms of the Bellak ratings, these are congruent findings. The stimulus barrier rating is a unipolar scale of adaptivity that was found by Bellak et al. (1973) to be associated with other measures of ego efficiency or successful coping. Duffy (1962) and Schmolling and Lapidus (1972) found that such linear measures were related to curvilinear measures of psychophysiological arousal such that optimal performance occurs at the moderate level of arousal and relatively poor performance occurs at both extremes. It would thus appear that stimulus barrier is an area of ego functioning in which the psychophysiological mechanisms associated with a particular psychodynamic construct are identifiable.

The results of the present study indicate that the schizophrenic is particularly deficient in dealing with stimulation—whether it is internal or external in origin. The selective filtering of stimuli, which is employed by the individual to achieve an optimal level of stimulation, is absent in the schizophrenic. Stimuli either elicit an unusually intense level of reaction, to which the schizophrenic is unable to become acclimated, or are virtually excluded from awareness. Similarly, schizophrenics exhibit two extremes of spontaneous responsivity in the absence of external stimulation, exhibiting an extremely abnormal excess or paucity of spontaneous fluctuations. Schizophrenics thus exhibit unproductive baseline levels of arousal: They are either hyperaroused or hypoaroused, depending on their overall pattern.

Overresponders react to the normal range of environmental stimuli (and by extrapolation from the findings concerning spontaneous fluctuations, they similarly react to internal impulses) as though they were all potential danger signals. Overresponders are more sensitive, more reactive, and less able to integrate their experiences in such a way as to enable them adaptively to modulate their reactions. Clinically, they are in a state of high anxiety.

Underresponders, on the other hand, are in an unusually low state of baseline arousal. They have reduced their contact with the stimulus-laden world and have ceased to exhibit the type of responsivity that is essential for adaptive functioning. Even their responsivity to their internal stimuli has been diminished, as reflected by the virtual absence of spontaneous fluctuations.

As predicted, certain schizophrenics alternated between response patterns, although in no instance did any schizophrenic exhibit a normal habituation pattern. Even the changers, who swung from one extreme of responsivity to the other, were unable to achieve a normal balance at any time. Nevertheless, it appears that the very existence of alternation between response patterns may represent an attempt on the part of the schizophrenics to modulate their responsivity to stimulation.

The comparison of changers and nonchangers yielded several results that support the conclusion that a changing response pattern may represent an adaptive attempt to compensate for otherwise impaired stimulus barrier functioning. In both the outpatient and inpatient samples, changers exhibited skin conductance levels that were indicative of more nearly normal baseline levels of arousal. An intriguing finding was that changers, when in their underresponder phase, in every case exhibited isolated Trial 1 responses. This extremely fast habituation appears to represent a somewhat less complete withdrawal from the world of stimulation than does the total absence of any response, characteristic of most nonchanger underresponders. The outpatient changers had a significantly shorter length of accumulated psychiatric hospitalization, and their inpatient counterparts showed a trend in the same direction. Thus, it would seem that such schizophrenics have a better prognosis than nonchangers. This possibility is reinforced by the fact that there were significantly fewer changers found among the chronically institutionalized patients who comprised the inpatient sample than among the outpatient sample.

In general, changers appeared to be more affectively alive than nonchangers, having been rated more anxious (both objectively observed on the SCI Fear–Worry Scale and subjectively reported on the TMAS) and more pathological on the Anger–Hostility and Self-depreciation Scales of the SCI. Nevertheless, changers were less pathological with respect to incongruous behavior, suggesting that they may use more direct, adaptive means of expressing their conflicts. They are more directly reactive to their environment and exhibit a broader range of active and emotional responses. By alternating between the two extreme patterns of schizophrenic stimulus barrier functioning, they accomplish some degree of modulation that might otherwise not be open to them.

The results of the present study support the view that central to schizophrenic pathology is a severe deficit in the individual's ability to modulate his or her basic responsivity to stimulation, and that stimulus barrier dysfunction and maladaptive patterns of arousal are two modes of viewing this phenomenon. It is further suggested that alternation between response patterns exhibited by changers represents an attempt to compensate for this deficit and is at least a partially successful mode by which these schizophrenics establish a degree of modulated responsivity to stimulation.

CONCLUSION AND SUMMARY

In conclusion, the present study provides a psychophysiological construct validation of the adaptive ego function of psychological stimulus barrier. The striking relationship found between patterns of modulation of arousal as reflected in the psychophysiological skin conductance (GSR patterns) and in the distinct levels of psychological stimulus barrier functioning [as measured by the Bellak et al. (1973), Stimulus Barrier ratings], supports the construct that these two different approaches describe similar aspects of human function: the individual's most basic patterns of responsivity to both the external world and his or her own internal impulse life. The normally functioning individual is able to screen and modulate the amount and type of stimulation that is admitted into his or her consciousness. The schizophrenics show impaired stimulus barrier functioning and maladaptive psychophysiological arousal which is over or underresponsive. Overresponders were slow to habituate and exhibited a high number of orienting responses, a high baseline skin conductance level, and a high incidence of spontaneous fluctuations. Underresponders exhibited low baseline skin conductance levels, few spontaneous fluctuations, and either an absence of orienting activity or only an isolated initial orienting response. As predicted, certain schizophrenics alternated between these response patterns, but they never showed the normal pattern of arousal. The schizophrenics, of both an underarousal and overarousal pattern of GSR activation, whether their psychophysiological pattern was stable or changing, exhibited an abnormal level of stimulation and pathologically maladaptive levels of psychological stimulus barrier functioning.

REFERENCES

American National Standards Institute. *American national standard for audiometers* (ANSI S3.6). New York, 1969.

American Psychiatric Association. *Diagnostic and statistical manual of mental disorders* (2nd ed.). Washington, D.C., 1968.

Appelbaum, M. L. *The MANOVA manual: Complete factorial design.* Chapel Hill: The L. L. Thurston Psychometrics Laboratory, University of North Carolina, 1974.

Beck, A. T., Ward, C. H., Mendelson, M., Mack, J., & Erbaugh, J. An inventory for measuring depression. *Archives of General Psychiatry,* 1961, *4,* 561–571.

Bellak, L. Acting out: Conceptual and therapeutic considerations. *American Journal of Psychotherapy,* 1963, *17,* 375–389.

Bellak, L., Hurvich, M., & Gediman, H. K. *Ego functions in schizophrenics, neurotics, and normals.* New York: Wiley, 1973.

Beres, D. Ego deviation and the concept of schizophrenia. *The psychoanalytic study of the child* (Vol. 2). New York: International Universities Press, 1956.

Braning, J. L., & Kintz, B. L. *Computational handbook of statistics.* Glenview, Ill.: Scott, Foresman, 1968.

Burdock, E. I., & Hardesty, A. L. *Structured clinical interview manual.* New York: Springer, 1969.

Claridge, G. S. *Personality and arousal.* Oxford, England: Pergamon Press, 1967.

Des Lauriers, A. M., & Carlson, C. F. *Your child is asleep: Early infantile autism.* Homewood, Ill.: Dorsey Press, 1969.

Duffy, E. *Activation and behavior.* New York: Wiley, 1962.

Engel, G. L. *Psychological development in health and disease.* Philadelphia: Saunders, 1962.

Freud, S. Extracts from the Fliess papers. In J. Strachey (Ed.), *The standard edition of the complete psychological works of Sigmund Freud* (Vol. 1). London: Hogarth Press, 1961. (Originally published, 1892.)

Freud, S. Beyond the pleasure principle. In J. Strachey (Ed.), *The standard edition of the complete psychological works of Sigmund Freud* (Vol. 18). London: Hogarth Press, 1961. (Originally published, 1920.)

Freud, S. An outline of psycho-analysis. In J. Strachey (Ed.), *The standard edition of the complete psychological works of Sigmund Freud* (Vol. 23). London: Hogarth Press, 1961. (Originally published, 1940.)

Gediman, H. K. The concept of stimulus barrier: Its review and reformulation as an adaptive ego function. *International Journal of Psychoanalysis,* 1971, *52,* 243–256.

Gruzelier, J. H. Investigation of possible limbic dysfunction in schizophrenia by psychophysiological methods. Unpublished doctoral dissertation, University of London, 1973.

Gruzelier, J. H., & Venables, P. H. Skin conductance orienting activity in a heterogeneous sample of schizophrenics: Possible evidence of limbic dysfunction. *Journal of Nervous and Mental Disease,* 1972, *155,* 277–287.

Gruzelier, J. H., & Venables, P. H. Skin conductance response to tones with and without attentional significance in schizophrenic and nonschizophrenic psychiatric patients. *Neurophychologia,* 1973, *11,* 221–230.

Gruzelier, J. H., & Venables, P. H. Bimodality and lateral asymmetry of skin conductance orienting activity in schizophrenics: Replication and evidence of lateral asymmetry in patients with depression and disorders of personality. *Biological Psychiatry,* 1974, *8,* 594–604.

Lapidus, L. B., & Schmolling, P. Anxiety, arousal, and schizophrenia: A theoretical integration. *Psychological Bulletin,* 1975, *82,* 689–710.

Lykken, D. T., & Venables, P. H. Direct measurement of skin conductance: A proposal for standardization. *Psychophysiology,* 1972, *8,* 656–672.

Prien, R. *Pharmacotherapy in chronic schizophrenia.* Washington, D.C.: Department of Medicine and Surgery, Veterans Administration, 1973.

Rubens, R. L. *Arousal patterns and stimulus barrier functioning and schizophrenia* (doctoral dissertation, Columbia University, 1976). *Dissertation Abstracts International,* 1976, *37,* 3626B. (University Microfilms No. 76-29, 857.)

Rubens, R. L., & Lapidus, L. B. Schizophrenic patterns of arousal and stimulus barrier functioning. *Journal of Abnormal Psychology,* 1978, *87,* 199–211.

Schildkraut, J. J., & Klein, D. F. The classification and treatment of depressive disorders. In R. I. Shader (Ed.), *Manual of psychiatric therapeutics.* Boston: Little, Brown, 1975.

Schmolling, P., & Lapidus, L. B. Arousal and task complexity in schizophrenic performance deficit: A theoretical discussion. *Psychological Reports,* 1972, *30,* 315–326.

Shader, R. I., & Jackson, A. H. Approaches to schizophrenia. In R. I. Shader (Ed.), *Manual of psychiatric therapeutics.* Boston: Little, Brown, 1975.

Taylor, J. A. A personality scale of manifest anxiety. *Journal of Abnormal and Social Psychology.* 1953, *48,* 285–290.

Venables, P. H., & Martin, I. Skin resistance and skin potential. In P. H. Venables and I. Martin (Eds.), *Manual of psychophysiological methods.* Amsterdam: North-Holland, 1967.

Wallerstein, R. S. Development and metapsychology of the defense organization of the ego. Panel report, American Psychoanalytic Association Meeting. *Journal of the American Psychoanalytic Association,* 1967, *15,* 551–583.

— CHAPTER THIRTY ————————————

Ego Function and Coping Response: A Framework for the Study of Adaptation to Life Transitions

SAMUEL OSHERSON

INTRODUCTION

This paper presents a framework for studying ego functioning and coping response in key life transitions during the adult life cycle. The framework has evolved from a series of studies we have been conducting as part of the Adult Development Project. The project has been examining how career and family pressures combine at different points in the life cycle to produce discrete life transitions. From this point of view career changes within or between discrete careers become marker events denoting deeper developmental dynamics at play. We focus in particular on young adulthood and midlife, examining the kinds of career transitions that take place at these two distinct stages of the adult life cycle. Our preliminary findings indicate that career and life-stage dynamics can combine to produce identifiable, expectable life transitions that can be understood in terms of a model of loss and grief. As such, adaptive response to career development and life transitions involves a number of psychosocial dimensions to which Bellak's model of Ego Function Assessment is a useful guide. The first two sections of this paper develop the relation between career and life-stage dynamics and the manner in which key life transitions approximate experiences of loss. The last section shows how we can study adaptive function in such experiences by integrating coping response theory with Bellak's empirical model of Ego Function Assessment.

PROBLEM STATEMENT

For reasons I will discuss below occupational changes encompass both shifts from one occupation to another as well as horizontal or vertical movements over time within a continuous career. Much of the vocational-educational literature in this area represents studies with a narrow contextual focus where attention is paid primarily to the role of vocational skills and job requirements. Although such approaches are valuable, we also see the need for studies with a broader contextual focus, and, specifically, one that both explores the demands and challenges that job or occupational changes make on the life situation of the individual and specifies the dimensions of adaptive response to such challenges.

It will be proposed that job changes within a specific career, or occupational changes from one career to another, involve significant life changes and stresses that demand a number of psychological skills and social resources for successful adaptation at work. I believe my own research, and that of others, indicates that occupational transfers contain the stress and challenges of transition and loss.

I plan to introduce into the analysis of occupational transfers information on the stage of life during which the transfer occurs, the particular type of transfer that takes place, how problems of work and career have been dealt with earlier in the individual's life, and the psychological and social resources facilitating occupational transfers. Through this I hope to enlarge and deepen the *contextual analyses* of adaptation to occupational transfers and work changes.

I propose to explore the problem in two ways: (1) by understanding the relation of adolescent career awareness and preparation to the pattern of subsequent career development at midlife and (2) by delineating the specific skills and abilities involved in successful and less successful adaptations to different kinds of occupational transitions at midlife, taken as a specific point in life development. To do this I will develop a model of the nature of occupational transfers, based on my work to date in this area. This model will specify the tasks and challenges in an occupational transfer as a *transitional event* in the life of the individual, and the kinds of educable affective, cognitive, and behavioral skills and social resources that result in successful adaptation and transfer of performance across vocational situations.

In our attention to adolescence I am concerned with the question of whether different patterns of self-awareness and career preparation prior to the career or work choice better prepare the individual for occupational transitions and changes at later points in his or her development. In other words, do adolescent educational experiences develop an individual's capacity to adapt and transfer at later stages of the career and life cycle?

I further focus on the process of occupational transition at a point emerging from recent research as crucial for individual development: midlife. In studying different career transitions at the same point in development I hope to be able to observe the manner in which occupational transfers affect, and are themselves affected by, concurrent life-stage demands and challenges. That is, are particular kinds of occupational transfers more difficult at midlife?

There are a number of different types of occupational transfer that could be studied at midlife: job changes, career changes, and so on. I have decided to focus on variations in career trajectories at midlife—that is, transitions in stages of career movement from one stage of a career to another—as our case of occupational transfer. I have chosen this focus because our model of transfer seems generalizable to other types of occupational transition as well, and because our cohort (see below) is ideally suited to the study of this specific type of occupational transfer.

During the years 1960 to 1964 the Harvard Student Study collected a broad range of detailed information on the attitudes, abilities, work adjustment, and career plans of a large sample of the class of 1964. These individuals have subsequently displayed a wide range of career trajectories in their work lives. By 1978 our samples were all approximately 35 years of age and were just entering a new developmental stage—that of midlife. During this time as well the subjects were transiting through various stages of their work careers. We thus had a cohort experiencing different types of occupational transfers during the same life stage, for which we had rich data already collected on their career preparedness at an earlier life stage. What seemed indicated was a detailed, finely focused study of these transitions in career trajectories, observing psychological and social processes of adaptation as they were occurring, and attempting to postdict successful and more inferior patterns of transfer at midlife from the adolescent data already collected (Osherson & Dill, 1983).

In a second project the investigator collected intensive interview data from a group of individuals who carried out a voluntary midlife career change from successful professional positions (e.g. law, medicine, business, science) into the creative and performing arts (two target groups: visual artists and actors). This "career-change" study has been discussed in a continuing series of reports (Osherson, 1980).

Twenty subjects who had successfully carried out such changes were interviewed at a period 3–10 years after the change. All subjects were between the ages of 35 and 50. Each subject was seen 5 times (each session lasting 1½ hours) within a 2-week period. All sessions were tape-recorded and later transcribed for analysis. Some important findings that emerged from this research were: (1) a clear link between adolescent career preparation and self-awareness and the transition into later stages of career development at midlife, (2) a picture of the kinds of stresses and challenges involved in both occupational changes and in midlife as a distinct developmental stage and (3) different patterns of adaptation during the career change itself.

I will at times draw on short sections of interview material from both projects to give some flavor of the richness and texture of this life history data. (The specifics of the interview methodology will be discussed in the last section of the paper.)

I. WHAT IS THE ROLE OF WORK IN THE RESOLUTION OF PARTICULAR LIFE-STAGE TASKS AND CHALLENGES?

Considerable research has appeared over the last decade indicating the general outlines of distinct stages to adult development, with stage-specific stresses and challenges. Levinson (1978) has presented perhaps the most clearly age-linked stage perceptions on adult development, presenting the adult years as a series of four stages with intervening transitional periods. Vaillant (1978) has recently presented a model of adulthood describing development in terms of the maturation of coping and defensive processes and emphasizing the role of separation issues throughout adult development, particularly the midlife years.

A key question involves how to link emerging knowledge about adulthood with that of career development and change. One way to understand the reciprocal relationship between career and life history is to reconstruct the links between events at work and these stage-specific stresses. For example, the career change research mentioned generated a frame of analysis focusing on career experiences and decision-making in the (1) adolescent–young adulthood period and (2) the midlife years. Our findings suggest that career choices in adolescence were clearly intertwined with problems of separation from parents and that the career change at midlife emerged from recurrent difficulties at home as well as at work. In sum, career-stage and life-stage issues seemed quite intertwined.

The analysis of adolescence–young adulthood in our group of career changers indicated clear problems around two key tasks at this point in the life cycle: separation from family of origin and the autonomous definition of self. Career choices represented attempts to "affirm" or "implement" a sense of self organized around idealized, grandiose parental models that were relatively undifferentiated from family of origin. This was reflected in difficulty with both the self-testing and role exploration of college and the career choices made early in young adulthood. There was a sense of external pressure from parents, teachers, or relatives and either a tone of inner uncertainty at the time with evidence of real exploration and information seeking *or* the rigid, somewhat brittle certainty that is characteristic of foreclosed identity resolutions. Work seemed to play an essential role for these men in resolving the very crisis of self-definition of late adolescence and in providing a means of "getting into the adult world." It is noted in the literature that career choices are often an important vehicle at this time for self-definition and identity achievement (Erikson, 1959; Goethals & Klos, 1976).

What we found in our sample of career changers is that their professional, socially sanctioned career choices in young adulthood contained at their core powerful expectations and assumptions as to *who they would be* in the profession or career. Goldsmith (1972) has used the phrase "identity appropriation"—as opposed to career choice through "identity approximation"—to describe this use of work to resolve problems around self-definition in adolescence. In the subjects' description of their initial career choices we often found indications of some confusion between idealized role attributes of a career and self-definition: "Science seemed like an ideal life," "the university seemed like a glorious world . . . the only place to exist in American society," "I wanted to redeem myself by becoming a teacher." These comments implied powerful expectations surrounding the initial career choices: Science—a career—is equated with one's life, a university with a world, teaching with redemption of the person.

The powerful fantasies associated with the career choice can be seen in the following memory, from a professor of history who left his position at midlife to pursue a career in pottery:

> I had so many expectations in graduate school. Part of that whole trip through the university was the need to justify my existence by being a hero of some sort. It was really spectacular. It was a terrific burden from my birth. To be recognized as someone special.

> I was very bitter (about experiences in the University). All that work hadn't given me what I wanted. (What was that?) I'm not sure. Success, the hero's welcome, trumpet's playing, for everyone to clap or something. Finally, getting my father's love.

To summarize, we find that work and family choices in young adulthood are heavily tied to conflict around "who one is" and in defining oneself separately from parents, tasks, and challenges characteristic of this point in the life cycle. At the same time, work and career choices were a means of remaining tied to idealized parents and of exiling or suppressing narcissistically devalued or anxiety-producing aspects of self.

At midlife, these problems around self-definition reappeared under the press of a variety of stage-specific challenges. The characteristic demands and challenges of the midlife years served to erode or call into question the self-definition expressed by work and marital choices effected in young adulthood. These demands typically included those of parenting, marriage, career socialization into new roles and responsibilities, death of parents, and altered time perspectives under the acknowledgement of personal "aging" (Neugarten, 1968). The work of Gould (1972, 1978), Vaillant (1979), and Levinson et al. (1975, 1978) indicate that the age range 35–50 is a time of potential stress related to a general questioning or "reevaluation" of the direction of one's life, resulting in either an adaptive recommitment to work or conflict and blockage in this area (Rapaport, 1970; Soddy, 1966).

For the men in the career change research these midlife-specific experiences were discrepant to, or at variance with, the sense of self organized around the marriage and career choices of young adulthood. The impact of these stage-specific challenges was to reopen those very questions only partially resolved in adolescence and young adulthood. The career changes in the sample came about after a considerable period of turmoil and difficulty and represented attempts to affirm or implement new identity patterns in response to the experience of self at midlife. Some subjects were able to define themselves in a more complete and gratifying manner, whereas others seemed to have replicated the foreclosed resolution of young adulthood. Further, we observed the impact of other life factors on career development at midlife. In particular, marriage and family were the source of a number of experiences that challenged the wished-for self embedded in the initial career choice. An example of the reverberation on self-definition between events at work and home comes from a research scientist, who I shall label "Mr. Markowitz."

Mr. Markowitz is a 50-year-old actor in New York who, 5 years ago, left his position as a microbiologist for the federal government in Colorado. His decision after college to pursue a career in science and to marry was related to his perception of himself as a rigidly responsible, controlled individual without antisocial motives, impulses, or "dangerous anger." And yet discrepant experiences began to accumulate during the midlife years that invalidated this very experience of himself. There was, first, a confrontation with the "real" nature of science; he found himself in a world where impulses, lying, cheating, and corruption did indeed exist. Although his descriptions of those years in science are marked by a sense of participating in an enterprise with dispassionate men in the midst of reassuring structure and control, as he progressed in his career a more differentiated view of the scientist's life appeared. This included bitter conflicts with colleagues, assistants who falsified data, and a sense of the not necessarily socially beneficial end products of science. Furthermore, he confronted the realization that not only science, but he himself, struggled with unruly human emotions. In his work not only were other scientists coming to be seen as "corruptible" and impulse-ridden, but he himself struggled with these difficulties. He, as well as others, participated in bitter laboratory struggles, and he found himself working on the manufacture of gas masks—a far cry from the fantasy of eliminating disease. It was in the areas of close interpersonal relationships, that Mr. M's self-definition received perhaps its most severe upheaval. He felt bitter anger and disappointment at his wife and children, as suggested in the following comments:

> Our oldest daughter left the house when she was sixteen or seventeen, we think. And the speech she made was, "I'm glad to be leaving this fucking house. The only regret I have [is that] I'm leaving these poor helpless children in your care." And as each one left they would repeat the same speech. . . . A man would have to be made of stone not to think "what the hell is going on?"

> Last summer [one son] wrote me a very disturbing letter in which he told me that he had very bad memories of his childhood. His memories were of like walking on egg shells when he was around me. I wasn't consistent, he never knew when I might fly off the handle and explode in rage. And he was finding things out about himself now, and he felt impelled to tell me this. So I wrote back, recalling my own memories which were just the opposite. Of course I lost my temper sometimes. But it wasn't an accurate impression of his childhood with me. I felt that if it were accurate I would have been behaving in a terrible way. That is, I'm not that kind of person. I don't think that's my picture of myself.

Note the sense of discrepancy and discontinuity in the representation of self, for example, "I don't think that's my picture of myself." In this case such discrepancies in experiences at work and at home called into question Mr. Markowitz's organizing definition of himself as a scientist and father who had banished impulse and affect and who was utterly respectable, intellectual, and dispassionate.

The initial question about the interrelation of career and life stages can now perhaps be seen as containing a number of more finely focused questions that emerge from the career change study and that are being pursued in current research:

1. Are there variant patterns of career choice in adolescence in which (a) work choices are embedded in problems around self-definition and separation from family of origin or (b) that emerge from a fuller resolution of the crisis of separation and autonomous self-definition at this time? Thus, the question raised is the degree to which work itself is embedded in developmental conflict. We are in fact currently examining different patterns of identity resolutions and self-exploration in adolescence (Marcia, 1967; Orlofsky et al., 1973).

2. We can ask a similar question for midlife, namely, what is the reciprocal impact of the stresses and challenges of this life stage and the work change that may occur at this time? One way to approach this is to examine the relationship between midlife and the quality of adaptation to different kinds of occupational changes that may occur at the time. Yet to do so we need a theory of career development not linked tightly to chronological age. In our current research we have developed such a model, integrating the work of Schein (1975), Levinson (1978), and Super (1976). This model de-

scribes the growth of a career in terms of a Preparatory, Establishment, and Continuation phases. For some men in our sample we observed career transition at early midlife into an Establishing stage, for others, out of it. Super (1957, 1976) describes the stages of a career in terms of Growth, Exploration, Establishment, Maintenance, and Decline. We have restricted the term Exploratory to refer to the initial (usually adolescent or college) experience of information gathering, self-testing, and role taking surrounding the career choice, and limit the Establishment stage to the posttraining or postapprenticeship period of greater autonomy and responsibility at the work place. In between we have identified a Preparatory or Apprenticeship stage in any work career, wherein the individual learns the required skills and abilities of work and how to take the worker role. Each of these career stages encompasses its own stage-specific demands and stresses. In the Preparatory stage for example, one is learning the role, apprenticing, and assessing responsibility for peripheral or secondary duties (e.g., salesman training program, law school). In the Establishment stage of a career the individual assumes more primary duties, often with greater autonomy and less direct supervision (one becomes a partner in a law firm, receives a promotion to account executive in an advertising agency, is put into a managerial position in business). In the Maintenance stage of a career duties and responsibilities again shift, the individual this time receiving a more advanced executive position, or becoming a supervisor or mentor to others, or as Super (1976) says, becoming suddenly preoccupied with "holding one's own against younger people, keeping up with new developments, forging ahead by breaking new ground 'and so on' " (1976, p. 23).

From this conceptualization of the course of a career, we can develop a typology of midlife career trajectories, in which particular occupational transfers (career stage transitions) are influenced by the distinct stresses and tasks of midlife. First, note that Super assigns age links to each of these stages: Exploratory, beginning in adolescence, Establishment in the midtwenties, and the Maintenance stage at about 45. However, if we look at the functions and demands of each stage we see that in different careers the precise time of particular stages may vary. Thus, for careers with extended training and preparation for practice (e.g., medicine and some of the very specialized sciences) the Establishment stage actually will not begin until the early thirties, when training and apprenticeship (e.g., residency) is finally completed. By age 35 (the beginning of midlife) these individuals would just be transiting from the Preparatory to Maintenance stage. On the other hand, some work careers have a relatively short Preparatory stage, with immediate entry after college (e.g., clerical and sales, business or managerial positions not requiring advanced degrees), and by age 35 the individual would have already transited into the Maintenance stage of his or her career. Finally, there are intermediate choices, such as the professions where some postgraduate training is required and the Preparatory periods extends into the late twenties. Examples of such careers are law, academics, and advanced

Type of Career

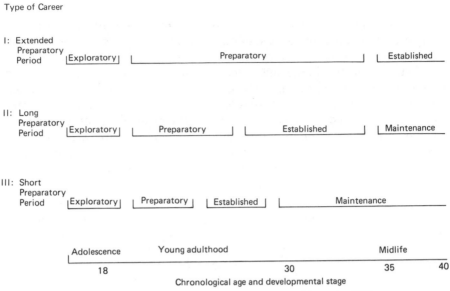

Figure 30.1.   Three different career-stage transitions at midlife.

executive/managerial positions, where LLBs, Ph.D.s, and MBAs are required. At 35 these individuals would be transiting from the Established to Maintenance Stage of their careers. Figure 30.1 summarizes these three different types of midlife career-stage transitions in our typology.

Separating career stages from chronological age, per se, opens up some important questions needing further research: How are adaptations to these different kinds of occupational changes effected by the specific life-stage issues and conflicts of midlife? What is the effect of transiting from the Preparatory into the Establishment stage during midlife as opposed to the transition out of the Establishment stage? How do the demands of parenting and the relationship with one's wife at midlife impact on these different types of transitions? Do the changes in personal time perspective generally identified with midlife suggest that a particular type of transition is more easily carried out? These are the questions to which our current work is addressed.

3. Finally, is there a relationship between the manner in which the problem of work and career have been dealt with earlier in the individual's life and the subsequent adaptation to work changes? Our focus is on the relationship of adolescent career preparation to the adaptation to occupational changes occurring during midlife. Also of interest here is whether work, when tied to developmental conflict in young adulthood, can alternatively achieve some relative independence from such conflict at midlife.

Theoretical perspectives on the career consequences of adolescent career decision-making and identity resolution are voluminous in the vocational literature. Most major vocational theorists, such as Ginzburg (1951), Roe (1956), Super (1957), Tiedemann and O'Hara (1963), and Holland (1966) imply—each from their own perspective—that the personality gains of late adolescence (usually conceived in terms of a self-concept or "identity" notion) and the degree of career preparedness (e.g., self-testing, vocational exploration, and the quality of career decision-making) play an important role in the pattern of subsequent career development. However, empirical support for this assumption is sparse. Our understanding of the relation of adolescent career preparedness to later career developments is hampered in general by a lack of carefully focused, longitudinal studies of adult career transitions through different points of the life cycle (McKinley, 1976). It is to this lack that the current study is addressed as the longitudinal nature of the current sample will allow for the testing of relationships between adolescent career choice and career development at midlife.

II. WHAT IS THE LIFE-SITUATIONAL IMPACT OF OCCUPATIONAL CHANGES? OCCUPATIONAL TRANSITIONS AS STRESSFUL EVENTS

Careers can be understood as a series of breaks and discontinuities in life structure. Although career trajectories have continuity to the external observer or to the individual retrospectively, to the person experiencing a career, work can often be a series of anticipated and unanticipated breaks, discontinuities, and irregularities. A major finding from career-change research demonstrates the closeness to experiences of loss and change of the complex challenges of career-stage shifts and distinctive developmental tasks of the midlife years. This was so because as stated the transitions involved in career development also involved fundamental alterations in how these subjects tended to define and understand themselves. There are a number of sources of such "discontinuity" in self-definition concomitant to occupational transfer (within or between jobs and careers): shifts in expectations for oneself from others; new job responsibilities and demands, changing patterns of friendship resulting from the job changes; altered time schedules; some fundamental alterations in personal habits and routines.

How are the challenges of loss involved in these changes? First, we note that the pattern of our subjects' midlife career development was marked by reports of intense and painful self-questioning, doubt, and depression, often with a sense of being "out-of-control." This period of "midlife crisis" was reported to extend over several years, beginning around age 35. To account for this interview data, we needed to refer to the recent empirical and theoretical work on loss and change as they relate to life-stage transitions as stressful events.

Both changes in jobs and occupation (from one stage of a career to another or from one career or job to another) and movement from one life stage to another (e.g., from young adulthood to midlife) contain the challenge of loss and transition, as fundamental ways of defining and understanding oneself are altered and must be reconstituted. For this reason, any occupational transfer, whether positive (e.g., promotions, raise in pay) or negative (e.g., unemployment), voluntary or involuntary, is generally considered as a stressful life event (Holmes & Masuda, 1974).

Recent work on loss has extended our concept of loss from that of separation from concrete attachments (e.g., death of a loved one) to situations that involve, fundamentally, the (actual or anticipated) invalidation of central interpretations of and assumptions about the world in which the individual lives (Carr, 1975; Marris, 1974; Weinstein & Platt, 1975). Thus, a variety of studies have found evidence of grief reactions among individuals in different situations of sharp transition and change (Marris, 1975; Fried, 1963). This developing perspective sees the fundamental substrate of all losses as that of a disruption in the individual's context of psychic stability by experiences fundamentally discrepant with trusted understandings of self-in-the-world. Within this context, urban relocation, immigration—and possibly unemployment, career development, or career change—all partake of losses because the continuity of expectation and assumption about oneself-in-the-world is dramatically altered. The experience of loss arises out of a confrontation with experiences sharply discrepant with one's understanding of the world, with a resulting "crisis of discontinuity" between the sense of "who one was" and "who one will be." From this perspective "loss" is of oneself, not of others, as the particular understanding of self that is organized around the lost attachments and commitments (e.g., to a marriage partner or career)— the fundamental markers of "who we are"—is threatened and must be reconstituted.

The career-change subjects' accounts of the year preceding the career change often contained a sense of gaps in their understanding of the world, with an uncertain searching for new explanations, as evidenced in the following excerpts.

> I had a profound philosophic crisis, maybe when I was 35 or 40. I realized that . . . the key I had been using was a key that didn't unlock anything really.

> Then began a whole period of trying to compartmentalize my life and keep things going, to be a teacher, an artist, a lover, a husband, and father, and they were all kind of separate worlds. . . . But when all the truths were out—and it did come out—I was faced with trying to bring it all together—or simplify it by throwing some of them out. . . . I got scared because I was really out-of-control.

Tiedemann (1965) has written of the "discontinuity" in the life of the individual resulting from transitions in employment, a problem that can be met with purposeful action or apathy or withdrawal. The "adaptive career task" (Kroll et al., 1970), involving the maintenance of a work relationship satisfying to the individual (given his or her needs and the demands of the environment) is thus a challenge to the psychological resources of the individual.

III. WHAT ARE THE DIMENSIONS OF ADAPTIVE PSYCHOSOCIAL RESPONSE TO BREAKS IN OCCUPATIONAL CONTINUITY THROUGH THE LIFE COURSE?

Coping response theory (Hamburg, 1974) offers some conceptual and empirical tools for understanding adaptive response to occupational transitions. I will initially present a model of adaptive response based on findings from the career-change project, and then integrate this model with recent work on coping and adaptation, and finally consider some social variables relevant to the process of adaptation.

If we take seriously this view of occupational shifts—career changes or movement from one stage of a career to another—as stressful life events, then we need to have a broader view of how individuals cope with and adapt to such experiences. Work changes can thus be conceived of as a transitional event in the life of the individual, in at least two ways: (1) separation from the work, and (2) separation from the expectations and assumptions that served to define "who I am" within the initial career.

Successful adaptive responses to occupational transfers involve the reconstitution of a reassuring sense of self through the period of "discontinuity" at work. In the career-change study a theoretical model of adaptation to transition was developed, with specific empirical dimensions delineated for the study of such adaptation. There is a form by which the process of adaptive responses proceeds, oscillating, over the course of months or years, between the desire to rigidly hold onto the past and letting go and rushing into the future—a process not dissimilar to that of mourning. Reconstitution can be seen as a process of moving between these poles in a series of attempts at gathering new information about self-in-the-world, "trying on" new roles and "testing possibilities" (Marris, 1975). When the process is not short-circuited, what can emerge is a restoration of the continuity of experience by reconstituting the sense of self independently of the past; one integrates who one was then with who one is now and will be in the future. However, when adaptive responses are unsuccessful, it usually reflects one pole of this ambivalent oscillation; either rigidly holding onto or abruptly letting go of the past (Osherson, 1980). We have indications that such unsuccessful reconstitutions can be marked both by difficulties at work and symptoms of personal disorganization (incipient alcoholism, depression, etc.).

In the current study we found three empirical dimensions of adaptive coping that could encompass and depict how well subjects coped with their work "crisis of discontinuity" and transition—namely, the affective, cognitive, and behavioral. Subjects who responded to the career-stage transitions of midlife with high anxiety and defensiveness (affective) also displayed patterns of poor decision making (cognitive) and relatively little information seeking or career exploration (behavioral). These subjects were characterized by poor adaptation to transitions, marked by work difficulty and personal disorganization. Subjects with good adaptation (little evidence of work difficulty or personal disorganization) showed less rigid defenses and lower anxiety, with greater reality testing and higher quality decision making, and greater amounts of information seeking and career exploration. Further, the same event—a career change—had a very different meaning for the person's subsequent development as a function of how adaptively or maladaptively the crisis was managed.

An adaptive response to occupational transitions can be further understood in terms of both psychological and social variables. In terms of individual responses to stress and change two convergent psychological theories can be of considerable help to vocational counselors and theorists: coping response theory (Hamburg & Adams, 1967) and recent work on ego functioning (Bellak et al., 1973). In terms of social variables, a key dimension was the social support system available to the individual (Cobb, 1978).

The theory of coping response and coping strategy emphasizes the individual's management of internal and external resources to deal with situations of challenge and stress. From effective use of coping strategies come active mastery and resolution of the problem situation. The variety of theoretical and empirical work in this area is united in viewing effective resource management as involving three tasks (Hamburg et al., 1974; White, 1974; Osherson, 1980):

1. Affective: the management of affect and anxiety. There are several dimensions to this task—preventing tension and emotional responses from interfering with an adequate assessment of the situation while remaining attentive to internal affective resources.

2. Cognitive: securing and utilizing adequate information about the environment (problem solving).

3. Behavioral: the capacity for autonomous action (e.g., presence of effective patterns of seeking and using help).

Effective response to a stressful situation depends on the ego's ability to defend against internal disruption, to interact with the environment to gain problem-solving information, and to take effective action. This approach to human behavior allows us to understand the major problems and crises faced by individuals at "nodal points and major transitions of the life cycle" (Hamburg et al., 1974, p. 437).

Although the general aspects of coping response have been well presented (Hamburg et al., 1974; White, 1974), systematic consideration of the specific coping functions underlying the affective, cognitive, and behavioral tasks involved has not—to my knowledge—yet appeared. However, some recent theoretical and empirical advances make further specification possible. We have seen that the theory of coping response has derived in large part from the work of the ego psychologists. And in the strategic management of internal and external resources coming to terms with reality within the context of the greatest possible need satisfaction, coping responses are a task of the ego, par excellence. The model of ego functioning developed by Bellak, Hurwich, and Gediman (1973) describes the range of cognitive, affective, and behavioral capacities available to the individual. Their model provides a way to elaborate and systematize the general model of coping response. Table 30.1 groups the 12 dimensions of ego functioning proposed by Bellak et al. according to the three dimensions of coping response to crises.

The three general dimensions given in Table 30.1 with their 12 component functions seem to allow for a systematic analysis of the dimensions of coping response to a "work crisis" with a strong theoretical lineage and research base. Thus, in relation to the affective dimension, White (1974) has pointed to the critical role of defense mechanisms (Function 1) in coping. It is likely that specific ego mechanisms serve defensive (maladaptive) or coping functions (Haan, 1963, 1969) in the process of occupational transfer. In relation to regulation and control of drives (Function 2) Zetzel (1949, 1963) has written of the importance of the capacity to tolerate anxiety and depression as a prerequisite to constructive growth and adaptation. Hamburg (1974) has noted similar processes in the coping reactions of patients with severe or prolonged injury or illness.

Cognitively, we have delineated five ego functions that give a broad view of the capacity of the individual to obtain, process, and utilize information in

Table 30.1. Ego Functions Grouped Along Three Dimensions of Coping Response

A. *Management of Affect and Anxiety:*
1. Defensive functioning
2. Regulation and control of drives, affects, and impulses
B. *Possession and Utilization of Cognitive Problem-solving Skills*
3. Reality testing
4. Thought processes
5. Judgment
6. Adaptive regression in the service of the ego
7. Synthetic–integrative functioning
C. *Capacity for Autonomous Action*
8. Object relations
9. Stimulus barrier
10. Autonomous functioning
11. Sense of reality of world and of self
12. Mastery–competence

Gould, R. The phases of adult life. *American Journal of Psychiatry*, 1972, *129*(5), 521–531.

Gould, R. *Transformations*. New York: Simon & Schuster, 1978.

Haan, N. Proposed model of ego functioning: Coping and defense mechanisms in relationship to I.Q. change. *Psychological Monographs*, 1963, *77*(8), 1–23.

Haan, N. An investigation of the relationship of Rorschach scores, patterns, and behavior to coping and defense mechanisms. *Journal of Projective Techniques*, 1969, *28*, 429–441.

Hamburg, D. Coping behavior in life-threatening circumstances. *Psychotherapy and Psychosomatics*, 1974, *23*, 13–25.

Hamburg, D., & Adams, J. A perspective on coping behavior: Seeking and utilizing information in major transactions. *Archives of General Psychiatry*, 1967, *17*, 277–284.

Hamburg, D., Coelho, G. V., & Adams, J. E. Coping and adaptation: Steps toward a synthesis of biological and social perspectives. In G. V. Coelho, D. Hamburg, & J. E. Adams (Eds.), *Coping and adaptation*. New York: Basic Books, 1974.

Hartmann, E. *Ego psychology and the problem of adaptation*. New York: International Universities Press, 1958.

Holland, J. L. *The psychology of vocational choice: A theory of personality types and model environments*. Waltham, Mass Blaisdell, 1966.

Holland, J. L. *Making vocational choices: A theory of careers*. Englewood Cliffs, N.J.: Prentice-Hall, 1973.

Holmes, T., & Masuda, M. Life change and illness susceptibility. In B. S. Dohrenwend & B. P. Dohrenwend (Eds.), *Stressful life events: Their nature and effects*. New York: Wiley, 1974.

Jacques, E. Death and the midlife crisis. *International Journal of Psychiatry*, 1965, *XLVI*, 502–513.

Kroll, A. M., Dinklage, L. G., Lee, J., Morley, E. B., & Wilson, E. H. *Career development: Growth and crisis. New York:* Wiley, 1970.

Kubie, L. *Neurotic distortions of the creative process*. Lawrence, Kansas: University Press, 1958.

Levinson, D., Darrow, C., Klein, E., Levinson, M., & McKee, B. The psychosocial development of men in early adulthood and the midlife transition. In D. Ricks et al. (Eds.), *Life history research in psychopathology*, Vol. 3. Minneapolis: University of Minneapolis Press, 1975.

Levinson, D., Darrow, C., Klein, E., Levinson, M., & McKee, B. *The seasons of a man's life*. New York: Knopf, 1978.

Liem, G. R., & Liem, J. H. Social support and stress: Some general issues and their application to the problem of unemployment. In L. A. Ferman & J. P. Gordus (eds.), *Mental health and the economy*. Kalamazoo, Mich.: Upjohn Institute, 1979.

Marcia, J. E. Ego identity status relationship to change in self-esteem, "general maladjustment," and authoritarianism. *Journal Personality*, 1967, *35*, 118–133.

Marris, P. *Loss and change*. New York: Doubleday, 1975.

McKinley, B. *Characteristics of jobs that are considered common: Review of literature and research*. Columbus, Ohio: Center for Vocational Education, Ohio State University, October 1976.

Murphy, L., & Moriarity, A. *Vulnerability, coping and growth: From infancy to adolescence*. New Haven: Yale University Press, 1976.

Neugarten, B. S. Adult psychology: Toward a psychology of the life cycle. In B. S. Neugarten (Ed.), *Middle age and aging*. Chicago: University of Chicago Press, 1968.

Orlofsky, J. L., Marcia, J. E., & Lesser, I. M. Ego identity status and the intimacy vs. isolation crisis of young adulthood. *Journal of Personality Social Psychology*, 1973, *27*(2), 211–219.

Osherson, S. *Holding on or letting go: Men and career change at midlife*. New York: The Free Press, 1980.

Osherson, S., & Dill, D. Varying work and family choices: Their impact on men's work satisfaction. *Journal of Marriage and the Family,* 1983, *45*(2), 339–346.

Rappaport, R. N. *Midcareer development*. London: Tavistock Publications, 1970.

Roe, A. *The psychology of occupations*. New York: Wiley, 1956.

Schein, E. H. Career development: Theoretical and practical issues for organizations. Paper prepared for Conference on Career Development, International Labor Office, Budapest, Hungary, 1975.

Soddy, D. *Men at midlife*. London: Tavistock Publications, 1966.

Super, D. E. *The psychology of careers: An introduction to vocational development*. New York: Harper & Row, 1957.

Super, D. E. *Career education and the meaning of work*. Washington, D.C.: U.S. Department of Health, Education, and Welfare, 1976.

Tiedmann, D., & O'Hara, R. *Career Development: Choice and adjustment*. New York: College Entrance Examination Board, 1963.

Tiedmann, D. V. Career pattern studies: Current findings with possibilities. *Harvard Studies in Career Development,* 1965, *40,* 101–133.

Vaillant, G. E. *Adaptation to life*. Boston: Little, Brown, 1978.

Weinstein, F., & Platt, G. *Psychoanalytic sociology*. Baltimore: John Hopkins University Press, 1973.

White, R. Strategies of adaptation: An attempt at systematic description. In G. V. Coelho, et al. (Eds.), *Coping and adaptation*. New York: Basic Books, 1974, pp. 47–100.

Zetzel, E. The significance of the adaptive hypotheses for psychoanalytic theory and practice. *International Journal of Psychoanalysis,* 1965, *46,* 39–52.

Zetzel, E. Anxiety and the capacity to bear it. *International Journal of Psychoanalysis,* 1949, *30,* 1–12.

— PART FIVE ——————————

Future Perspectives
——————————

CHAPTER THIRTY-ONE

The Flexibility of EFA

LEOPOLD BELLAK

To some extent the usefulness of EFA has been demonstrated. Some of the papers in Part 2 have, among other things, confirmed the reliability and validity of the measures, while others have also illustrated the clinical usefulness of EFA for diagnosis, prognosis, and treatment.

For most of the research presented, the original Ego Function Assessment Scale served as the concrete basis for assessment (see Appendices), though some investigators modified the questions, abbreviated the scale, and so on.

In this final chapter an attempt is made to indicate trends for further development and application of EFA, particularly in two directions. One is to further make clear that it is an instrument that can be used in an open-ended and free-wheeling way: Clinicians may not want to do more than keep the 12 ego functions in mind in the context of evaluating patients and articulating treatment recommendations.

In another direction, the hope is that EFA will continue to stimulate research and further codification and perhaps crystallize, in the manner of the Wechsler Adult Intelligence Scale, into devices that permit the testing of specific processes via criterion measures.

Given the model of the WAIS, it is clear that EFA still needs to be validated on a larger population than has been done so far. Of particular note is that to be useful broadly and practically, EFA not only has to be neatly "packaged"—in terms of time for administration, criterion scores, and so on—but must also be usable by people other than those with the highest clinical skill.

One temptation has been to simplify assessment via a questionnaire method. Especially in American psychology, the preferred method of testing has, in fact, been by questionnaire method. This held true once even for intelligence testing (e.g., the Army Alpha of World War I) and also played a role in the early personality questionnaires (such as the one by Bell and the one by Bernreuter). The pitfalls of these questionnaires were readily recognized in that people would only too readily guess what the right answer *should* be, rather than responding with what *actually* occurred to them. For example, if the question was, "When you see a friend approaching on the street, do you usually cross the street to avoid him?" most people were quite aware of the fact that the "healthier" thing to do was to answer "No," irrespective of what they in fact might do in that situation. If there were a matter of rating involved, most people chose—or were likely to choose—a central tendency for their rating. For example, if asked, "Do you do this often, sometimes, or never," the temptation was to hedge and say "sometimes."

Various techniques were then devised to try and deal with these methodological shortcomings of the questionnaire method. Possibly the most ambitious approach, and one still in use, is Stephenson's Q sort technique (1953), which forced the subject to rank-order items. The Q technique probably gets somewhat more valid data than a paper and pencil questionnaire. The most popular and widely used of all questionnaires is the MMPI, the Minnesota Multiphasic Personality Inventory, which attempts to deal with the possibility of faking results by testing the internal consistency of the replies and adding the L Scale, or Lying Scale.

Questionnaire methods have a tremendous attraction for several reasons: First, they are easy to administer, especially if one can hand them to the subject and have them self-administered. Second, they can be machine scored. Both procedures make them economical and lend themselves to easy quantification. A critical problem remains in that one loses the unique qualities and details and nuances in the person's functioning.

Still, the questionnaire method is attractive enough to have tried it for EFA. This author therefore developed a questionnaire form for ego functioning. As it was primarily used in a pilot study to differentiate schizophrenics from patients with psychosis and attention deficit disorder (ADD), the items tended to be more discriminating on the lower end of the scale. Supervising the administration of the questionnaire showed that even a questionnaire method produces different results in different hands, depending to a large extent on the skill of the administrator. A skilled psychologist who sees that a patient cannot handle a question can learn a great deal from how the patient handles this inability. That information is lost if only a score is recorded by the administrator. Thus, I reverted to a variation of the interview technique that underlies the original scale.

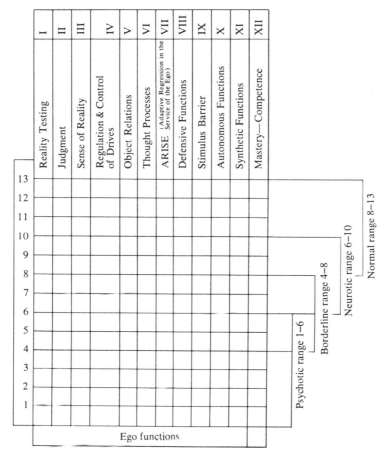

This entire questionnaire is to be seen by the clinician only, not by the patient.

Using the questionnaire as a *starting point* and enriching it by personal observations of how the patient deals with the questions, and, in turn, modifying the questions when necessary, it was possible to make the questionnaire a more useful instrument. The scoring is used as a rough guide, not yet validated, and, as stated earlier, is more useful for psychotics than for better-functioning patients.

With these reservations, the questionnaire is presented herewith, as are preliminary attempts at modifying EFA. It is best preceded by the history questions asked in the section dealing with the modified interview document.

REALITY TESTING

Patient _____ Date _____

Interviewer _____ Patient's Age _____ Sex _____

		At Admission						*At Discharge*	
Rarely (2)	Some-times (1)	Often (0)	NA				Rarely (2)	Some-times (1)	Often (0)
_____	_____	_____	____	1.	Do you have trouble deciding whether something really happened or was a dream or just in your mind?		_____	_____	_____
_____	_____	_____	____	2.	Do you see things that other people can't see?		_____	_____	_____
_____	_____	_____	____	3.	Do you hear things that other people can't hear?		_____	_____	_____
_____	_____	_____	____	4.	Do people tell you that you are confused about where you are?		_____	_____	_____
_____	_____	_____	____	5.	Do people tell you that you are confused about who you are?		_____	_____	_____
_____	_____	_____	____	6.	Are you confused about who you are?		_____	_____	_____
_____	_____	_____	____	7.	Are you confused about where you are?		_____	_____	_____
_____	_____	_____	____	8.	Do people misunderstand what you are trying to tell them?		_____	_____	_____
_____	_____	_____	____	9.	Do people tell you that what you say doesn't make sense?		_____	_____	_____
_____	_____	_____	____	10.	Do people tell you that you are imagining your complaints?		_____	_____	_____

Total Score: _____   Total Score: _____

At Admission: Interviewer's 1 2 3 4 5 6 7
               Global Rating: _____
               (circle number   poor   excellent
               that applies)

At Discharge: *Global Rating:* 1 2 3 4 5 6 7
               (circle number _____
               that applies)   poor   excellent

456

JUDGMENT

Patient _____ Date _____

Interviewer _____ Patient's Age _____ Sex _____

At Admission						*At Discharge*		
Rarely (2)	Some-times (1)	Often (0)	NA			Rarely (2)	Some-times (1)	Often (0)
_____	_____	_____	_____	1.	Do you do dangerous things?	_____	_____	_____
_____	_____	_____	_____	2.	Do you do things other people consider dangerous?	_____	_____	_____
_____	_____	_____	_____	3.	Do you become disappointed in the friends you make?	_____	_____	_____
_____	_____	_____	_____	4.	Do things not work out the way you expected?	_____	_____	_____
_____	_____	_____	_____	5.	Do you find yourself in dangerous situations?	_____	_____	_____
_____	_____	_____	_____	6.	Do people misunderstand the things you do?	_____	_____	_____
_____	_____	_____	_____	7.	Do you feel you can get away with things that other people can't?	_____	_____	_____
_____	_____	_____	_____	8.	Do you find that you take a lot of risks?	_____	_____	_____
_____	_____	_____	_____	9.	Are you surprised to find that you've rubbed people the wrong way?	_____	_____	_____
_____	_____	_____	_____	10.	Do you feel that you are too trusting of people?	_____	_____	_____

Total Score: _____   Total Score: _____

At Admission: Interviewer's   1 2 3 4 5 6 7
                Global Rating: _____
                (circle number   poor   excellent
                that applies)

At Discharge: Global Rating: 1 2 3 4 5 6 7
                (circle number   _____
                that applies)   poor   excellent

457

SENSE OF REALITY

Patient _____ Date _____

Interviewer _____ Patient's Age _____ Sex _____

	At Admission						*At Discharge*		
Rarely (2)	Some-times (1)	Often (0)	NA				Rarely (2)	Some-times (1)	Often (0)
_____	_____	_____	_____	1.	Do you feel that parts of your body don't belong to you?		_____	_____	_____
_____	_____	_____	_____	2.	Do familiar surroundings seem strange to you?		_____	_____	_____
_____	_____	_____	_____	3.	Do you think of yourself as two or more people?		_____	_____	_____
_____	_____	_____	_____	4.	Do you get the feeling that the world will be destroyed or blown apart?		_____	_____	_____
_____	_____	_____	_____	5.	Do you have the surprising feeling that something that happens has happened to you before?		_____	_____	_____
_____	_____	_____	_____	6.	Do parts of your body feel strange or unreal to you?		_____	_____	_____
_____	_____	_____	_____	7.	Does your head or other part of your body feel larger or smaller than usual?		_____	_____	_____
_____	_____	_____	_____	8.	Do you feel as if your body is empty?		_____	_____	_____
_____	_____	_____	_____	9.	Do you feel that life is like a dream or a movie?		_____	_____	_____
_____	_____	_____	_____	10.	Do you feel you are not the same person today as you were yesterday or the day before?		_____	_____	_____

Total Score: _____   Total Score: _____

At Admission: Interviewer's   1 2 3 4 5 6 7
               Global Rating: _____
               (circle number   poor   excellent
               that applies)

At Discharge: *Global Rating:*   1 2 3 4 5 6 7
               (circle number   _____
               that applies)   poor   excellent

REGULATION AND CONTROL OF DRIVES, AFFECTS, AND IMPULSES

Patient _____ Date _____

Interviewer _____ Patient's Age _____ Sex _____

At Admission					*At Discharge*		

Rarely (2)	Some-times (1)	Often (0)	NA		Rarely (2)	Some-times (1)	Often (0)
_____	_____	_____	_____	1. Do you have a strong urge to be physically active?	_____	_____	_____
_____	_____	_____	_____	2. Do you have to be on the go all the time?	_____	_____	_____
_____	_____	_____	_____	3. Do you tend to be emotional and excitable about things?	_____	_____	_____
_____	_____	_____	_____	4. Do you have rapid changes in your moods?	_____	_____	_____
_____	_____	_____	_____	5. Are you an impatient person?	_____	_____	_____
_____	_____	_____	_____	6. Do you feel so angry that you wish you could kill someone?	_____	_____	_____
_____	_____	_____	_____	7. Do you feel an overwhelming urge to commit suicide?	_____	_____	_____
_____	_____	_____	_____	8. Do you have the urge to do certain things sexually that you consider wrong?	_____	_____	_____
_____	_____	_____	_____	9. Do you feel unable to control any of your urges or impulses?	_____	_____	_____
_____	_____	_____	_____	10. Do you have rages that you can't seem to control?	_____	_____	_____

Total Score: _____   Total Score: _____

At Admission:	Interviewer's *Global Rating:* (circle number that applies)	1 2 3 4 5 6 7
		poor excellent
At Discharge:	*Global Rating:* (circle number that applies)	1 2 3 4 5 6 7
		poor excellent

OBJECT RELATIONS

Patient _____ Date _____

Interviewer _____ Patient's Age _____ Sex _____

<table>
<tr><td colspan="4" align="center">At Admission</td><td></td><td colspan="3" align="center">At Discharge</td></tr>
<tr>
<td>Rarely
(2)</td>
<td>Some-
times
(1)</td>
<td>Often
(0)</td>
<td>NA</td>
<td></td>
<td>Rarely
(2)</td>
<td>Some-
times
(1)</td>
<td>Often
(0)</td>
</tr>
<tr>
<td>_____</td><td>_____</td><td>_____</td><td>_____</td>
<td>1. Do you feel that nobody is really your friend?</td>
<td>_____</td><td>_____</td><td>_____</td>
</tr>
<tr>
<td>_____</td><td>_____</td><td>_____</td><td>_____</td>
<td>2. Do you feel that other people aren't really necessary to you?</td>
<td>_____</td><td>_____</td><td>_____</td>
</tr>
<tr>
<td>_____</td><td>_____</td><td>_____</td><td>_____</td>
<td>3. If you become close to some-one, does the relationship quickly fall apart?</td>
<td>_____</td><td>_____</td><td>_____</td>
</tr>
<tr>
<td>_____</td><td>_____</td><td>_____</td><td>_____</td>
<td>4. Do you wish, in general, that people would stay emotion-ally far away from you?</td>
<td>_____</td><td>_____</td><td>_____</td>
</tr>
<tr>
<td>_____</td><td>_____</td><td>_____</td><td>_____</td>
<td>5. Do you become attracted to the same sort of person that you have had trouble with before?</td>
<td>_____</td><td>_____</td><td>_____</td>
</tr>
<tr>
<td>_____</td><td>_____</td><td>_____</td><td>_____</td>
<td>6. Are you able to put yourself in the place of others and feel what they feel?</td>
<td>_____</td><td>_____</td><td>_____</td>
</tr>
<tr>
<td>(0)</td><td>(1)</td><td>(2)</td><td></td>
<td></td>
<td>(0)</td><td>(1)</td><td>(2)</td>
</tr>
<tr>
<td>_____</td><td>_____</td><td>_____</td><td>_____</td>
<td>7. Do you feel that when some-one important to you is ab-sent from you he or she is gone forever?</td>
<td>_____</td><td>_____</td><td>_____</td>
</tr>
<tr>
<td>_____</td><td>_____</td><td>_____</td><td>_____</td>
<td>8. Are you overdependent or clinging in a relationship?</td>
<td>_____</td><td>_____</td><td>_____</td>
</tr>
<tr>
<td>_____</td><td>_____</td><td>_____</td><td>_____</td>
<td>9. Do you feel rejected if some-one important to you is not giving you all his or her at-tention?</td>
<td>_____</td><td>_____</td><td>_____</td>
</tr>
<tr>
<td>_____</td><td>_____</td><td>_____</td><td>_____</td>
<td>10. Do you get personal satisfac-tion out of helping others?</td>
<td>_____</td><td>_____</td><td>_____</td>
</tr>
<tr>
<td>(0)</td><td>(1)</td><td>(2)</td><td></td>
<td></td>
<td>(0)</td><td>(1)</td><td>(2)</td>
</tr>
</table>

Total Score: _____   Total Score: _____

At Admission: Interviewer's   1 2 3 4 5 6 7
               Global Rating: _____
               (circle number   poor   excellent
               that applies)

At Discharge: *Global Rating:*   1 2 3 4 5 6 7
               (circle number   _____
               that applies)   poor   excellent

THOUGHT PROCESSES

Patient _____ Date _____

Interviewer _____ Patient's Age _____ Sex _____

	At Admission					*At Discharge*		
Rarely (2)	Some-times (1)	Often (0)	NA			Rarely (2)	Some-times (1)	Often (0)
_____	_____	_____	_____	1.	Do you find events or other thoughts interfering with your ability to concentrate?	_____	_____	_____
_____	_____	_____	_____	2.	Do you find it impossible to remember even simple things?	_____	_____	_____
_____	_____	_____	_____	3.	When you are emotionally upset, do you find it difficult to remember things?	_____	_____	_____
_____	_____	_____	_____	4.	Do you find it difficult to pay attention to things?	_____	_____	_____
_____	_____	_____	_____	5.	Do you find yourself using words that other people can't understand?	_____	_____	_____
_____	_____	_____	_____	6.	Do you find yourself shifting from one topic to another in your conversations?	_____	_____	_____
_____	_____	_____	_____	7.	Do your thoughts seem to run on by themselves without your control?	_____	_____	_____
_____	_____	_____	_____	8.	Do you feel that thoughts are being put into your head from outside?	_____	_____	_____
_____	_____	_____	_____	9.	Do you have thoughts you think other people would not understand?	_____	_____	_____
_____	_____	_____	_____	10.	When you are speaking, do you have trouble finishing what you are trying to say?	_____	_____	_____

Total Score: _____   Total Score: _____

At Admission: Interviewer's   1 2 3 4 5 6 7
               Global Rating: _____
               (circle number   poor   excellent
               that applies)

At Discharge: *Global Rating:* 1 2 3 4 5 6 7
               (circle number   _____
               that applies)   poor   excellent

461

ARISE

Patient _____ Date _____

Interviewer _____ Patient's Age _____ Sex _____

	At Admission					*At Discharge*		
Rarely (0)	Some-times (1)	Often (2)	NA			Rarely (0)	Some-times (1)	Often (2)
_____	_____	_____	_____	1.	Are you able to let go and think strange thoughts without being upset or frightened?	_____	_____	_____
_____	_____	_____	_____	2.	Do you have fantasies that can be used as the basis for artistic productions or activities?	_____	_____	_____
_____	_____	_____	_____	3.	Do you relax and have a good time without worrying that you're not doing anything important?	_____	_____	_____
_____	_____	_____	_____	4.	Do you enjoy daydreaming?	_____	_____	_____
_____	_____	_____	_____	5.	Do you act spontaneously?	_____	_____	_____
_____	_____	_____	_____	6.	When you are working on a hobby (cooking, carpentry, model building), do you enjoy deviating from the instructions?	_____	_____	_____
_____	_____	_____	_____	7.	Do you enjoy doing creative things (e.g., painting, clay modeling, creative writing)?	_____	_____	_____
_____	_____	_____	_____	8.	Do you think situations are funny or humorous?	_____	_____	_____
_____	_____	_____	_____	9.	Do you enjoy playing games?	_____	_____	_____
_____	_____	_____	_____	10.	Do you find it easy to laugh when someone tells a joke?	_____	_____	_____

Total Score: _____   Total Score: _____

At Admission: Interviewer's   1 2 3 4 5 6 7
                Global Rating: _____
                (circle number   poor   excellent
                that applies)

At Discharge: *Global Rating:* 1 2 3 4 5 6 7
                (circle number   _____
                that applies)   poor   excellent

462

DEFENSIVE FUNCTIONING

Patient _____ Date _____

Interviewer _____ Patient's Age _____ Sex _____

At Admission

At Discharge

Rarely (2)	Some-times (1)	Often (0)	NA		Rarely (2)	Some-times (1)	Often (0)
___	___	___	___	1. Do things easily upset you?	___	___	___
___	___	___	___	2. Do you feel restless or jumpy and not know why?	___	___	___
___	___	___	___	3. Are you an anxious person?	___	___	___
___	___	___	___	4. Do you feel as if you were falling apart?	.	___	___
___	___	___	___	5. Do you have difficulty getting the point of jokes you hear?	___	___	___
___	___	___	___	6. Do you have nightmares?	___	___	___
___	___	___	___	7. Do you worry about what other people are saying about you?	___	___	___
___	___	___	___	8. Do strange or frightening thoughts cross your mind?	___	___	___
___	___	___	___	9. Do you feel you cannot handle the problems that come up in your life from day to day?	___	___	___
___	___	___	___	10. Do you believe that if you don't think about problems, they will go away by themselves?	___	___	___

Total Score: _____

Total Score: _____

At Admission: Interviewer's *Global Rating:* (circle number that applies)   1 2 3 4 5 6 7
_____
poor   excellent

At Discharge: *Global Rating:* (circle number that applies)   1 2 3 4 5 6 7
_____
poor   excellent

STIMULUS BARRIER

Patient _____ Date _____
Interviewer _____ Patient's Age _____ Sex _____

	At Admission					*At Discharge*		
Rarely (2)	Some-times (1)	Often (0)	NA			Rarely (2)	Some-times (1)	Often (0)
____	____	____	____	1.	Are you especially sensitive to light, sound, or temperature changes?	____	____	____
____	____	____	____	2.	Are you irritable or jumpy when there's a lot of noise around you?	____	____	____
____	____	____	____	3.	When things get too much for you, do you go off by yourself?	____	____	____
____	____	____	____	4.	Does your skin feel particularly sensitive?	____	____	____
____	____	____	____	5.	Does the slightest sound or light keep you awake at night?	____	____	____
____	____	____	____	6.	Do you have minor physical aches and complaints?	____	____	____
____	____	____	____	7.	Do you get headaches?	____	____	____
____	____	____	____	8.	Do you get easily rattled when lots of things are going on at once?	____	____	____
____	____	____	____	9.	After a vacation, does it take you a long time to get back into your job?	____	____	____
____	____	____	____	10.	Are you a light sleeper?	____	____	____

Total Score: _____   Total Score: _____

At Admission: Interviewer's   1 2 3 4 5 6 7
                 Global Rating: _____
                 (circle number   poor   excellent
                 that applies)

At Discharge: *Global Rating:* 1 2 3 4 5 6 7
                 (circle number   _____
                 that applies)   poor   excellent

AUTONOMOUS FUNCTIONING

Patient _____ Date _____

Interviewer _____ Patient's Age _____ Sex _____

At Admission						*At Discharge*		
Rarely (2)	Some-times (1)	Often (0)	NA			Rarely (2)	Some-times (1)	Often (0)
____	____	____	____	1.	Do you get tongue-tied?	____	____	____
____	____	____	____	2.	Does your speech get mixed up when you are embarrassed?	____	____	____
____	____	____	____	3.	Do you feel so lacking in energy that you cannot do things you usually do?	____	____	____
____	____	____	____	4.	Do you find it hard to get started on something you want to do?	____	____	____
____	____	____	____	5.	Do you consider yourself to be lazy?	____	____	____
(0)	(1)	(2)	____	6.	Can you stay in control of yourself when other people seem to be going to pieces?	(0)	(1)	(2)
____	____	____	____	7.	Do you bump into objects?	____	____	____
____	____	____	____	8.	When you are doing something, do you have difficulty finishing it?	____	____	____
____	____	____	____	9.	Do you have problems paying attention to someone or something (television, book) for any length of time?	____	____	____
____	____	____	____	10.	Do you forget things like names and places?	____	____	____

Total Score: _____   Total Score: _____

At Admission: Interviewer's *Global Rating:* (circle number that applies)   1 2 3 4 5 6 7
poor   excellent

At Discharge: *Global Rating:* (circle number that applies)   1 2 3 4 5 6 7
poor   excellent

SYNTHETIC–INTEGRATIVE FUNCTIONING

Patient _____ Date _____

Interviewer _____ Patient's Age _____ Sex _____

At Admission						*At Discharge*		
Rarely (0)	Some-times (1)	Often (2)	NA			Rarely (0)	Some-times (1)	Often (2)
____	____	____	____	1.	Do you adapt easily to changes in your routine?	____	____	____
____	____	____	____	2.	Can you do things you are supposed to do even though you don't feel like it?	____	____	____
				3.	Do you often change your feelings about people or ideas?			
(2)	(1)	(0)				(2)	(1)	(0)
____	____	____	____	4.	Are you predictable in the things you do or say?	____	____	____
____	____	____	____	5.	Are you organized in your daily life?	____	____	____
____	____	____	____	6.	Do you like to plan for the future?	____	____	____
____	____	____	____	7.	Are you able to handle more than one task at a time?	____	____	____
____	____	____	____	8.	Can you organize your life so there are no loose ends?	____	____	____
____	____	____	____	9.	Do you learn from your past mistakes?	____	____	____
____	____	____	____	10.	Are you able to carry out your plans?	____	____	____

Total Score: _____   Total Score: _____

At Admission: Interviewer's *Global Rating:* (circle number that applies)   1 2 3 4 5 6 7

poor   excellent

At Discharge: *Global Rating:* (circle number that applies)   1 2 3 4 5 6 7

poor   excellent

MASTERY–COMPETENCE

Patient _____ Date _____

Interviewer _____ Patient's Age _____ Sex _____

At Admission					**At Discharge**		
Rarely (0)	Some-times (1)	Often (2)	NA		Rarely (0)	Some-times (1)	Often (2)

At Admission					At Discharge		
_____	_____	_____	_____	1. Do you function as well as you believe you are capable of functioning?	_____	_____	_____
_____	_____	_____	_____	2. Do you like to be in charge of things?	_____	_____	_____
_____	_____	_____	_____	3. Do you live up to your own expectations of yourself?	_____	_____	_____
_____	_____	_____	_____	4. Do you feel that you can do things as well as most people?	_____	_____	_____
_____	_____	_____	_____	5. Do you feel that you can change things that happen to you that you don't like?	_____	_____	_____
_____	_____	_____	_____	6. Do you make decisions without much difficulty?	_____	_____	_____
_____	_____	_____	_____	7. When you have bad luck, do you feel you can do something to help yourself?	_____	_____	_____
_____	_____	_____	_____	8. Do people praise you for doing a good job?	_____	_____	_____
_____	_____	_____	_____	9. Do you or did you set goals for your life?	_____	_____	_____
_____	_____	_____	_____	10. Do you think one is master of one's own fate?	_____	_____	_____

Total Score: _____   Total Score: _____

At Admission:	Interviewer's Global Rating: (circle number that applies)	1 2 3 4 5 6 7	
		poor	excellent
At Discharge:	Global Rating: (circle number that applies)	1 2 3 4 5 6 7	
		poor	excellent

TOWARD A FURTHER MODIFICATION OF EFA

The foregoing questionnaire, enriched by observations on how the subject handles the inquiry, is one attempt to modify the interview technique as originally described.

It must be remembered that from the start of the original EFA research, multiple avenues for assessment were attempted from which the interview emerged, for the time being, as the most useful. We did, however, use psychological testing as well as psychophysical methods, employing the pursuit rotor to test a type of frustration tolerance or the GSR for assessing anxiety levels and a large number of other procedures.

I have attempted to modify the EFA currently by enriching it from other sources, for example, the WAIS, the TAT, and other tests, while maintaining the original ego functions as the framework for assessment.

The WAIS, in fact, had struck me as useful for such a purpose as early as 1958. The idea of using the WAIS for personality assessment actually must be credited to Rapaport and co-workers as early as 1946.

The Comprehensive Scale of the WAIS, for instance, involves judgment to a large extent. When we ask, "If you are the first person to discover a fire in a movie theater, what is the first thing for you to do?" we are assessing a person's judgment. Of course, we know that persons who answer us very reasonably, saying that they would quietly get up and inform the usher, may indeed, when faced with that situation, not react that way at all but instead yell "Fire!" and storm out and cause a panic. In that sense, this may not be a good *operational* test. Thus, it still shares some problems typically seen with the questionnaires. The task is different if we actually ask someone to arrange the Kohs Blocks, and find that his or her synthetic functioning, at least of the kind used in arranging Kohs Blocks, is excellent, good, fair, or poor: In such situations the test task itself is the operational criterion.

The following material then presents a few concrete suggestions, offered only tentatively, with the hope that such formulations will result in a more systematic and valid measurement instrument, in the spirit of the WAIS.

Incidentally, for some subjects the order of inquiry into the particular ego function does seem to have an effect; for example, asking persons about their reality testing alarms them much more than inquiring about their object relations, as Goldsmith, Charles, and Feiner (see Chapter 25, this volume) found in their research on borderline patients. These suggestions are incorporated in the following proposal.

A MODIFIED VERSION OF EGO FUNCTION ASSESSMENT

BRIEF GENERAL HISTORY

1. What is your full name, your age, your address?
2. How long have you been living there?
3. Who else lives in your household?
4. How does that work out?
5. Where are you originally from? What was your neighborhood like?
6. Who is in your family? (If any deaths, determine time, circumstance, causes and reactions)
7. How long have you been married? (If appropriate)
8. What kind of work do you do?
9. Your education? (If any degree or school not completed, ask why)
10. How do you feel about your work? (If any discrepancy between education level and nature of job, inquire about it)
11. Have you had any major illnesses or operations?
12. Were you sick at all when you were little?
13. Have you ever had any accidents? Injuries?
14. Have other people in your family been sick?
15. What kinds of problems bother you typically?
16. How do these problems affect your regular activities, such as work, taking care of the house, and so on?
17. How do you spend a routine day?
18. What did you dream last night? Do you have any recurrent dreams? Do you remember a recurrent dream from your childhood?
19. What brought you to the clinic/office? (Pursue presenting complaint, focusing especially on all information about ego function, strength and deficiency)

Each inquiry starts with a history broadly based on items from the interview guide. Then one proceeds with the TAT and other supplementary methods and, if necessary, later rounds out the inquiry with parts of the highly structured EFA questionnaire.

Object Relations

In addition to the inquiry, I would also, in testing for patterns in object relations, want to use at least one TAT picture, specifically Card 2 (country scene: in the foreground is a young woman with books in her hand; in the background a man is working in the fields and an older woman is looking on). I consider this picture an excellent indicator of object relations, though several other TAT pictures could also be used. In connection with TAT stories, it is also often easy to ask for dreams, using them also mostly to study object relations.

ARISE

To test ARISE, Card 1 on the TAT (a young boy is contemplating a violin that rests on a table in front of him), Card 8BM (an adolescent boy looks straight out of the picture; the barrel of a rifle is visible at one side, and in the background is the dim scene of a surgical operation, like a reverie image), and Card 11 (a road skirting a deep chasm between high cliffs; on the road in the distance are obscure figures) may be particularly useful.

One might also be able to use a technique like Weisskopf's Ambiguity Index to get a measure of Adaptive Regression in the Service of the Ego. Weisskopf has established what might be called a popular response index for each TAT card, and then compared individual variations to that popular interpretation. She counted the number of new objects introduced, as well as objects omitted, and thus determined how much an individual subject transcended the norm she had computed. Thus, somebody relating a completely unusual story would have a large transcendence index, while somebody remaining with the popular responses would have a very small transcendence index. To a considerable extent, the degree of the transcendence index might indicate originality and creativity. Of course, it might also be a function of disturbance. Some psychotic patients pay little attention to the stimulus in elaborating their responses. One would therefore have to note qualitatively the extent to which the subject takes sufficient heed of the stimulus in creating his stories.

Reality Testing

The Picture Completion Tests from the WAIS, especially Cards 16 and 18, constitute challenging tasks in the area of Reality Testing. These could be supplemented by TAT Card 18BM (a man is clutched from behind by three hands; the figures of his antagonists are invisible), which is a difficult picture to deal with realistically. Acuity of form perception on the Rorschach (F + %) is also a useful indicator.

Judgment

To test judgment, I would suggest using all or most of the Comprehension Subtest of the WAIS, as already mentioned. It is virtually ready-made to test judgment, while also giving clues as to superego and drive control.

"What's the thing for you to do if you find an envelope that is stamped, addressed and sealed?"

"Why do we have to pay taxes?"

"Why does the state require a license in order to marry?"

In short, nearly every one of the questions of this subtest could be adapted to test judgment very effectively.

Sense of Reality of the Self and of the World

The Draw a Person Test may elicit some material reflective of the body image and the sense of self.

A brief operational task might be to tell the testee: "Close your eyes until I tell you to open them. How did you feel during that time?"

1. I felt very relaxed.
2. I was feeling relaxed, but had some slight feeling of lightheadedness.
3. I was feeling a little dizzy, and had to touch my leg (or other part of the body) to feel all right.
4. I experienced a feeling of floating.
5. I was feeling anxious and didn't know where I was. I had a feeling of being one with space.

Otherwise, the questions from the Interview Guide and those from the Questionnaire will have to suffice. Experimental techniques could be developed, but would be too cumbersome for the clinical situation.

Regulation and Control of Drives, Affects, and Impulses

Regulation and control of drives can be studied very effectively through an analysis of TAT stories. The testee may either tell a story of losing control over aggressive, sexual, or other drives, or the story, conversely, may be cohesive with an appropriate balance between drives and ego forces.

Aggressive themes are typically elicited on Card 8BM of the TAT (an adolescent boy looks straight out of the picture. The barrel of a rifle is visible at one side, and in the background is the dim scene of a surgical operation, like a reverie image). The same card, because of its complexity, also elicits information about synthetic functioning, namely, how well the testee incorporates the gun in the left corner of the card into a story that includes an operation. Similarly, TAT Card 13MF (a young man is standing with downcast head buried in his arm; behind him is the figure of a woman lying in bed, her breasts nude) is useful in assessing problems in the control of drives of both an aggressive and sexual nature. Both Card 18BM (a man clutched from behind by three hands—the figures of his antagonists are invisible) and Card 12M (a young man is lying on a couch with his eyes closed; leaning over him is the gaunt form of an elderly man, his hands stretched out above the face of the reclining figure) give one an idea of how the subject handles passivity and fear of attack.

Synthetic–Integrative Functioning

As suggested, the Synthetic–Integrative function can be assessed by TAT Card 18BM as well as Card 13MF. The Rorschach inkblots also lend themselves to this task; for example, the question of how well the subject can integrate form and color draws on synthetic functioning. If someone sees the classical "green grass bear," then there obviously are problems in synthetic functioning, whereas a "chamelion" may be the end product of better synthesizing.

Thought Processes

To test thought processes, the similarity items from the WAIS are ideal, as are the interpretation of proverbs, for example, "What is the meaning of the proverb, 'You can catch more flies with honey than with vinegar'?"

Mastery and Competence

To a certain extent, the way in which the subject approaches the test situation as a whole provides data as to how challenges are managed and adaptively negotiated. These may be assessed not only in terms of the subject's overall behavior during the evaluation, but also in response to the specific questions designed to tap this function.

Autonomous Functioning

The Digit Span test of the WAIS is a good test of recent memory; the Digit Symbol test a good indicator of eye–hand coordination; and the Bender–Gestalt and Bender Recall tests are good indicators of form perception and memory.

Stimulus Barrier

In the testing situation one might observe whether the testee is disturbed by sound, light, or time pressure. While one could design a great many experimental techniques, they would most likely be too cumbersome for the clinical situation, so the EFA Questionnaire and EFA Interview Guide will have to suffice.

Defensive Functioning

An inquiry with regard to nightmares, temper outbursts, and difficulty in concentration as well as eliciting any kind of symptomatology may be helpful.

Card 3BM of the TAT may be helpful in judging defenses regarding aggression and intraggression, 8BM for aggression, and number 13MF for defenses concerning sexual drive and aggression.

EFA can be an exquisitely sensitive, operational technique for assessing subtle personality characteristics within the matrix of psychoanalytic theory. One can only hope that the preliminary notions outlined here will help in the development of a practical instrument, neatly packaged, and with as good reliability and validity as the WAIS.

REFERENCES

Bellak, L. *Schizophrenia: A review of the syndrome*. L. Bellak (Ed. and contributor). New York: Logos Press, now distributed by Grune & Stratton, 1958.

Bellak, L. *The schizophrenic syndrome*. L. Bellak and L. Loeb (Eds.). New York: Grune & Stratton, 1969.

Bellak, L. *The T.A.T., C.A.T., and S.A.T. in Clinical Use*. Third ed. New York: Grune & Stratton, 1975.

Bellak, L., Hurvich, M., & Gediman, H. K. *Ego functions in schizophrenics, neurotics, and normals*. New York: Wiley, 1973.

Kohut, H. *The analysis of the self*. New York: International Universities Press, 1971.

Rapaport, D., Gill, M., & Schafer, R. *Diagnostic psychological testing*. Chicago: Year Book, 1946.

Stephenson, W. *The study of behavior*. Chicago: University of Chicago Press, 1953.

Weisskopf, E. A. An experimental study of the effect of brightness and ambiguity on projection in the Thematic Apperception Test. *Journal of Psychology*, 1950, *29*, 407–416.

Appendices

APPENDIX A

An Interview Guide for the Clinical Assessment of Ego Functions

INTERVIEW GUIDE

CONTENTS

GENERAL ORIENTATION FOR INTERVIEWS

Questions Coordinated to Rating Scales

This guide contains 12 sets of specific questions, each set keyed to its corresponding ego function scale as specified in the Manual for Rating Ego

Reproduced from Bellak, L., Hurvich, M., & Gediman, H. D. *Ego functions in schizophrenics, neurotics, and normals: A systematic study of conceptual, diagnostic, and therapeutic aspects*. New York: Wiley, 1973. By permission of John Wiley & Sons, CPS, Inc., and the authors.

Functions from a Clinical Interview. Wherever possible, the specific component factors will be designated in the margin. Where the interview questions could not be specifically tailored to the rating-scale format, the interviewer is expected to do this job by himself, by his clinical skills, judgment, *thorough knowledge of the Rating Manual and its relation to the Interview Guide*, and the aims of the raters. The major purpose of the clinical interview is to provide data on the 12 ego functions and their components such that they can be reliably rated.

Rigor and Flexibility

These suggestions are not intended to inhibit the interviewer in using his own clinical style, but rather to help him in furthering the major purposes of the interview.

Ingenuity (which at times may have to include direct departures from the suggested questions) will be required, especially when a subject dodges the questions being asked. Some firmness and control will also be necessary to limit the extent of digressions. At other times, the interviewer may devise shortcuts to condense areas of questioning. Parsimony is always desirable.

Ingenuity and flexibility will also be required in probing for specific details whenever a subject reveals any information crucial to rating any aspect or component of any of the ego functions, no matter what function is being formally pursued at the time. At some places in the Interview Guide there are parenthetical remarks directed to the interviewers to do specific probing. Such standard interviewing directions as "Tell me more," "When did it start," "Give a specific example," "Do you still feel that way," will not be included. Interviewers will be presumed to be experienced and skilled enough to probe at their own discretion.

By and large it is best to follow the guide, function by function, but occasional patients with communication difficulties might best be interviewed in a more flexible way, following their own leads as to what function gets covered at what point.

Present and Past Status of Ego Functioning

While we want to know the current (often acute) status of any ego function being rated, we are equally interested in what a person's *characteristic level* of adaptation-maladaptation with respect to each function has been, as well as his highest and lowest level. When the Interview Guide does not explicitly direct the interviewer to obtain such information, the interviewer should nevertheless attempt to discover (a) when the person began to have trouble with respect to the function and what level of development was reached prior to illness; (b) to what extent the difficulties interfered with adaptation; (c) how long the interference lasted; (d) how often it tended to recur; and (e) how easily the person recovered after a disturbance. We are also interested in determining the status of ego deficits at critical phases in the life cycle – infancy, childhood, adolescence, adulthood, old age – as well as in response to specific stress or trauma. Although the questions are not always specifically geared to tap these areas, the interviewer is advised to obtain the information whenever it is appropriate during the interview: in the initial section dealing with presenting complaints and history of illness or during the questioning about specific ego functioning. Obtaining a clinical history should thus be limited to relevant ratable yield of information about ego functions, especially with the aim of rating current characteristic, highest, and lowest levels of functioning.

Miscellaneous Issues

If, while obtaining information about a specific ego function, you discover that the subject offers information on other ego functions, do not hesitate to follow up on the other functions at that time, as well as when the guide explicitly directs you to do so. Remember also that from the rater's point of view, any responses may be pertinent to one or more ego functions.

Although the guide offers specific questions worded in a particular way, you need not desert your usual attempt to gear your verbalization of the questions to the particular subject's background and intelligence. If you judge something in the guide to be worded in a way that is either too sophisticated or might sound too patronizingly naive for the subject you happen to be interviewing, feel free to substitute a more appropriate terminology.

INITIAL RAPPORT

What is your full name, please?

Your age?

And your address? How long have you been living there? Who else lives in your current household? Where are you originally from?

What kind of work do you do? And your education? (If any degree or school not completed, ask why.) (If any discrepancy between education level and nature of job, inquire about it.)

What brought you to the hospital (treatment)? (Pursue presenting complaint, focussing especially on all information about ego function strength and deficiency.)

I. REALITY TESTING

a   1.   Do you ever have trouble deciding whether something really happened or if it was a dream?

a   2.   Have you ever wondered if a thing only happened in your mind?

a,b 3.   Have you ever been surprised to find that what you thought was going on really wasn't?

b   4.   Do you sometimes feel that you see what you want to see rather than what's really there? Like an ostrich burying his head in the sand?

b   5.   Do you ever read into other people's behavior things that really aren't there? Has anyone ever told you that you do this?

b   6.   Do you have the feeling that you're out of touch? Is it important for you to be in touch with everything about you? (Or: Does it upset you when you don't know what's going on?)

b   7.   Have you ever been confused about things? Have people ever told you you're confused about things? Do you get confused easily? Disoriented? (Time, place, people)

a,b 8.   Have others ever told you that you're not with it? Out of step with the
c   rest of the world? Do you think they're right?

b   9.   Do people often misunderstand what you are trying to tell them?

a,b 10.   Have you ever been told by people that what you say doesn't make sense? That your ideas are way off?

a   11.   Have you ever been convinced of the reality of something even though everyone around you disagreed? Has this been about things you saw? heard? thought?

c   12.   When you distort and misinterpret things, are you able to correct those notions?

a,c 13.   Have you ever heard strange sounds in your ears that you couldn't account for on a physiological basis? Ever heard voices? What about visual experiences? In such cases, have you known that the voice (or whatever) couldn't be real even though it seemed real at the time?

a   14.   Have you ever hallucinated?

c   15.   How did you eventually find out that you had been hallucinating?

c   16.   Do you pay attention to what goes on inside of you, like emotions, aches and pains? Possibly too much attention?

II. JUDGMENT

c   1.   What are some of the things you've done which have shown poor judgment?

c   2.   Do you care what other people think of you?

c   3.   Have you ever felt awkward socially? Have you ever put your foot in your mouth or offended someone without intending to?

a,c 4.   Are you good at sizing people up? At anticipating their responses to you?

c   5. Have you had the experience of being shocked or surprised that something you did had rubbed people the wrong way? Or when you thought you were being pleasant, you had actually annoyed someone or made him angry?

c,a 6. Do you ever find that you misjudge people?

a,b 7. Are you ever too trusting of people?

a   8. How do you go about making decisions? (Like taking a new job, quitting school, breaking up with a girlfriend/boyfriend, getting married?) Do you consider all the angles or do you act without thinking too long about things?

a   9. Are you a planner in that you think a lot about the consequences of what you might do? Do you have trouble estimating how long it would take or how much work is required in getting something done?

a,b 10. Are you an impulsive person? Are you careless with yourself or your health?

b   11. Are you a daredevil? Do you like to take chances? What if other people are involved?

a,b 12. Have you ever felt that you could get away with things that the average person couldn't? Like doing something risky that could get you into trouble? Like applying for a job for which you had no proper skills or training? Like speeding or driving without a license? If you get away with it, is it luck or something else?

b   13. Do you ever do dangerous things, like walking around the city at night (unaccompanied)? Opening your door to strangers before you know what they want? Riding in a car with defective brakes?

III. SENSE OF REALITY

a   1. Most people sometimes have the experience that things are happening that have happened before, like a déjà vu. Have you ever had this experience? Like you had been to a certain place before, or heard, thought, or said something, even though you knew it couldn't possibly be so? Did you wonder if it really happened or was just your imagination?

a   2. Do people and things around you sometimes feel unreal to you? As though they really weren't there, or couldn't have happened?

a   3. Do people and things sometimes look foggy or as though seen through a haze, or perhaps as though there were a glass wall between you and the rest of the world?

a   4. Have people and things ever looked closer or further away, larger or smaller than you know them actually to be?

b   5.   Have you ever felt as though you were walking around in a trance?

b   6.   Have you ever felt that you were not real?

b   7.   Have you ever had strange feelings in various parts of your body that there was no physical explanation for? (As if electricity was going through you; as if your head, tongue, or some other part of your body was feeling much bigger or smaller than usual; as if some part of your body is changing shape; or as if you were literally physically empty or had a hole in your stomach?)

a   8.   Have you ever had a physical subjective feeling or sensation as though the world were going to collapse or fall apart? As though you could cause it, for example, by some act, thought, dream?

c   9.   Do you spend much time thinking about the question "Who am I?"

d   10. Have you ever had trouble feeling yourself to be a person separate and independent from other people?

c,d 11. Describe yourself.

c   12. Do you have special ways to make yourself feel good about yourself?

c   13. What kinds of things make you feel humiliated?

c,d 14. Are you more affected in your opinions about yourself if someone says you're great or if someone says you're doing terribly?

c,d 15. Can you tell me of any times when you feel important or good living through someone else's accomplishment? Because they are perhaps intelligent, good-looking, popular, or very successful? When they're not around, do you get depressed or feel generally bad?

d   16. Is it very important for you to feel as though you were in special communication with someone else? Feeling merged or fused together? Do you feel you can read someone's mind, or they yours? Have you ever believed you possessed a capacity for ESP?

a,b, 17. Do you smoke pot or take other drugs? What kinds of feelings does
c,d   this give you? Do they effect any of the things we've just discussed? Even after the effect of the drug has worn off?

IV. REGULATION AND CONTROL OF DRIVE, AFFECT, AND IMPULSE

a   1.   Do you have a lot of drive to be physically active? Do you have to be on the go all the time? Or do you ever find it hard to get going?

a,b 2.   Do you tend to be emotional and excitable about things, or are you relatively calm and detached? Do you consider yourself to be an undercontrolled or an overcontrolled person? What do other people think about you?

b   3.   Do you ever have rapid changes in your mood – going from high to low rather quickly?

b   4. Have other people ever told you that you were overdramatizing or overreacting to something?

a,b 5. Are you a defiant or rebellious person? Are you spiteful? Do you tend to be well behaved? Polite?

b   6. Are you a patient or impatient person?

b   7. If you don't get your way or what you want immediately, how do you react? Are you easily frustrated? Can you stand frustration for any length of time?

b   8. How well do you think you tolerate feelings of anxiety when there is no immediate way of getting rid of them? How do you get relief from anxiety?

a,b 9. Do you feel much inner pressure to act? Pressure to talk?

a   10. Do you find it hard to be frank and direct about the way you feel? About something you want?

a   11. Do you spend much time daydreaming about things you want or about things you'd like to be? Do you find daydreaming more pleasant or satisfying than reality?

a,b 12. What sort of things make you angry? How angry do you get?

   A. How are these feelings expressed? Do they come out directly or do you do something else with them? Think? Dream? Daydream?

   B. Do you argue? Throw things? Hit people? Ever wanted to kill someone?

   C. Do you think you control these feelings too well or not enough?

a,b 13. What sort of things make you sad, blue, depressed? Are you sad a lot or a little?

   A. What do you do when you are feeling depressed?

   B. Do you cry a lot? Ever wish you would die? Did you ever think about committing suicide? Ever actually try it?

   C. How well or poorly do you think you control emotions like these?

a,b 14. A. What are the usual outlets for your sexual feelings? How frequently does this occur?

   B. How often do you masturbate? Under what circumstances? Any fantasies?

   C. In general, do you think a lot or a little about sex? Do you dream or daydream about sex? Do these thoughts or feelings ever worry you?

   D. Under what circumstances have your sexual urges been stronger than is usual for you? Weaker?

   E. Have you ever had the urge to do certain things sexually that you've thought it would be better not to do? Or that you wouldn't dare do?

F. Do your sexual feelings ever get out of control? Or do you feel that you control them too much?

V. OBJECT RELATIONS

a,b 1. What was your father like? Your mother? How was your home life?
c,d   Your current home life?

a,b 2. How do you get along with your girlfriend/spouse/boss/parent?
c,d

b   3. Have you discovered that no matter how hard you try to avoid them, the same difficulties crop up in most important relationships?

b   4. Do you keep getting involved with the same kind of person? Like even when you thought he/she was going to be different?

a,d 5. Do you generally prefer to be close to people or keep your distance? How do you feel most comfortable, with intense relationships or cool ones? Which kinds for which sorts of things?

a,d 6. Is it hard to get close? To stay close? What are the kinds of things that make you want to retain distance? In close relationships do you often reach a point where things are getting too intimate? So that you've wanted to or actually have broken it up?

a,d 7. Have you ever run away from or broken up a relationship for fear of getting hurt if you got too close? Or do you find it hard to let go even when things are going bad?

d   8. Did you ever feel that someone rejected you or a friend abandoned you?

d   9. How easily are your feelings hurt? Are you sensitive to criticism? To being left out of things? Do you often feel you've been rejected or abandoned?

a,d 10. Have you been hurt a lot in your life? Have you felt it's your fate to always be on the losing end? When you are hurt, do you have ways of trying or wishing to get back?

a,d 11. Have there ever been times in your life when you had to live alone? Or wanted very much to live alone? How do feel when "X" (whomever patient lives with) is away for the weekend? Or longer?

a,d 12. Have you ever gone to a restaurant or movie alone?

c   13. How well do you understand other people? How well do they understand you?

c   14. Have you felt that things would be all right if only he/she/they would change?

c   15. Do you try to change the way people are and how they act so that they'd be the way you'd like them?

c   16.   How do you get what you want from other people?

c   17.   What kinds of things do you do to make people pay attention to you? (Life of the party, crying, temper, dressing well, etc.)

c   18.   Do you enjoy exercising power over other people? Is that a secret pleasure?

a   19.   Who handles what in your household? Like making major decisions. (Who's responsible for the caring of children? Who handles finances?) Who *really* runs things?

a   20.   Who usually makes the initial approaches for sex, you or your girlfriend/boyfriend/spouse? Immediately after sex, what do you like to do?

a   21.   Have you ever been involved in love affairs or involved sexually with more than one person at a time? Is this (or would this be) difficult for you to sustain emotionally, or do you (or do you think you would) prefer it that way?

      22.   Do you play games like "cat and mouse" with people close to you?

VI. THOUGHT PROCESSES

a   1.   Do you have trouble keeping your mind on what you're doing? For example, when reading a book or newspaper, do you find yourself being distracted by noises or find your attention wandering?

a   2.   How well do you concentrate? Is it ever difficult for you? When? Do you ever find that you have so many thoughts racing through your mind that you can't concentrate on any particular thing?

a   3.   Do you ever think of yourself as a forgetful person?

a   4.   If you think as far back as you can, what's the earliest thing you remember? What are the most significant things you remember about your early years?

a,b   5.   Are you ever troubled by thoughts that seem to stick in your mind so that you can't get rid of them? Do they ever seem to run on by themselves without your control? Tell me about them. What ideas do you have about how they got there?

b   6.   Do you ever have thoughts that you think others would not understand? Tell me about them.

b   7.   What's foolish, or does not make good sense, about these:
      A. They put a cake of ice on the stove to keep it from melting.
      B. As he crossed the finish-line ahead of his rivals, he saw them still running in front of him.

a,b   8.   What are these sayings supposed to mean?
      A. You catch more flies with honey than with vinegar.

B. Strike while the iron is hot.

9. In what way are an orange and a banana alike? A coat and a dress? An axe and a saw? A dog and a lion? North and West? Eye and Ear? Air and Water? A table and a chair? An egg and a seed? A poem and statue? Wood and alcohol? Praise and punishment? A fly and a tree?

VII. ARISE

a,b 1. What do you do when you're alone and have nothing to do?

a,b 2. Do you daydream? What about? Are they more like fantasies, or do they involve thoughts and plans about actual things you may be doing?

a,b 3. Describe one of the most creative ideas you've ever had.

a   4. Are you ever able to let go and think strange and "nutty" thoughts without being upset or frightened? Describe one of the wildest, most fantastic ideas you've ever had. Do you ever get so carried away by your own ideas that it's hard to come back "down to earth"?

a,b 5. What is one of the most creative things you've ever done? What is the most spontaneous thing you've ever done? Are you generally spontaneous?

a,b 6. When you listen to the kind of music you enjoy, what's it like? What about art? Poetry? Literature? Making things? Inventing things?

7. Do you like to cook? Do you usually follow recipes or do you prefer making things up as you go along?

VIII. DEFENSIVE FUNCTIONING

b   1. Do things easily upset you? Which things? Do you ever feel restless or jumpy and not know why? How long do these feelings last? Do you have any special ways of getting rid of such feelings?

b   2. Are you an anxious person? Describe your feelings.

b   3. Do you feel you have ways to protect yourself from too many worries and anxieties?

b   4. Have you ever felt that you were falling apart? Rocky? Cracking up?

a   5. When things throw you, how well are you able to pull yourself together afterwards?

a   6. Do you ever find that you don't catch on to jokes that everyone around you is laughing at? Or that you miss the point of things?

b   7. Do you ever have strange or frightening thoughts? Nightmares? Tell me about them.

a   8.   Do you have any special fears? Like claustrophobia, fear of travel, fear of crowds?

a   9.   Have you ever been concerned about what other people are saying about you?

IX. STIMULUS BARRIER

a   1.   Are you especially sensitive to anything like light, sound, or temperature?

b   2.   Have you ever been irritable or jumpy when there's too much noise around you?

b   3.   What do you do if you are bothered (by the above)? Accept it? Grin and bear it? React in some way to show how uncomfortable you are? Tune it out yet still not leave the scene?

b   4.   Do you ever seek solitude when outside irritants get to be too much?

b   5.   Do you ever feel like "jumping out of your skin" if things get too much for you?

a   6.   Do you have particularly sensitive skin? Any itching that nobody found a satisfactory explanation for?

a,b   7.   How long does it usually take you to fall asleep? What seems to keep you up? Anything like light or sound or things outside of yourself?

a,b   8.   Are you easily awakened by traffic noises? Lights if the shades aren't down all the way? Any other sleep problems?

a,b   9.   (For women) Just before your menstrual periods, do you ever feel particularly bad? (Tense, depressed, irritable?) What do you do about it? (Go about your business? Stay in bed? Keep away from people as much as possible?)

a,b 10.   Are you sick often? Can you feel an illness coming on, or does it usually get pretty advanced before you realize that you are sick?

a,b 11.   Do you get headaches often? What brings them on?

a   12.   Have you ever been regarded as the "Princess on the Pea" (or male equivalent) — extremely sensitive, fragile, delicate, to be treated with kid gloves?

a   13.   Do you get bored when things aren't exciting enough? Does excitement rattle you?

a,b 14.   After being in some peaceful state (like being away in a quiet place, as for a weekend or a vacation) how do you feel getting back to the pace, din, noise of everyday life?

X. AUTONOMOUS FUNCTIONING

a   1. Does reading ever make you tense? Have you ever had trouble with hearing or vision that you know is not caused by any physical illness or defect? When you are upset or excited, do you forget things that are ordinarily easy to remember?

a   2. Do you ever get tongue-tied? Does your speech ever get garbled when you are self-conscious or embarrassed?

a   3. Are you physically awkward? Is this generally true or only in special situations?

a,b 4. Have you ever had trouble with routine things, like getting dressed, walking down steps, or carrying on with your usual work routine?

a   5. Do you ever get lost in the middle of what you're doing so that you have to stop and think about what the next step is?

a,b 6. How is your energy or drive level? Have you ever felt so lacking in energy that you couldn't carry through with things that you ordinarily do? Have you ever had any work blocks?

b   7. Is it hard to get going on something that you want to do? Are you at all lazy? About what sort of things?

b   8. When you get some free or leisure time, do you get to carry out the things you had just thought about when you were too busy or do you procrastinate?

XI. SYNTHETIC-INTEGRATIVE FUNCTIONING

b   1. Can you adapt easily to change or does it throw you out of gear? Like changes in your usual routine, or where you suddenly have to change plans?

a,b 2. When you're busy doing one thing and then something else comes up that needs to be done, can you continue doing what you were originally doing? Can you do both at once?

a   3. Do you think it's only possible to do one major thing well? For instance, can a person be both a leader and a follower? A student and a teacher? Can you imagine being both a leader and a follower yourself?

a   4. (For women) Can you imagine (How do you find) being a mother and holding down some job? How might you accomplish this?

a   5. (For men) Can you imagine being in charge of things at home but mostly following instructions at work? Can a man really be both ways? How might you accomplish this?

a   6.   Can you imagine a serious job being fun, or do you think that work is work and play is play?

a   7.   Do you often find yourself doing or saying things that seem very unlike you? When you don't really feel or act like yourself? Do you feel surprised?

b   8.   How well organized are you in your daily life? What sorts of things disorganize you?

b   9.   Do you like to live from day to day or do you prefer planning for the future? To what extent?

b   10.   Are you bothered by having bits and pieces or loose ends around? To what extent do you need to tie things together and how well are you able to do this? How well can you stand things being left undone and up in the air?

XII. MASTERY AND COMPETENCE

a   1.   Do you function as well as you believe you are capable of functioning? If not, what do you think gets in the way?

a   2.   Do you feel that you generally stay on top of things? Do you like to be in charge of things?

a,b   3.   Do you live up to your own expectations of yourself? Have you ever felt that you could make more of yourself and your life than you have thus far?

b   4.   Do you ever feel that you are missing out on life? Why do you think this is so?

b   5.   Do you feel very much at the mercy of events, or do you feel that you are master of your own fate? Do you feel that you could effectively alter your life or influence the people around you to get what you want and need?

SUPEREGO QUESTIONS

1. Does your conscience bother you a lot or a little? Are you strict with yourself or lenient?
2. Do you feel guilty a lot or a little? Do you sometimes feel guilty about things that you know aren't your fault?
3. Do you often stew over something you have said or done and wished you had not said or done it?
4. How often do you get feelings of unworthiness or of being just no good?

5. What are your expectations of how you ought to be? Are you a person who expects too much of yourself? Too little? Do you live up to the expectations of your parents?
6. Are you particularly concerned about the meaning of right and wrong? Whether a thing is moral, ethical, proper?
7. Do you think people are generally responsible?
8. Do you believe our society permits too much or too little sexual expression? What about expression of angry feelings?
9. To what extent would you be willing to step on others' toes to achieve something really important?

APPENDIX B

Manual for Rating Ego Functions From a Clinical Interview

CONTENTS

GENERAL GUIDE FOR USE OF THE MANUAL

The Manual consists of scales for rating each ego function, id, and superego. "Instructions to Raters" precede each scale. They explain each particular ego function in terms of the component factors and suggest ways to interpret and apply each scale.

Ordinal Scales

Each of the 12 ego function scales is an ordinal scale. The variables are dimensionalized on a seven-point continuum and are numbered 1 to 7. Raters are encouraged to score a subject 1.5, 2.5, and so on when the relevant data seem to fall between any two defined scale points, here called modal stops. Modal stop 1 represents the most maladaptive manifestation of the function being rated, and modal stop 7 represents the most adaptive.[1] Each ego function scale is also broken down into separate scales representing the "component factors" of the function being rated.

Although the scales are ordinal and not equal-interval, an attempt has been made to peg all stops across scales so that they reflect about the same degree of adaptation at any given stop. That is, stop 3 on any given scale is *approximately* equal in maladaptiveness to stop 3 on other scales, but this can only be approximate. While stops 1 and 7 serve primarily as anchor points to orient the rater with respect to the two extremes of the dimension(s) he is rating for each function, they may infrequently apply literally to a subject, such as a "back-ward" patient of many years standing or an unusually well-functioning individual.

A final point about the rank ordering of modal stops involves the scale placement of "average" functioning. It was decided to consider stop 6 as average. Thus, the meaning of "average" as used here has less to do with the statistical norm of functioning of some known population group and more with a meaning denoting the sense of absence of any notable maladaptation or pathology, yet short of optimal.

Global Ratings

The rater's major task is to make a global rating on a 13-point scale (1 through 7 with "half" points) for each of the 12 ego functions. The global rating will be influenced by his separate ratings of each component factor for each ego function.

In the absence of statistical weighting of the contribution of each component factor to the overall ego function score, the latter must be obtained from a global clinical estimate of the overall adaptive level of that function.

An attempt has been made to describe the function each scale represents, both abstractly (as in accordance with the component-factor definitions) and concretely (with illustrative descriptive material for each stop).

Concerning characteristic, current, highest, and lowest ratings, the frequency, intensity, and pervasiveness of any phenomenon being rated cannot be accounted for adequately in any one given rating. Thus, we need four separate ratings for each component factor and for each ego function. All of the qualities listed above would constitute the characteristic rating for a given subject(S). We

---

1. The defined scale points plus the undefined stops add up to 13. If the user of this scale desires to work with whole numbers, any score on the above scale can be converted to a 13 full-point scale by multiplying by two and then subtracting one.

must also obtain assessment of S's current level of functioning at the time of the interview, an assessment of S's lowest level of functioning, and his highest level of functioning (often highly inferential if we are dealing with hospitalized patients).

For any scale it is important to note whether the evidence for some given item of pathology is observed only currently or whether it has been noted throughout the life history. That is, the distinctions between acute, in remission, and chronic should influence the rating assigned. That is, one episode would be distinguished from episodic occurrences. The latter would score lower on characteristic level, whereas the former might conceivably rate lower on current level. Adaptive resilience and rate of recovery after temporary lapses in functioning should also be considered. For lowest level, we would not usually score a one-time lapse or regression. "Lowest" ordinarily applies to functioning during a reasonable time period, but there are exceptions here.

With respect to the type of data gleaned from interviews, some scales lend themselves best to global ratings from the subject's responses to the questions *designed specifically* to tap information pertinent to the function being rated (e.g., stimulus barrier). Other scales are applied most effectively to the person's *general style* of answering all *interview questions* (e.g., defensive functioning).

Another factor for the rater to keep in mind in making his final assessment is the congruence between degree of actual disruption in behavior at any level of ego functioning and the degree of disturbance reported as such. Thus, a person may report no difficulty in certain areas, but the interviewer can infer from other interview data that there is a greater disturbance in functioning that the subject either does not experience or does not report. Such a disturbance would be rated lower than a mere acceptance of the person's self-report would superficially suggest.

Rating Procedure

The following sequential approach has been found useful by our raters:

(1) The rater should familiarize himself with all scales, the component factors and the implied psychological dimensions upon which the modal stops of each have been ordered.

(2) The rater should be familiar with the interview questions. This will be of great help in identifying the function about which any particular interview segment provides information. In the Interview Guide, questions are organized according to function, and component factors are designated in the margin.

(3) The rater should read through, or listen to, the complete interview, making *notes* as he goes along, indicating on his rating sheet what ego function and what component factor of that function (not necessarily what stop) is reflected whenever such a judgment is possible from the material.

(4) The *rating sheets* provide sections for recording evidence for each component factor of each ego function. The rater enters on the rating sheets each bit of evidence that represents the function being rated. If he is listening to a tape, he can insert the pertinent evidence in its proper place as he goes along. For each function, the component factors are designated on the rating sheet so the rater can immediately record his data under the component factor to which it pertains. The rater then picks the scale point that most closely reflects the subject's characteristic and current levels for the given component factor, basing the rating on the specific data he has recorded on the rating sheet, qualified by his overall impression from the entire interview. When the subject falls between two defined (modal) scale points, then the rating should be made at the nondefined stop falling between the two (i.e., 1.5, 2.5, 3.5, etc.). Finally, he makes four overall global ratings (highest, lowest, characteristic, and current) for the ego function as a whole. In the absence of statistical weighting of the contribution of each component factor to the overall ego function score, the latter must be arrived at from a global clinical estimate of the adaptive capacity of that function and not from an arithmetic mean of the component scores.

I. REALITY TESTING

Instructions to Raters. The ability to differentiate between *inner and outer stimuli* involves continuous selective scanning and matching contemporary percepts against past percepts and ideas. Reality testing here also involves checking data from one sense against data from other senses. Social contexts and norms will always be relevant in assessing reality testing.

Inner-reality testing is included in this scale insofar as it refers to a person's subjective sense of the accuracy of his perceptions. Another way of stating this is the relation between the observing and participating aspects of ego functioning or the extent to which the ego is free to perceive itself. Inner-reality testing is also reflected here in the degree to which the person is in touch with his inner self. Stated another way, this implies "psychological-mindedness" or "reflective awareness."

The most maladaptive end of the scale includes those disturbances of reality testing involving delusions and hallucinations, severe disturbances in orientation with regard to time, place, and person, in general, the encroachment of drives and regressive ego states upon perceptual functioning. These disturbances become less severe, less pervasive, and less frequent at stops 2 and 3, which represent transitional states between hallucinations and optimal perception. At stops 4 and 5 perceptual vigilance is included, as well as less pathological forms of the sorts of inadequate reality testing described in stops 1 and 3. Optimal reality testing is defined along these dimensions as sharp, automatic, and flexible, including some lowering of vigilance in the service of overall adaptation.

Reality Testing
(a, b, c-components

Stop	a	b	c
	Distinction between inner and outer stimuli	Accuracy of perception of external events including orientation to time and place.	Accuracy of perception of internal events. Includes reflective awareness or extent to which person is aware of accuracy/distortions of inner reality.
1	Hallucinations and delusions pervade. Minimal ability to distinguish events occurring in dreams from those occurring in waking life; and between idea, image and hallucinations. Perceptual experience, especially, is grossly disturbed (e.g., moving things look still and vice versa).	Extreme disorientation or confusion with respect to time, place and person (e.g., inability to identify current year, month, or day). Interpretations of the meaning of events are extremely inaccurate and subject to severe distortion. This may accompany either poor attention to internal and external stimulation or hypervigilance, which could cause "overinterpretation." Thus, often highly inaccurate interpretations of perceptions. General failure to recognize familiar people, objects, and places. Frequent attribution of familiarity to strange (unfamiliar) objects, people, and places.	Minimal reflective awareness. Virtual inability to provide reasons to explain feelings and behavior. Almost no psychological mindedness (e.g., when S is sad, he may have little awareness of it).
2	Hallucinations and delusions are severe but limited to one or more content areas. May show considerable doubt about distinguishing whether an event really happened or happened in his mind or a dream.	A high degree of disorientation to time, place and person. Feels confused. A goodly amount of distortion in perceptions and in interpretation of	Subjective awareness of inaccuracies of perception is largely absent. Even long after the fact, S may not realize that a hallucination was a hallucination.

Stop	a	b	c
2 (cont)		their meanings. Distortions are limited to selected areas and thus do not pervade in all areas of functioning.	
3	Illusions are more likely to be found than hallucinations. S may be aware that he sees and hears things that are not there, but he knows that others don't see or hear them.	Distortions and misinterpretations of reality are likely, but occur mostly under provoking circumstances like the influence of drugs, alcohol and fatigue, or charged emotional situations. Failures in orientation are also sporadic here and only moderatbly pronounced.	Beginning emergence of some subjective sense of one's misperceptions, but usually after the fact, (e.g., "I realize now that I wasn't understanding things correctly last year when I was so upset". S may know that he feels bad but cannot say why, in terms of his own inner states.
4	Projection of inner states onto external reality is more likely than frank hallucinations or delusions. A "stimulus-bound" reality testing may occur at the cost of libidinal investments and gratifications.	Reality is distorted to conform to strong need states. When the latter are absent, perceptions are reasonably accurate, despite occasional cases of misinterpretations. There might also be perceptual vigilance that interferes moderately with adaptation. May be very upset when not in touch with everything.	Can usually recover from distortions when not in the situation that precipitated them. Moderate degree of awareness of feelings as emanating from self; occasionally may be a hypervigilance toward inner states, interfering some with adaptation.
5	Confusion about inner and outer states occurs mainly upon awakening or going to sleep.	Relatively minor perceptual inaccuracies. Minor, sporadic difficulties with orientation. Selective perception notable.	Resiliency is noted in ability to recover to a state of objectivity after certain perceptual inaccuracies. Can correct distortions fairly easily. With most inaccuracies, S is aware of his deviant perceptions at the time they occur. Mostly aware of inner states or overly

Reality Testing (Continued)

Stop	a	b	c
5 (cont)			attuned to own feelings and their possible meanings.
6	Inner and outer stimuli are well distinguished. Occasional denial of external reality in the service of adaptation.	Accurate perception of external events prevails.	Has good subjective awareness of accuracies and inaccuracies. Can correct distortions easily. Well in tune with inner states.
7	Clear awareness of whether events occurred in dreams or waking life. Correct identification of the source of cognitive and/or perceptual content as being idea or image and accurate identification of its source as internal or external. Distinction between outer and inner percepts holds up even under extreme stress. Checking one's perceptions against reality occurs with a very high degree of automaticity.	Sharp and flexible, thus extremely accurate attributions of meaning to reality, even in stressful and emotionally burdensome circumstances. Interpretive distortions are minimal. Orientation is excellent, with virtually no social contagion when there might be attempts to influence orientation or perception.	Reflective awareness and psychological-mindedness are optimal. Subjective sense of accuracy of his own perceptions is great, and corresponds to inner and outer reality. This is often gleaned from excellent use of consensual validation: checking one's own perceptions against those of others. Highly in touch with own feelings.

II. JUDGMENT

Instructions to Raters. Ratings for judgment are based on interview data indicating comprehension and appraisals of hypothetical and real situations, and S's evaluations of the consequences of action or other behavior related to these situations. Contemplated future judgmental activity and answers to questions about hypothetical "what would you do if" type situations should be taken into account, noting especially any discrepancies between what S says he will do in the future (or in a hypothetical situation) and what he in fact is doing or has done.

A guideline to rating here is that *activity* based on poor judgment will get a more maladaptive rating than either poor evaluations made *short* of action or poorly contemplated future activity. For example, the college student who actually cheats on an exam in full view of the proctor and is convinced that he will not be caught would be rated lower than the student who either merely announces that he plans to cheat in the future or one who makes the statement that if he were to cheat in this situation, he would not be caught.

An expansion and guide for use of two of the component factors follows:

(a) At the maladaptive end of the scale, there is no cognizance of actual dangers inherent in dangerous situations, and poor anticipation of garden-variety threats. Toward the middle of the scale, S may be aware of consequences of extreme dangers but not of more moderate ones. Overestimation as well as underestimation of real dangers must be evaluated.

(b) Here we have to consider how *behavior* is related to the anticipation of consequences of dangers. Ratings would tend toward the maladaptive end when behavior is congruent with extremely poor anticipations of its consequences and would tend toward the somewhat more adaptive if behavior were appropriate despite poor anticipations. Degree of repetition of behavior involving defective judgment must also be assessed.

This scale differs in one crucial respect from reality testing: anticipation of the consequences is the central dimension for judgment, together with a sense of appropriateness, whereas degree of distortion in perceptions and so on is crucial for reality testing. It differs from regulation and control in that judgment must be independently assessed, although drives and urges are the predominant basis for inappropriateness of behavior.

Judgment

Stop	a	b	c
	Anticipation of likely consequences of intended behavior (e.g., anticipating probable dangers, legal culpabilities, social censure, disapproval or inappropriateness, and physical harm).	Extent to which manifest behavior reflects the awareness of its likely consequences and the extent to which behavior expressing maladaptive judgment is repeated.	Appropriateness of behavior, extent to which person is able to attune himself emotionally to relevant aspects of external reality.
1	S minimally aware of consequences of his behavior. S may believe he is invulnerable or supervulnerable to anticipated dangers. Little awareness of severe dangers (e.g., consequences of jumping from 20-story building; (S may think he is	S acts in accordance with his faulty anticipations so that there is real danger to life and limb. Such behavior tends to be repeated with no regard for the reality of the situation. May act on belief	Behavior may be extremely inappropriate, socially and otherwise, and remains uncorrected. May disrobe in public, dance at a funeral, come to church clad in a bathing suit.

Stop	a1	b	c
1 (Cont)	too well padded to get hurt). Also, the most benign situations may seem extremely dangerous (e.g., a threat to life). Extreme "infantile omnipotence" may be a prominent feature. Among the situations highly misjudged are other people's intentions and behaviors.	that he is invulnerable (e.g., attempting to jump from 20-story building; giving himself the protection of an amulet or of his belief in his exceptional powers). May show no effective learning from past, identical errors in judgment.	
2	A history of inappropriate judgments involving moderate danger to life and limb. Awareness of consequences is quite defective. S may not anticipate, for example, that a prolonged starvation diet will affect his health; or that disrobing in park will lead to arrest; or that driving with very defective brakes could lead to an accident.	S actually does take unnecessary risks; has a history of behavior showing poor judgment. (e.g., will actually drive with defective brakes; is very negligent with respect to his health; socially may be quite bizarre, unwittingly provoking others to do him harm, or jail him).	May have strong conviction that cracking jokes out loud during funeral services will ease people's grief, and act accordingly. Soldier sticking tongue out at a general.
3	Anticipation of consequences of behavior is faulty (e.g., in an advance course requiring very technical and specialized knowledge, S may believe he could get an A without ever studying because his I.Q. is high). May often misjudge other people's intentions.	Behavioral consequences of defective judgment are present but not so severe as to cause serious danger to life, but could endanger health, work, and interpersonal relationships. Might repeatedly take exams without studying despite history of failure.	Inappropriate social-emotional responses might include repeated errors in appraising how a relationship might work out (e.g., after strong relationships with an alcoholic mate, S still chooses alcoholics, "feeling" it will work out O.K. this time).
4	Awareness of consequences fluctuates from one situation to another. Fairly encapsulated areas of faulty anticipation overestimation of dangers is limited to specific phobiclike reactions (e.g., person who has been a relative	Moderate behavioral manifestations of moderately poor judgment are observable mainly in relation to specific types of situations (e.g., although a person may continue to look for	General attempts to be friendly may alienate people. Inappropriateness may take the form of chronic intrusions on others privacy with belief that this is just being friendly.

Stop	a	b	c
4 (Cont)	failure in his chosen field of work believes that it is all caused by fate and he hasn't received enough lucky breaks). In overestimating, S may feel a symptom is inevitably a dangerous sign, despite reassurance to the contrary (moderate hypochondriasis). Lacunae in judgment (e.g., may be excellent in professional sphere but relatively poor in others).	jobs in a field where he has attained only marginal success and does not prepare to work in a more suitable area, he still responds with relatively good judgment in other areas of life. Misjudging people's ability to handle jobs.	Or having frequent contacts with people making sexual advances, yet feeling outraged when a "pass" is made.
5	Occasional errors in appraising his own and others' intended behavior. Trouble in estimating time and work to be done in meeting a deadline.	Behavior related to the more garden variety of situations may be inappropriate, reflecting minor, circumscribed errors in judgment (e.g., S puts off medical checkup for one inconsequential reason or another). May walk through dangerous areas of the city at night unaccompanied or may be overcautious in day-to-day routine behavior.	Social-emotional judgment approaches appropriate levels with lacunae limited to a few areas where inappropriateness may be moderate to pronounced (e.g., presumptuousness in calling a very formal person by his first name; being overly ebullient to a reserved person).
6	Average. Very few errors in anticipation of consequences. Appraisals of his own and others' intended behavior are pretty accurate and anticipated in advance. Estimation of time and resources required to complete tasks is good.	Behavior shows quite good judgment in all spheres. Past errors in judgment are only occasionally repeated. Pretty good ability to apply past learning to current behavior involving judgment.	Mostly in tune emotionally so that virtually no inappropriateness results. Emotionally out of tune only in alien situations and initially, before there is time for good judgmental appraisals to occur.
7	S shows sound awareness of the consequences of his behavior. Very fine appraisals of his own and others' intended behavior. Consequences of planned behavior	Behavior shows extremely sound judgment in all spheres: social physical, work, etc. This results from careful planning and decision-making and	Outstanding emotional intuneness to reality. Affective responses and appropriate behavior occur automatically and flexibly even in new

Judgment (Continued)

Stop	a	b	c
7 (Cont)	are very well thought out and anticipated in advance. Consequences of more immediate, spontaneous behavior are grasped with a very high degree of automaticity, with conscious awareness not necessarily intervening.	more rapid, automatic decisions about sound, appropriate actions. Past errors in judgment are almost never repeated, because of excellent ability to apply past learning to current decisions involving judgments about reality.	situations and alien surroundings.

III. SENSE OF REALITY OF THE WORLD AND OF THE SELF

Instructions to Raters. This scale assesses disturbances in the sense of one's self, as it relates to the outside world. It refers, on the optimally adaptive end, to a subjective experience, usually preconscious, of one's unique, dynamic wholeness, mentally and physically, as defined by clearly delimited self boundaries from other people and the general physical and social environment.

IV. REGULATION AND CONTROL OF DRIVES, AFFECTS, AND IMPULSES

Instructions to Raters. This function refers to the extent to which delaying and controlling mechanisms allow drive derivatives to be expressed in a modulated and adaptive way, characterized, optimally, by neither under- nor overcontrol.

Evidence here is from overt behavior, associated or indirect behavioral manifestations, fantasies and other ideation, dreams, and inferences made from symptoms, defenses, and controls. (For drive strength per se, we use ratings from the id scales.)

Regulation and control might very well be regarded as one aspect of defensive functioning, but since our concerns here are limited to behavioral and ideational indices of impulse expression and since drives and impulses may be controlled and channeled by ego structures other than defenses, regulation and control would appear to merit a scale of its own. Defensive functioning also relates in its own way to dealing with anxiety and intrapsychic conflict, thus differing from regulation and control.

Among the drives under consideration are the libidinal and aggressive, in both their developmentally earlier and more advanced forms. Included also are

Sense of Reality of the World and of the Self

Stop	a	b	c	d
	The extent to which external events are experienced as real and as being embedded in a familiar context.	The extent to which the body (or parts of it) and its functioning and one's behavior are experienced as familiar and unobtrusive and as belonging to (or emanating from) S.	The degree to which S has developed individuality, uniqueness, a sense of self, a stable body image, and self-esteem.	The extent to which the ego boundaries are clearly demarcated between the self and the outside world.
1	Extreme derealization. Feels the world as being a completely strange place. Otherwise familiar objects and events appear alien. Extreme déjà vu experiences. Surrounding people and things feel unreal, changed in appearance, as though they weren't there or couldn't have happened. All of the above are experienced as subjective sensations. May feel the world is in chaos or disintegrating (very prominent "world-destruction" fantasies). Very slight environmental changes may produce strange sensations.	Extreme depersonalization. May be oceanic feeling of nothingness, feeling dead, inanimate, selfless. Parts of body may feel unreal, extremely strange, or disconnected from the rest of the body (e.g., head or tongue or other part feels very much bigger or smaller than usual; the shape of some part feels changing). Feeling literally or physically empty inside. Feeling literally like two or more different people.	Identity grossly distorted and unstable: esteem is so low that S may feel extremely worthless. Or extreme grandiosity may be apparent. Unsuccessful and pathological means of regulating self-esteem are repeated ineffectually. Continuous feedback from external sources is ineffectual in helping the individual to establish a stable sense of self. There is virtually no continuity in self-feeling from past to present, moment-to-moment. Self-evaluations practically never correspond to realistic aspects of the self. Indications of excessive departures of body image from actual bodily configurations. Enormous discrepancy between sense of self and ego-ideal.	May experience states of extreme fusion or merging with others, suggesting near-total loss of boundaries between the self and the outside world. Opinions about self may be affected in a chameleonlike fashion, depending on what S knows others feel about him. S may believe he possesses mystical powers of communication with others, such as exceptional talent for ESP. At this stop, body boundaries may be extremely fluid and permeable, or else S erects firm or hard, nonpenetrable, exaggerated barriers.

2	Somewhat less than extreme derealization. Trances, fugues, and other dreamlike states. Outer reality often seems unfamiliar and produces feelings of confusion and estrangement. May feel as though a glass boundary separates him from his surroundings.	Strong feelings of depersonalization. Some major dissociations. Body and its functioning are often experienced as strange, peculiar, and unfamiliar. Things may seem to be happening to "someone else" rather than to own self. Many strange and peculiar feelings, like hole in stomach, electricity sensations.	Strong, unrealistic feelings of unworthiness. Or strong feelings of grandiosity. Marked use of pathological self-esteem regulators. Feedback from external sources is rarely effectual in establishing stable sense of self. Large discrepancy between self-image and ego-ideal.	Fusion phenomena are prominent, without total loss of distinction between self and outer reality. May also be overreaction to fusion needs by exaggerating separateness: as in severely overprotesting one's integrity as a person.
3	Marked but partial derealization likely to be less pronounced than depersonalization.	Marked but partial depersonalization. Parts of body may seem somewhat bigger or smaller than usual.	Self-esteem is quite poor. Identity is fragmented, unintegrated, and not very stable. Insatiable quests for money, status, assurance of sexual attractiveness. May often ruminate, "Who am I."	Self-image usually dependent on external feedback. Where feedback is negative or absent, sense of self as a separate entity falters. Often feels in "special communication" with others.
4	Very occasional signs of derealization, such as being in a fog or at sea. Seeing people through a haze. May sometimes feel on the outside looking in.	Occasional signs of depersonalization, usually under stressful circumstances. Some moderately unrealistic feelings about the body (e.g., becoming too bloated, fat, or thin when actual changes are in fact minimal).	May be "as-if" personality, or other manifestations of role-playing at identity rather than experiencing it from within. Often feels humiliated.	Sometimes dependent on external feedback to maintain identity. Under relatively stable conditions he is not dependent on outside support and can maintain a feeling of separateness.

Sense of Reality of the World and of the Self (Continued)

Stop	a	b	c	d
	Altered views of external reality are the exception rather than the rule, occuring primarily with radical environmental changes.	Depersonalization phenomena are fairly rare and limited to unusual conditions: falling asleep; waking up; drugs producing altered ego states.	More or less stable identity, self-image and self-esteem noted here. Identity sense may falter when external circumstances and people are unfamiliar or novel. Often feels important through significant others' accomplishments.	There are signs here of an independent sense of self, with a moderately good sense of inner reality, continuity, and internalized self-representations. Only sometimes does S depend on external cues for his full sense of individuality.
6	Derealization occurs only under conditions of extreme environmental alteration. It disappears with restoration of average expectable conditions.	Depersonalization occurs only under conditions of extreme environmental alterations. It disappears with restoration of average expectable conditions.	Stable identity, a distinct sense of self, and self-esteem are well internalized.	Requires only occasional feedback to maintain a sense of one's self as solidly separate from others.
7	Under average expectable environmental conditions or under conditions of extreme change and stress, experience of the world remains stable.	No disturbances in the sense of reality of the self, the body, or the body image.	Stable identity, distinct sense of self, and self-esteem are so well established and solid that they remain intact even under conditions of unusual stress or of minimal external cues ordinarily required for self-anchorage points.	S is exceptionally well able to differentiate between his own feelings, thoughts, and motives, and those of others. Minimal feedback from external sources is required for him to delineate his own self-boundaries. While S may enjoy temporary regressed states of fusion, merging, and unusual communication with others, he does not require them for the maintenance of his own sense of separate identity. Virtually no confusion between experiences emanating from within one's self and phenomena with points of origin outside the self.

impulse expressions deriving from superego pressures such as guilt and self-destructive urges, ranging from suicidal tendencies to less extreme manifestations of depression, then moral and instinctual masochism. Where relevant, we would also include pressures from the ego-ideal, such as "driving ambition," which, when it regulates self-esteem, may reflect varying degrees of impulse control.

It is important for the rater to distinguish between what the regulation-and-control scale measures and what the id scales of libidinal- and aggressive-drive components measure. The former concerns itself with the ego aspects pertaining to adaptation — the way that drive, affect, and impulse are controlled relevant to environmental context. The latter focuses on *strength* of drive, rather than the fate of the drive with respect to behavioral and ideational adaptation.

The rater will find it useful to think of degree of directness or sublimation as a relevant dimension for scaling regulation and control but not for scaling id scales of drive strength. For example, a person can have a high drive strength whether or not that drive is culturally adaptive.

Regulation and Control of Drive, Affect and Impulse

Stop	a	b
	The directness of impulse expression (ranging from primitive and psychopathic acting out, through activity of the impulse-ridden character, through neurotic acting out, to relatively indirect forms of behavioral expression). Maladaptiveness would be a function of the extent to which awareness of drive, affect, and impulse is experienced and expressed disruptively.	The effectiveness of delay and control mechanisms (including both under- and over-control); the degree of frustration-tolerance and the extent to which drive-derivatives are channeled through ideation, affective expression, and manifest behavior.
1	Aggression, and/or depression and/or sexual manifestations at their most disruptive extreme. Persons may have committed or attempted murder, suicide, or rape. Indirect or associated drive behavior is not observed at this stop, as impulses achieve full discharge through direct expression. Polymorphous perverse behavior in the extreme and in many areas (e.g., feces-smearing).	Extreme lack of control. Minimal frustration-tolerance inferable from inability to restrain impulse-dominated behavior. When thinking is at all rational, there is no evidence to show that this rationality exercises any delay or control over impulse expression. Weak controls in relation to the experience of extreme drive pressure leave physical or externally imposed constraints as about the only effective way to curb most urges. At times, no matter how hard the person tries to control urges, he cannot.
2	Aggression, depression, and sexual manifestations are quite disruptive. May be impulse-ridden personality.	S has great difficulty holding back sexual, aggressive, or other urges because of weak controls in relation to the experience of

Stop	a	b
2	Psychopathic behavior may be quite pronounced. Assaultive-type acts short of homicide. Sadistic superego pressure against the self could include serious self-inflicted injury short of suicide. Fantasy content would vary only a little from actual sexual or aggressive behavior, hardly ever as substitute formations at this level. May be rapid mood changes from one extreme to the other.	drive pressure. Physical constraints are the most effective way of curbing most urges. Frustration tolerance is almost always poor. Very little tolerance for anxiety or depression.
3	Strong urges are usually acted upon. Sometimes, although present, they are not experienced at all, and knowledge of them can only be deduced from behavior. There may be sporadic rages, tantrums or binges, as with alcohol, food, or sex. Affects and moods may be very labile, crying one moment, laughing the next. May be psychopathic personality. May be hyperkinetic, or need to be physically on the go all the time.	Urges are controlled either very poorly or excessively (overcontrol is first scored here). Excessive controls would be of the extremely rigid or brittle sort so that periods of overcontrol alternate with flurries of impulsive breakthroughs or psychosomatic spill-over. Where urges are extremely low (as in prolonged depressive states), few overt outlets are available. In cases of overcontrol of strong urges, sexual and aggressive preoccupations receive outlets in areas other than overt behavior. With strong urges and undercontrol, outlets might be voyeurism, promiscuity, "addiction" to pornographic material.
4	Drive-dominated behavior shows a few signs of adaptive directedness here. Aggressive behavior is more often verbal than physical, sometimes quite disguised and indirect, as in occupational choice of correction officer, butcher, photographer's model. May be overeating or have excessive interest in collecting and neatness. Acting out of unconscious wishes and fantasies may be quite prominent. May be general rebelliousness. Moderately high general excitability.	Controls may appear reasonably good but are of the "grit-your-teeth" or "count-to-ten" variety rather than of the smooth, automatic sort. Attempts to keep a rein on drive expression may also lead to a somewhat rigid picture. May involve overreacting, overdramatizing.
5	Drives, etc., are experienced and expressed either somewhat more	Controls are somewhat less than automatic but may be automatic in conflict-free areas.

Stop	a	b
5 (Cont)	or somewhat less than average. Irritability, arousability, or impulsivity in behavior tend to be responses to specific or conflict-ridden areas or to situational stress and external provocations. Associated, indirect behavior and interests may include mild teasing, sparring repartee, mildly inappropriate flirting or secualization of work. Some symptomatic acting out of unconscious conflicts. Moderate depressions (disappointments).	When not automatic, they can be mustered on the spot with moderate effort. Occasional work or social inhibitions.
6	When general behavior and interests are aggressively and sexually oriented, it is with effective sublimnation and neutralization (e.g., physical assaultiveness occurs only in the interest of survival of self and others when there is no other alternative). Intercourse is preferred outlet for sexual urges. Unusual sexual or aggressive behavior is seen only under extreme provocation or prolonged stress.	Reasonably smooth expression of urges, behaviorally, with the aid of fairly flexible controls. Degree of tightening or relaxing of controls is appropriate to the situation and is generally volitional and/or fairly automatic.
7	Overly aggressive behavior or its derivatives are seen only when there is no alternative, as in the interest of survival and the regulation of self-esteem along effective, adaptive lines. Effective action, whether automatic or by conscious choice in mastering tasks and achieving life goals, makes unnecessary any sort of aggressive behavior short of that mentioned above. Preferred sexual behavior is sexual intercourse. Depression and related states are limited to sadness, grief, and mourning in response to expectably provocative losses.	Control of urges to motility, etc., comes fairly quickly, calmly, and automatically. Flexibility of delay and control mechanisms allows S to respond according to his own choice rather than to pressures beyond his control. A minimum of subjective and automatic difficulties with automatic regulation and control of drive expression, such that the person functions extremely smoothly in work, sex, play, and object relations generally.

V. OBJECT RELATIONS

Instructions to Raters. Optimal relationships are relatively free of maladaptive elements suggesting patterns of interaction that were more appropriate to old situations than to the present ones. The most pathological extreme would be essentially an absence of relationships with any people; next would be present relations based on early fixations, unresolved conflicts, and very hostile, sadomasochistic relationships. Optimal relations would be the most mature, relatively free of distortions, and gratifying to adult libidinal, aggressive, and ego needs.

Intensity, diversity, and pervasiveness are not always essential components to span the entire scale, but to make global ratings, the rater is instructed to keep in mind the *quality* of the person's relationships to central and peripheral people. For more pathological adaptations the disturbances in object relations will be assumed to extend to a broader range of contacts than they would in the moderately maladaptive categories, where pathology might be limited to one or two significant relationships.

VI. THOUGHT PROCESSES

Instructions to Raters. Ratings will be based to a great extent on formal questioning, but person's overall style of language and other communications to interviewer in general will also be determining factors in evaluating this function.

VII. ARISE

Instructions to Raters. Adaptive regression in the service of the ego (ARISE) refers to the ability of the ego to initiate a partial, temporary, and controlled lowering of its own functions (keep in mind here the component factors of the other 11 ego functions) in the furtherance of its interests (i.e., promoting adaptation). Such regressions result in a relatively free, but controlled, play of the primary process.

The two components together make up what is known as the "oscillating function" — or the alterations between regressions — on the one hand, and integration into new configurations, on the other.

It will be important to assess manifestations of ARISE in the middle ranges of the population, that is, nonartists who make up the bulk of any sample to be studied. ARISE may be difficult to rate accurately in many people.

In this scale, the oscillating function can be reflected in the global ratings of the function as a whole. The general rationale for the ARISE scale is as follows:

Object Relations

Stop	a	b	c	d
	The degree and kind of relatedness to others (taking account of narcissism, symbiosis, separation-individuation, withdrawal trends, egocentricity, narcissistic object choice, or extent of mutuality, reciprocity, empathy, ease of communication). Degree of closeness-distance and degree of flexibility and choice in maintaining object relations.	The primitivity-maturity of object relations. Includes the extent to which present relationships are adaptively or maladaptively influenced by, or patterned upon, older ones.	The extent to which the person perceives and responds to others as independent entities rather than as extensions of himself.	The extent to which he can maintain object constancy, i.e., can sustain both the physical absence of the object and the presence of frustration or anxiety related to the object. Degree and kind of internalization (the way S perceives and responds to people who aren't physically present).
1	Essential lack of any object relatedness. Withdrawal, as into stupor or muteness; or living like a hermit or recluse. "Relationships" are presymbiotic, mostly autistic. When rudiments of relationships are present, they are fraught with turmoil, struggle, and other near total disruptive elements, deteriorating quite rapidly. "Distance regulators" are poor. S can tolerate little stimulation from other people.	Because of impoverishment and essential lack of relatedness, only the most primitive early elements characterize "relationships."	Minimal ability to perceive people in their own right. Extreme "parasitism," or narcissism.	Not developed enough even for separation anxiety. Bland withdrawal in response to "object loss." People do not "exist" when not present.

Object Relations (Continued)

Stop	a	b	c	d
2	Considerable withdrawal-schizoid detachment rather than total withdrawal. Severely narcissistic, parasitic, or symbiotic relationships; folie à deux, vicarious objects, intensely sadomasochistic binds. Either overattachment or underattachment of an infantile nature.	Present relationships characterized by transference based on very early fixations and may reflect disturbances in early mother-child relationships. Recurrent difficulties are the rule rather than the exception.	People's feelings, motives and beliefs are rarely understood from the other's point of view, but mostly in terms of the direct impact they have upon S. Exceedingly difficult for S to ignore his own needs as he responds to others primarily from an egocentric frame of reference. Derives pleasure from exercising "power" over others.	Separation anxiety may be prominent and may be maladaptive reaction to object loss, loss of love, or narcissistic injury. Reactions to loss still tend to be fairly catastrophic.
3	Relationships may be characterized by detachment or else by some overdependence and clinging. Considerable difficulty striking a comfortable balance between distance and closeness. Prefers either very intense or very cool relationships. May be distant for fear of a close relationship breaking up.	Present relationships are quite childlike and bear marks of earlier, similar ones. Expects to be "fed" emotionally. May wait for things to get better.	Other people only very occasionally are perceived and responded to as existing in their own right. Many "self-references" in responding to others. Own identity overly dependent on perception of others. Inordinate attempts to "change" others with belief that this will crystallize self-identity. May use and exploit people to satisfy own ambitions, oblivious to how others feel about this.	Inordinate strivings for either dependence on, or independence from, significant others, exaggerated attempts to prove one's self sufficiency. Or S may feel quite easily hurt or rejected. Representations of significant people still not too well internalized—over reactions to loss and separations. Virtually unable to live alone; or else distinctly prefers isolation from people in living arrangement.

510

4	Relations with significant others are characterized by neurotic-type interactions. Can be of withdrawn, narcissistic, or symbiotic types, but such manifestations are more complex than primitive. Examples would be Don Juanism, more "advanced" forms of sado-masochism, where usually just significant relationships are of this sort. Also includes the fringe, hanger-on person, most of whose relationships are superficial. "Game-playing."	Contains elements of conflicts characterizing early childhood, including relationships with both parents. In this sense they are a step more mature than relationships reflecting only the earliest ties to the mother, alone.	Other people can be responded to in their own right in situations that are not too emotionally charged or are neutral or nonstressful. Under more difficult circumstances, emphasis may be on trying to get other people to change in order to promote a stable self-feeling.	Sensitive to potential rejections and abandonments when not being clearly focused in others' attention. Loneliness, living alone are not tolerated very well.
5	Disturbed interactions with only a few people, and sporadically rather than chronically. Object choice and behavior with significant people shows some important degree of flexibility, but under stress becomes more compulsive or less free.	Transference and repetitions of early patterns of relating are the exception rather than the rule in everyday encounters, but may persist under very charged conditions. Some recurrent difficulties in important relationships.	Others are perceived as separate and well differentiated from the self, except under rather stressful or charged circumstances. E.g., S may recognize the other person's feelings, understand them, and respond appropriately, but when threatened, may have unreasonable expectation of what others urge and can do.	Internalization of objects is evident, but under severe or prolonged stress, absences and losses are overreacted to. May have some difficulty living alone, but finds ways to compensate for loneliness.
6	Flexibility of choice and mode in most relationships,	Tending toward mature object relations with goals that	S is usually responsive to other people as separate individuals	Object constancy is well developed, as important people are internalized.

Object Relations (Continued)

Stop	a	b	c	d
6 (Cont)	with conscious and automatic maintenance of optimal distance.	are mutually satisfying to self and significant others.	in their own rights. A reasonably good degree of empathy, but not so much as to get "lost" in the other person's feelings or point of view.	Losses separations, and other such potential traumas are weathered without undue strain. Thoughts about, reactions to, and respect for others continue whether or not the others are physically present.
7	Relationships are characterized by mutuality, reciprocity, depth, and extensivity. They maintain smoothness and stability despite stresses that might otherwise threaten them. They are flexibly maintained out of choice, as opposed to compulsion. "Distance regulators" are optimal. S functions adaptively even with maximal stimulation and excitement generated by other people.	No substantial evidence of fixations or distortions from early relationships. Maturity nearly completely replaces primitivity. Gratifications in relationships are in response to current adult needs. Flexibility and choice characterize object relationships.	Person responds to others as people in their own right, empathetic to their needs as separate people. Understands people for what they are and not from an egocentric frame of reference. Person can temporarily ignore his own needs in an effort to respond primarily to the other person. High degree of "field independence."	Object constancy excellent as judged by easy adaptations to separations, adaptive resiliency following loss of important objects. Relationships to significant others are highly viable, even when those people are not physically present.

512

Stop	a	b	c
	Degree of adaptiveness in memory, concentration, and attention.	The ability to conceptualize. The extent to which abstract and concrete modes of thinking are appropriate to the situation.	The extent to which language and communication reflect primary- or secondary-process thinking.
1	Memory, concentration and attention are grossly disturbed.	Person rarely, if ever, can conceptualize, generalize, or use abstract thinking in problem-solving or other tasks. Either the extremely concrete or the extremely syncretistic (overinclusive) modes of categorizing objects and experiences predominates. Person cannot understand metaphors or similes, is unable to grasp the general meaning of proverbs, and may show excessive literalness. No distinction is made between the object and the sign or symbol that represents the object. Capacity for syllogistic reasoning is nil.	Minimal ability to communicate verbally, owing to either mutism, extreme autism, word salad, flood of loosely or barely associated sounds, words, and phrases. Neologisms and clang associations. Practically no ability to comprehend the meaning of what other people are saying. Verbalizations contain fragmentation, primary-process influenced condensations, and contradictions. Extremely queer and peculiar expressions prevent meaningful verbal exchange.
2	Memory for only stereotyped content such as name, colors. Attention and concentration poor — very easily distractible. Foggy "sensorium."	Prominent failures of abstract reasoning. Overly concrete or overly general, with little ability to see relationships between discrete events.	Some autistic and many peculiar ideas. Thinking may sometimes be fragmented. Rigid or loose thinking often prevents adequate communication. Blocking and peculiarities in verbal expression. Thinking frequently illogical.
3	Large gaps in memory. Easily sidetracked by own thoughts and external distractions	Episodic failures of abstract reasoning and conceptualization.	At times, thoughts are organized and difficult to follow. Some

Stop	a	b	c
3 (Cont)	when attempting to concentrate. Attention and concentration remain unimpaired only if there are no competing distractions. Some trouble with remote and current memory.	Relies heavily on concrete or overideational or overinclusive modes of thought. Some little ability to see relationships and differences between events. Sometimes, difficulty in making distinctions between gradations and subtleties leads to "all-or-none" type thinking. When rigidity of thinking is present, it is difficult to entertain more than one possibility.	peculiar and queer ideas. Frequent but circumscribed disruptions in communication, possibly caused by intrusions of fantasy and drive-related thoughts that impede the flow of thought through language. Questionable logic.
4	Memory, attention, and concentration show periodic lapses, as in emotionally charged situations and with mildly compelling competing distractions. Great effort often required to exercise these functions effectively.	Occasional manifestations of flexibility in conceptualization, but under stress concrete or syncretistic modes of thought emerge. Thinking may be disordered or illogical while under stress.	Some rigid or meticulous modes of communication or else moderate degrees of looseness and disorganization. Some doubting and blocking. Occasional peculiar ideas. Mildly imprecise substitutions, expressions, or malapropisms. Some distractibility of intruding thoughts resulting in disruptive communication, particularly under stress. Some rigidity or looseness may interfere with free exchange and exploration.
5	Moderately strong competing stimuli cause lapses in memory, concentration, and attention, but mild distractions generally do not affect these functions. Moderate effort generally required to mobilize these functions.	Minor failures of conceptualization. Under stress there may be a tendency toward concreteness or overgenerality, but S can correct these lapses when asked to expand or delimit concepts.	Occasional vagueness, unclarity, or obsessionally overprecise thinking under stress. Occasional inability to stick to trend of thought because of pressure from intruding associations. Few peculiarities,

Thought Processes (Continued)

Stop	a	b	c
5 (Cont)			personalized associations, rigidity, looseness, or inability to go beyond the objective facts.
6	May forget names or be distracted from attending and concentrating when bored, sick, or upset, but otherwise, no substantial lapses in memory, concentration, or attention.	Satisfactory use of conceptualization. Evidence of flexibility in willingness to entertain and explore new ideas and in shifting back and forth between abstract and concrete modes.	More often than not, communication is clear, precise, and flexible. Possible egocentric modes of expressions, but no serious peculiarities in language. Thinking is for the most part logical and ordered.
7	Can concentrate exceptionally well even with strong distractions. Recent and remote memory is excellent for all kinds of events. These functions and attention are automatic and resistant to intrusions.	Conceptual thinking developed to its highest degree. Person shifts appropriately from abstract to concrete modes, and vice versa, when necessary.	Associations are meaningfully integrated into precise, but not overprecise, communications. No significant peculiarities of expression. Excellent ability to shift levels of discourse. Communications are unambiguous and reflect shared meanings of words and idea.

at the most maladaptive end, one sees only a primarily primitive or uncontrolled regression. In the "middle," one sees the oscillating function only with great difficulty or else a general absence of regression in the context of overcontrolled defensiveness. At the most adaptive end of the scale, one finds smoothly oscillating and flexibly controlled regressions in the service of new awareness and new integrations.

The rater is instructed to consider the final product (e.g., the work of art, the solved problem, the creative act) only insofar as it reflects the *process* of regression in the service of the ego. It is conceivable that a lesser work of art could involve more adaptive use of controlled regressions than a greater work of art. Raters should also keep in mind creative problem-solving in nonartistic areas: scientific and everyday resourcefulness.

Stop	a	b
	First phase of an oscillating process: degree of relaxation of perceptual and conceptual acuity with corresponding increase in awareness of previously preconscious and unconscious contents and the extent to which these "regressions" disrupt adaptation or are uncontrolled.	Extent of controlled use of primary-process thinking in the induction of new configurations. Extent of increase in adaptive potential as a result of creative integrations produced by ultimately controlled and secondary-process use of regressions.
1	Regressions are extremely prominent and primitively disrupt adaptive behavior (e.g., "wild" fantasies intrude willy-nilly and may either be distressing or disabling, creating confusion and chaos).	New configurations are largely absent, or when they do occur, they are not a product of controlled regressions but may be a result of "rote" learning or other very simplified, uncreative processes. No oscillating function is observed. Artistic productions might be aimless smearing or "tracing" with a stencil.
2	Regression phenomena are still fairly primitive and do not afford pleasure and enjoyment. Disruptions in adaptation may be seen in being "carried away" by one's own fantasies; highly regressed use of artistic materials (e.g., clay used only for kneading or throwing).	Occasionally, elements from dreams, fantasies, or other regressed states may be discovered in planned activities. Their effect, however, is not very marked, and thus their influence on new or creative ways of looking at things to promote adaptation is nil. Unimaginative approach to problem-solving leads to sterility and stereotype.
3	Regressive phenomena may be observed here, but so, too, may be a virtual absence of regressive phenomena. Specifically, there might be a relative inability to loosen or relinquish the more constricted types of control that one sees in unimaginative or obsessional people, who find it difficult to engage in playful fantasy or humor. Regressions of all ego functions in that instance are experienced as ego-alien threats. Or, regressive behavior is enjoyable but may be overly prolonged and resistant to recovery.	The transition from regression to adaptation is hampered by difficulties in smoothly emerging from the regressed state. Regressions and controls work separately, not together, so that creative efforts are still not aided by controlled regressions (e.g., humor may be silly, products may be sloppy or uninspired because of lack of coordination between the two phases of the oscillating function).
4	S may be able to enjoy primitive thoughts, feelings, fantasies, and regressed ego states generally. The regressions are only somewhat controlled. Or, S may be quite controlled,	S has some difficulty in adaptively channeling the outcomes of regressively based enjoyments (e.g., fantasies or daydreams may be reasonably rich but not often carried over

ARISE (Continued)

Stop	a	b
4 (Cont)	so that playful regressions and their enjoyment are somewhat difficult to achieve.	into productive activity). May never deviate from recipe when cooking.
5	Enjoyment of regressions may be fairly high, possibly owing to an acceptance of temporary passivity. S demonstrates a fair amount of control in initiating and in emerging from regressed states. Can be somewhat playful in attempting to solve a problem, but may feel compelled to return to a serious stance a bit prematurely.	Regressions are employed fairly adaptively. The oscillating function, however, lacks the sustaining power and smooth operation that would ensure truly creative-adaptive uses of regression in the service of the ego. Can be playful one moment, serious the next, without the smooth transition needed for optimal productivity.
6	Regressions to primary-process thinking and activities are well controlled and pleasurable. S may be silly, humorous, playful, fantasy-ridden — but can usually engage in and suspend these activities at will.	The adaptive-creative uses of regressive content are quite highly developed. Achievement of new integrations is often arrived at by regressive detours (e.g., controlled use of regressive humor or self-analysis may be put to use in a well-constructed story or autobiography).
7	Regressions are "controlled" and promote maximal enjoyment of and/or active participation in art, humor, play, sexuality, imagination, and creativity. The regressions "oscillate" with component b. S enjoys the absurd, and is spontaneous in producing and/or enjoying jokes.	Achievement of adaptive, integrative, creative ego function is arrived at by a regressive detour. The role of the oscillating function in this achievement is maximally observable. The adaptive-creative uses of regressive content are maximally developed, and the oscillation leading to the creative channeling of regressions is flexible and automatically controlled.

VIII. DEFENSIVE FUNCTIONING

Instructions to Raters. Defenses protect preconscious and conscious organizations from the instrusions of id derivatives, unconscious ego, and superego tendencies. They aid adaptation by controlling the emergence of anxiety-arousing or other dysphoric psychic content, such as ego-alien instinctual wishes and affects (including depression), which conflict with reality demands. Any function may at specifiable times be erected defensively against any other ego function, and a drive derivative (e.g., aggression) may defend against another (e.g., passivity).

This scale differs from the regulation-and-control-of-drives scale in that the latter measures the degree of impulse expression and motor discharge in behavior. Defensive functioning is not a scale of impulsivity but of measures employed to deal with disturbing elements of mental content, anxiety, and intrapsychic conflict.

Formation of a hierarchical ordering of the specific, classic 10 or 12 defenses with respect to pathology is an issue that has yet to be resolved in psychoanalytic theory, so the basis for ordering the scale will mainly be a dimensionalization of the efficacy of defensive functioning rather than an attempt to order specific mechanisms along an adaptive continuum. While certain stops explicitly list certain defenses and not others, the rater is to rate according to the overall rationale of the scale.

Excessive use of defenses is added at stop 3 in addition to relative failure of defenses. Stops 4 and 5 illustrate defenses as they are used in symptoms or compromises; stops 6 and 7 delineate circumstances where the defenses operate optimally to accomplish the most adaptive aims of the ego, and not as intrusions.

In making his ratings, the rater is instructed to rely not only on the specific questions designed to tap defensive functioning but on the person's *style* of responding to all questions throughout the interview. For example, pedantry in verbal behavior generally might tell more about how excessive the person's defensive functioning is than would a direct answer to a specific question about defenses.

Defensive Functioning

Stop	a	b
	Extent to which defense mechanisms, character defenses, and other defensive functioning have maladaptively affected ideation, behavior, and the adaptive level of other ego functions.	Extent to which defenses have succeeded or failed (e.g., degree of emergence of anxiety, depression, and/or other dysphoric affects).
1	Defense mechanisms and elements are among those in the general hierarchy of defense mechanisms that reflect least adaptation or are most pathological. Might be projection at its most extreme, manifest in broad delusional systems. Massive repression and denial might rule out any reflective thinking. Splitting mechanisms are prominent.	Massive failure and/or pathological misuse of defensive functioning, so that there is emergence of id derivatives and unconscious contents producing extreme anxiety, depression, or other dysphoric affect. Degree of anxiety and panic is extreme.
2	Rather extensive and inflexible use of primitive defenses (denial, splitting)	Considerable failure of defenses. Anxiety likely to be free-floating and unbound thus interferes with adaptive functioning to a

Stop	a	b

2 (Cont) are generalized in character and behavior. Affect storms usually defend against reflective thinking since thoughts may be potentially disturbing. Extreme uses of projection. Socially pathological forms of identification with the aggressor. Functioning has a highly defensive quality which interferes considerably with general adaptation.

significant degree. May be chronic depressive states. Feels as though he is falling apart.

3 Defenses analogous to "overcontrol" score here. May be extreme overideational defenses, such as isolation and intellectualization, where thought predominates over affect. May also be fairly pervasive projections, quasi delusions, perceptual vigilance, avoidance, evasions, severe inhibitions and ego restriction. Whatever the defenses, their effect is more maladaptive than adaptive.

Frequent breakthroughs of anxiety, depression, drive-related material, ego-alien thoughts, parapraxes. Free-floating anxiety of the sort seen in agoraphobia or claustrophobia. A pervasive feeling of vulnerability.

4 S may show evidence of rationalization, reaction-formation, transient projections, occasional parapraxes, and malapropisms. Also, symptomatic acting out (where action is a substitute for a repressed thought). Generally defensive behavior is fairly prominent.

Anxiety more likely to be bound in symptoms than free-floating. Tolerance for anxiety and other dysphoric states is not very good. When jumpy, upset, or anxious, means of protection and recovery do not come easily.

5 Some ability to adaptively relinquish or adaptively employ defensive operations, whatever they may be, except in situations that are characteristically conflictual for the individual.

Anxiety is present to a moderate degree; there is some tolerance for it, so that while it sometimes interferes with functioning, it need not do so markedly. May feel temporarily thrown but shows some adaptive resilience in recovery.

6 Defensive functioning, or the lack of it, is employed primarily in the service of adaptation with good resilience and recovery to nondefensive modes. An absence of excessive or insufficient use of defenses.

Anxiety present only when appropriate to situational stress and is well tolerated.

Defensive Functioning (Continued)

Stop	a	b
7	Only the most adaptive defensive elements are present (e.g., denial when in the service of adaptation to reality). The warding off of painful or dysphoric material is accomplished by recognizing, considering, making judgments and taking appropriate action about it. Defensive functions observable at this stop are in the service of adaptation to external events as well as involved in the resolution of intrapsychic conflict. Under conditions of stress, there is minimal disruption of other ego functions by defensive functioning.	Access to unconscious contents and id derivatives does not produce disruption and/or anxiety.

IX. STIMULUS BARRIER

Instructions to Raters. Both thresholds and responses to stimuli contribute to adaptation by the organism's potential for responding to high, average, or low sensory input, so that optimal homeostasis (as well as adaptation) is maintained. Stimulus barrier determines, in part, how resilient a person is or how he readapts after the stress and impingements are no longer present.

Thresholds, as described in component a, refer not only to reaction to external stimuli but also to internal stimuli that provide proprioceptive cues or those originating within the body but eventually impinging on sensory organs. Light, sound, temperature, pain, pressure, drugs, and intoxicants are the stimuli to be considered relevant to assessing thresholds. Responses to varying degrees of stimulation from people are assessed in the object-relations scale. Stimulus barrier focuses on inaminate stimuli.

Responses other than sensory threshold (component a) include motor responses, coping mechanisms, effects on sleep, and mood (component b).

Stimulus Barrier

Stop	a	b
	Threshold for, sensitivity to, or registration of external and internal stimuli impinging upon various sensory modalities (corresponds to "receptive function").	Degree of adaptation, organization, and integration of responses to various levels of sensory stimulation. The effectiveness of "coping mechanisms" in relation to degree of sensory stimulation—whether observed in

Stop	a	b
		motor behavior, affective response, or cognition.

Stop	a	b
1	Extremely low thresholds to most or all sensory stimuli. Awareness of sensory impingements may be hyperacute. Sensitivity to subliminal incidental or peripheral stimulation is also extremely acute. Or thresholds may be exceedingly low with no awareness (i.e., S is hypersensitive, but doesn't know to what, such as noise, that he doesn't hear").	Coping modes reflect vulnerability and lack of ego integration through hyperkinetic or chaotic type of motor discharge patterns. May be aimless flailing about under conditions of even mild sensory stimulation. Sensory stimulation may lead to sleep disturbances, "psychosomatic spill-over" or possibly migraine headaches. Excessive response to drugs and intoxicants. Noise, light, crowds, multiple stimuli produce disorganized reactions.
2	Very low thresholds to most sensory stimuli. Quite aware of minor bodily changes. High, low, and relatively small changes in temperature produce considerable discomfort. Noise may produce a diffuse excitability, and too much light may cause agitation. May or may not know source of discomfort.	S often feels like "jumping out of his skin." Adaptive efforts at keeping stimulation low or minimizing one's reactions to it are very poor. Severe insomnia may reflect poor response to high sensory stimulation. Women may experience high degree of premenstrual tension and agitation. Adaptive behavior is largely immobilized because attention and efforts are riveted on the experience of overstimulation. The fabled "princess and the pea."
3	Thresholds to most sensory stimuli are quite low. About average sensitivity to "irrelevant," peripheral, or incidental stimuli. Cold, heat, noise, bright lights are very bothersome. May hear, see, and smell things that the average person would not be aware of. There may be a stimulus-seeking or stimulus-hunger. Paradoxically, S may enjoy being "turned on" despite his hypersensitivity and excitability.	Less chaotic motor discharge and more general irritability. Adaptive efforts at "filtering" stimulation are relatively ineffective. Disorganization or withdrawal may follow upon exposure to strong stimuli. Can stick with adaptive tasks for only a short time with sensory overload. Sleep patterns are irregular. May react with headaches in response to stimuli. Adaptive efforts while "turned on" are not very effective. In women, premenstrual tension may take the form of extreme irritability
4	Thresholds to sensory stimuli from fairly low to average and a bit above. S may be sensitive to specific noises but not to others or to light. Or flashing lights would be bothersome but steady daylight quite tolerable. Specific stimulus hungers	While occasionally irritable, grumpy, or annoyed by the circumscribed range of distressing stimuli, S is able to contain his responses to stimulation fairly adaptively. He may grin and bear it despite inner irritability, although the effort thus expended may lead to fatigue and/or relatively poor recovery and

Stimulus Barrier (Continued)

Stop	a	b
4 (Cont)	may be noted. May or may not be aware of source of stimulation.	adaptive resilience. Adaptive behavior is only moderately disrupted by peripheral or incidental stimuli. May seek solitude and then have some difficulty returning to a more stimulating environment.
5	S has moderately high sensory thresholds in most modalities. Only very strong central or focal stimuli would be bothersome. Peripheral and average range of light, sound, temperature, inner states would not be experienced as troublesome or offensive. When stimuli are bothersome, S tends to be aware of what the stimuli are.	A reasonably good balance between discharge and control patterns in the face of high levels of stimulus input. When there are motor-discharge reactions, they may be fairly even, or when more explosive, S is resilient and able to compose himself relatively soon after exposure to strong, potentially disruptive stimuli. Many adaptive activities can be carried out despite level of sensory stimulation. Appears to "ride the waves" somewhat comfortably, even in the middle of "5 o'clock mayhem" or a boisterous party.
6	Somewhat flexible and automatic fluctuations in thresholds to stimuli within a reasonably high range. Good "screening mechanism" to permit adequate input and avoid sensory overload (e.g., S is receptive to mild noises, unruffled by loud ones. Sensitivity to subliminal and peripheral stimuli varies adaptively with the situation.	Coping modes, including motor discharge patterns, are reasonably flexible. Sleeps well without need for oblivion and defensive withdrawal from stimuli.
7	Very flexible, automatic fluctuations in thresholds to stimuli. Thresholds appear to be high. There is an optimal "screening mechanism."	Flexible, automatic responses to all degrees of stimulation. There is an optimally smooth operation of responses. Person is reasonably comfortable with what to others is "sensory overload"; he sleeps well, adapts flexibly to all sensory impingements.

X. AUTONOMOUS FUNCTIONING

Instructions to Raters. Intrusion of conflict, ideation, affect, and/or impulse upon functioning is a major criterion for determining impairment of either the primary or the secondary autonomy.

The basic apparatuses and functions of primary autonomy are

perception   memory   language
intentionality   hearing   productivity
concentration   vision   motor development and
attention   speech   expression

Secondarily autonomous functions are more numerous and include most of the ego functions in this manual. We are therefore focusing the scoring of autonomous functioning on habit patterns, skills, routines, hobbies, and interests.

Autonomous Functioning

Stop	a	b
	Degree of freedom from impairment of apparatuses of primary autonomy (attention, concentration, memory, learning, perception, motor function, intention).	Degree of freedom from impairment of secondary autonomy (disturbances in habit patterns, learned complex skills, work routines, hobbies, and interests).
1	Severe interference with the functioning of one or more of the "apparatuses" of primary autonomy. Inability to concentrate or attend no matter how much effort is expended. Word use and pronunciation may be markedly impaired. Perceptually, there may be tunnel vision, loss of ability to estimate seen distances correctly. Motor coordination may be poor or interfered with. Efforts at willful performance are virtually ineffective.	Habit patterns, work habits, and/or learned skills of any kind are massively hampered so that person is unable to utilize most of these (e.g., a previously skilled worker who cannot carry out his job because the component activities have taken on sexual and aggressive meanings to a marked extent, showing minimal resistance to intrusions from instinctual drives or from the environment)
2	Interference with primary autonomous functions is significant. Examples may be selective visual scotoma; serious interference with intentionality or "will"; grave difficulties in motor coordination or in mobilizing one's self to exercise ordinary motor functions. Attention, concentration, and learning suffer considerable impairment.	Complex skills and habits are interfered with to a serious degree (e.g., a housewife's previously automatically accomplished routine tasks are no longer carried through effectively). Even with maximal effort, performance in learned, automatic tasks falls short of minimal adequacy. "Writer's cramp" might be another example if it is severe without being totally disabling. Experience of extreme lack of energy.
3	Interference with primary autonomous functions is moderately high. Illusory experiences may be fairly prominent in thinking and perception. There may be blurred vision when reading school assignments, novels with general sexual	Skills, habits, and automatic behavior are interfered with to a moderately high degree, so that much effort must be expended to perform tasks previously automatic and routine. Ongoing complex behavior may be easily disrupted when drive-related ideas,

Autonomous Functioning (Continued)

Stop	a	b
3 (Cont)	content, or whatever material may be upsetting to the particular individual concerned. Similarly, concentration and attention may be impaired while reading any emotionally charged material.	affects, or stimuli intrude. Work may be impaired by intruding sexual or aggressive fantasies. Some difficulty with routine activities like dressing or walking.
4	Disturbance of primary autonomous functions to a moderate degree. Vision, motor behavior, language, intention, etc., could suffer from the intrusion of circumscribed aggressive and sexual thoughts, feelings, and fantasies.	Secondary autonomous habits, patterns, and skills are interfered with to a moderately low degree. Greater than usual effort must be expended to carry out routine tasks and work only when these become associated with circumscribed conflict areas. Such conflict-related intrusions do not occur frequently. S may sometimes get tongue-tied, physically awkward.
5	Primary autonomous functions may be interfered with by drive derivatives to a mild, but noticeable, degree (e.g., occasional stuttering, mind-wandering, forgetting of names and some remote and recent events.	Moderate resistance to intrusions upon secondary autonomous habits and skills. When interferences do occur, some extra effort is required to perform work previously done with little strain. Occasionally, it may be hard just to "get going."
6	Structures of primary autonomy are interfered with rarely or only to a minor degree, as under extreme stress. Might stumble over words when in a hurry or under great pressure.	Habit patterns and skills are utilized with relative ease or with relatively minor interference except under extreme stress. Good resistance to intrusions upon skills and work patterns, when these intrusions have the potential to interfere with ongoing work. Energy level is reasonably high.
7	Minimal interference with structures of primary autonomy by drive interference or other intrusions. Attention, concentration, memory, perception, and will function optimally in accordance with the person's potential.	There is high resistance to intrusions from instinctual drives and environmental influences among secondary autonomous functions. Habits and skills are carried on with ease and flexibility despite inner and outer pressure. Great energy level and productivity.

XI. SYNTHETIC-INTEGRATIVE FUNCTIONING

This ego function fulfills one of the major tasks of the ego as defined by Freud, in terms of reconciling the often conflicting demands of the id, superego, and outside world, as well as the incongruities within the ego. We focus on the reconciling of areas that are in conflict and also on the extent of relating together areas that are not in conflict.

Synthetic-Integrative Functioning

Stop	a	b
	Degree of reconciliation or integration of discrepant or potentially contradictory attitudes, values, affects, behavior, and self-representations.	Degree of *active* relating together (i.e., integrating) of both intrapsychic and behavioral events. These events may or may not be conflict-ridden and are not necessarily limited to behavior.
1	S has minimal ability to reconcile contradictions (e.g., the content of his thought may remain opposite to the quality of the accompanying feeling, and S is at best puzzled by the discrepancy). Certain aspects of identity and self-feeling may be dissociated from others, as in multiple personality. Maximal intolerance for ambiguity or incongruity in external events might be seen in adopting extremist points of view that oversimplify, in accordance with the S's inability to grasp a unity underlying surface contradictions. May be large discrepancy between affect display and behavior or thoughts (e.g., laughing when telling bad news).	S cannot cope with more than one task at a time. He needs to stay on "one track." If he is absorbed in one simple task and a second is introduced, he cannot cope with the second: he might either cling rigidly to the first or become so disorganized that any active coping behavior is minimal. Active, adaptive connection-making among different aspects of experience is nil. For example, S is virtually unable to utilize relevant past experience toward the solution of current problems. The ability to first plan and then carry out activities according to that plan is nil, especially when that planning and activity involve the organization of two or more elements of behavior. There might be rapid fluctuation of moods due to poorly integrated sense of continuity about what produced one mood or another. Fragmentation in the extreme.
2	Only a slight degree of synthesis and integration of disparate aspects of experience, behavior and self-representations, S experiences most events as fragmented, ambiguous and contradictory. He may say that he opposes violence yet regularly engage in violent behavior. Apparent contradictions are experienced as very distressing.	Only a small degree of active effort can be expended in relating different aspects of experience. The relation of past experience and events to present experience and behavior is rarely used in solving current problems. Disorganization in daily living is typical. Life is a lot of bits and pieces and loose ends that S cannot tie together.
3	Significant indications of unintegrated ego functioning. May be no consistent life goals, very divergent sets of career and future plans. S is puzzled by apparent contradictions	Quite difficult to carry out more than one project or activity at a time—even simple ones. Not adequately organized in daily life, but simple activities can be carried out reliably enough. Organizational efforts show

Stop	a	b
3 (Cont)	and ambiguities. May belong to or support "extremist" political groups. May be breakthroughs of opposing attitudes and beliefs.	fragmented or piecemeal results (e.g., living from day to day rather than following an overall directional plan).
4	Some areas of potential contradiction are reconciled while others remain unintegrated (e.g., may be moderately difficult to tolerate feelings of love and hate directed at the same person or to integrate disparate aspects of his personality into a unified identity). Outbursts reflecting lack of integration may occur (e.g., uncontrollable laughing during a tragic time).	Active efforts to relate different aspects of experience are only moderately successful. Purposeful, planned activities can be carried out, but considerable trouble results in S's attempts to keep up with the demands of everyday life for organization. Because of a defect in carrying through, or in tolerating unexpected intrusions into routines, he may be chronically quite far behind in meeting obligations and deadlines. Things are often left undone, S may either not care or be extremely concerned because of his difficulties in getting them done.
5	Major areas of the personality show a fair degree of consistency (e.g., there may be reasonable harmony between behavior and affect), but there are periodic exceptions of inconsistent attitudes, values, affects, and behavior. The inconsistencies are occasionally experienced as troublesome (e.g., some conflict in adopting apparently contradictory roles: being a follower one day, a leader the next.	Active efforts to reconcile different areas of experience in the service of adaptation show periodic lapses, as does carrying out purposeful activities and meeting demands and commitments. May be thrown out of gear when unexpected demands for changes in routine occur but does eventually recover equilibrium.
6	Consistency and a fair degree of integration in the major sectors of the personality are found. There may be a few minor inconsistencies, as in behavior, affect, and thinking. Good tolerance for the inevitable inconsistencies and incongruities that may occur. Can retain sense of humor while doing serious work.	S shows effective, successful efforts to make causal connections between the different areas of his experiences. Behavior is generally well organized and S deals with integrative requirements with relatively little stress and strain. Social, sexual, and vocational areas are satisfactorily integrated. Can tie loose ends together but has no compulsion to do this, which may disrupt adaptation.
7	S shows high, but flexible, consistency and integration in thinking, feeling, and behavior. His attitudes and values cover a wide range of feeling and opinion, yet despite	S actively makes connections, causal or otherwise, between different aspects of his experience. He responds flexibly to complex problems and can cope with a great variety of tasks simultaneously, alternately and

526

Synthetic-Integrative Functioning (Continued)

Stop	a	b
7 (Cont)	apparent disparities, possess an underlying consistent unity.	automatically in both thought and behavior employed in the service of active problem-solving. He can easily shift "set" when required to do so. Plans are carried out with minimal stress, with the aid of rapid, automatic shifts in orientation (e.g., when things are not going according to a prearranged "blueprint". That is, when a second or unexpected "track" is introduced, the person can automatically incorporate its demands into goal-oriented behavior. He has a good sense of continuity about what caused one mood or another (e.g., he would stay in a bad mood for an appropriate time).

XII. MASTERY COMPETENCE

Instructions to Raters. Raters are asked to score competence and sense of competence separately, since a number of different relationships between the two are possible: (1) they may be congruent; (2) actual performance may exceed the sense of competence; (3) sense of competence may exceed mastery-competence. In addition, score -, =, or + for discrepancy score.

The specific environment and the limitations it imposes on the *form* of a person's competence should be carefully considered. A highly intelligent minority group person, for example, from a truly restrictive environment who performs a menial task skillfully would receive a higher score than his counterpart from an "advantaged" group performing the same work. Similarly, a well-educated housewife, realistically restricted to the rearing of four young children, would be rated in the context of competence within that role.

(1) Component c, the discrepancy score, reflects an aspect of self-esteem: that which has relevance only to actively mastering and affecting the environment. Thus, it should not overlap with all the other aspects of self-esteem, which are scored under the appropriate component factor of the ego function, sense of reality.

(2) The scaling of this ego function does not involve the desired degree of independence of all components. While component factors a and b are independent in the same manner as all other ego function components, component c differs radically. Component c, by definition, is the degree of dependence and *interaction* between the other two components. It perhaps will be the best indicator, among the three components, of mastery-competence as a whole.

There will be no global rating for mastery-competence. Each component *must* be rated separately, in order to get a discrepancy score (component c).

Mastery-Competence

Stop	a	b	c
	Competence. How well S actually performs in relation to his existing capacity to interact with and *actively* master and affect his environment.	The subjective role, or S's feeling of competence with respect to actively mastering and affecting his environment. S's expectations of success or actual performance (How he feels about how he does and what he can do). Sense of competence is scored *at face value* (e.g., higher than actual competence if there is an exaggerated sense of competence).	The degree of discrepancy between component a and component b (i.e., between actual competence and sense of competence). It may be negative (−), as when actual competence exceeds sense of competence. It may be equal (=), when actual competence and sense of competence are congruent. It may be positive (+), when sense of competence exceeds actual competence, as in a grandiose, exaggerated sense of competence compared with performance.
1	S does almost nothing with respect to altering, affecting, or interacting with his environment, because he is largely unable to utilize abilities and capacities in relation to reality. What minimal apparently effective action might be seen results merely from passive reacting rather than active coping.	The sense of competence is almost nil, and S feels powerless to act effectively in most ways, independently of his actual performance.	Discrepancy score may be either −, =, or +. Minus or plus discrepancies would be extremely high. Where +, sense of competence is grossly overinflated.
2	S is able to make only minimal efforts in coping with the environment. Prototypically, he waits for things to happen, rather than take an active role in effecting their occurence	Sense of competence is only minimally or sporadically present, so that any realistic effectuality is experienced as "luck" or "fate."	Discrepancy score may be −, =, or +; when + or − it will be so to a very high degree.
3	Successful interactions with the environment	A rather low sense of competence, as among	Discrepancy score may be −, =, or +. When − or + it

Stop	a	b	c
3	come primarily from passive mastery or passive manipulation of people. Typical might be the "underachieving" college student with very high aptitudes who has coasted along and then falls progressively **lower** in his achievements as more active efforts to master are actually required. Tools and skills have been poorly mastered.	severely masochistic people who suffer ego restrictions and the concomitantly low sense of effectuality (e.g., S may seek employment for which he is overqualified).	will be so to a rather high degree.
4	Mastery is partial: sometimes passive, sometimes active. Active efforts, however, will probably be directed toward getting others to achieve the desired outcomes rather than through direct coping or altering. Other stumbling blocks to mastery might be caused by restricting activity due to fears of failure, rejection, risk-taking, etc.	Sense of competence may be somewhat low because S devaluates his own efforts, no matter how effective they actually are. This devaluation may be caused by low esteem, guilt, masochism, poor sense of reality, fear of envy.	Discrepancy score may be −, =, or +. When − or + it will be so to a somewhat high degree.
5	Performance level is high a good part of the time, but in limited areas there may be some underachievement and lapses in competence (e.g., S in psychotherapy might have achieved maximal insight about conflict areas but delays exerting his own energy to actually work through and resolve the conflicts). At this level might also be the exaggerated "do-it-yourself" person whose need for active mastery is inordinate	Sense of competence is somewhat more likely to be high than low.	Discrepancy score may be −, =, or +. More likely to be = at this level than at previous ones. When − or + it will be so to a small degree. When −, poor self-appraisal in relation to actual effectiveness.

Mastery Competence (Continued)

Stop	a	b	c
5 (Cont)	and who fears relinquishing overcompensated efforts because he feels the competing passive tendencies.		
6	Actual competence and efforts at active mastery of the environment are quite high with only occasional lapses.	Sense of competence is usually quite high. S is aware of the successes he achieves in altering the environment in his own interests.	Discrepancy score is most likely to be =. Any + or − score is very slight.
7	The prototype here is the "do-it-yourself" person who is unusually resourceful at actively coping with, mastering and altering the environment effectively in the service of adaptation. He performs appropriately in his environmental context, or in harmony with the facilities and limitations of his environment and constitutional endowment.	Subjective sense of competence is maximally high. S feels extraordinarily able to affect and master his environment.	Discrepancy score will be =.

SUPEREGO SCALES

General Considerations

Below you will find three sections relating to superego functioning:

(1) a listing of how superego factors may interfere with each of the ego functions;

(2) a description of the dimension inconsistency-consistency of superego functioning;

(3) a scale of overall superego adaptation (13-points with half stops).

The rating sheet will provide a 4-point scale for rating interference with ego functions; a 7-point scale for rating adaptation; and a 4-point scale for rating consistency.

It seemed important enough to rate interference with ego functions specifically and also to evaluate the dimension consistency-inconsistency.

The third scale represents superego adaptiveness-maladaptiveness from an overall viewpoint. Adaptiveness-maladaptiveness is for practical purposes identical with strength of the superego. It is important to keep in mind the difference between strength and severity in this context. An overly severe superego is often maladaptive and, from that standpoint, not better than a very weak superego (compare the fact that excessive defenses are as pathological as defective ones).

Rating interference of the superego with ego functions and consistency-inconsistency should make overall superego rating easier. A superego that interferes with ego functions and is inconsistent is hardly a strong or adaptive superego. In that sense, the overall rating should reflect the detailed ratings, above and beyond the specification in the rating stops provided for general guidance.

Interference of Superego Factors with Ego Functions

Reality Testing
Strong underlying hostility, in conjunction with a superego that "prevents" direct awareness of the hostility, can result in projection of the hostility and thereby interfere with reality testing.

Judgment
Judgment can be interfered with by a mechanism similar to that described above for reality testing, as when action is taken relevant to defective awareness.

Sense of Reality
(1) Feelings of depersonalization, an important disturbance in the sense of self, can result from underlying guilt over strong hostility. (2) Both guilt and shame can affect S's sense of self.

Object Relations
(1) Projection of severe superego attitudes – blaming, faultfinding, and so on – can vitally affect object relations. (2) A weak superego, associated with irresponsibility, unfairness, cheating, taking advantage of, and so on, also can be seen to vitally affect an individual's interpersonal relations. (3) A superego response-prohibition to experienced aggression can result in withdrawal from another person.

Thought Processes
(1) Obsessive thought mechanisms may be a result of superego prohibition of aggressive and/or sexual drive derivatives. (2) Indecisiveness or obsessive doubting can result from the unconscious idea that decisiveness constitutes destructive aggressive behavior.

ARISE
This function requires becoming aware of more primitive, sexual, aggressive, and

forbidden contents. Individuals with severe superego would be expected to have difficulty in controlled regressions.

Defensive Functioning

A severe superego will tend to be associated with excessive use of defensive operations. Some defensive maneuvers are directed primarily against superego contents.

Stimulus Barrier

(1) Strong voyeuristic trends, when "disapproved" by a superego, can result in disturbances in vision and headaches (Greenacre, 1947). The same appears to be true in the auditory sphere. (2) High hostility in conjunction with superego blocking can result in projection of hostility and consequent vigilance and sensitization. Depressives often manifest high sensitivity to noise, which may reflect the above mechanism. Insomniacs may also illustrate the above mechanism: fear of aggression and of being attacked at night is often found.

Autonomous Functioning

Reading disabilities may involve an invasion of voyeuristic trends. Writing cramp can occur where phallic or hostile trends intrude. The general formulation here is (1) the autonomous functioning becomes libidinized, (2) superego prohibitions ensue, and (3) ego functioning is interfered with or inhibited by superego prohibitions.

Synthetic-Integrative Functioning

Superego gaps will be manifest in low synthetic functioning.

Interference of superego factors with ego functions will be rated on a four-point scale: severe (1), moderate (2), mild (3), negligible (4).

Scale of Superego Adaptation

Stop	a	b
	Guilt and blame, including: 1. degree of self-directed punishment for aggressive and libidinal drive expression; 2. transformations and displacements of unconscious guilt; 3. degree of blame-avoidance; 4. degree to which talion principle (desire for revenge for wrongs) operates; 5. extent to which guilt feelings are reality-based.	Ego-ideal status, including: 1. extent of realistic evaluation of ego goals and strivings; 2. sense of worth; 3. self-esteem regulation.
1	Highest degree of self-punishment	Ego's goals are excessively disproportionate

Stop	a	b

1 (Cont)	for aggressive and libidinal drive expression. Suicidal behavior may be associated with extreme depression. Transformations of guilt may be seen in extreme projection, reaction-formation, and denial of wishes. Placing and avoiding blame are paramount characteristics of life style. Demands for strict conformity to rules may be as high for others as for self. Guilt is predominantly unrealistically based.	to S's abilities. Extreme self-criticism where S regards himself and his actions as bad and unworthy. Standards for performance and achievement are archaic and ruthlessly primitive. Examples are strivings for ultimate perfection in all areas without regard for whether such maximal performance can be realistically expected of him or anyone.
2	*For severe superego*: Self directed punishment short of suicidal behavior. May be self-mutilation, conviction that he has an incurable disease. Real source of guilt may be masked by delusional guilt, as of chronic, undeserved persecution by others. Delusions about committing unpardonable sins. *For weak superego:* No conscience or guilt feelings, whether realistic or not. Psychopathic personality or impulse ridden personality in the extreme. Lax or indulgent standards of responsibility to self and others.	*For severe ego-ideal*: Overly strict and unrealistic standards of goal achievement for self and others. Poor sense of worth may be manifest in great self-abnegation and denial. *For weak ego-ideal*: Highly indifferent as to own performance, strivings and life goals.
3	*For severe superego*: Rigid, authoritarian attitudes about sex and aggression in self and others. Guilt may be transformed into experiences of fear and hate. Characteristically attributes blame to self and others, and tries to avoid inner and outer signs of it. May be over concerned with minutiae in assuming obligations in order to avoid blame and criticism. *For weak superego*: Quite lax with respect to impulses and urges. May be concerned with consequences to self but not to others. More likely to see evidences of shame than guilt.	*For severe ego-ideal*: Unrealistically critical self-observations with respect to achievements and successes. Severe self-criticism could alternate with overinflated sense of worth. Generally hypercritical of others in areas of achievement and ideals. *For weak ego-ideal*: Self-indulgence and careless self-evaluations. Overly lax and lenient about standards for self and others.

Stop	a	b
4	*For severe superego*: Sizable "puritan" streak in moral judgments of self and others. May be "do-gooder" type of person as reaction-formation against opposite wishes. Overconscientious; seeks moderate infractions of rules and standards. Tendency to protest innocence and blamelessness too much. *For weak superego*: Happy-go-lucky type; overly glib when can't meet responsibilities. Somewhat too casual.	Perfectionism in many areas of self and self-goals often interferes with adaptation.
5	S overcautiously anticipates or offers criticism for mistakes. Some guilt feelings can be tolerated or lived with. Some occasional alteration of behavior or environment to eliminate the source of guilt feelings may occur. Occasional defensive behavior (e.g., compulsiveness, displacement, projection) to deal with guilt over impulses, wishes, and deeds. Or, can role play acceptable, responsible behavior without much internal pressure to do so.	Somewhat perfectionistic or somewhat lax in living up to ideals. Sense of worth may suffer only with respect to a feeling of falling short of own (and others') expectations in circumscribed areas. The areas may have to do either with work, certain social relationships, marriage, but never all of them.
6	Reasonably strong superego—neither too strict nor too lenient. Realistically based guilt feelings serve primarily as a signal to reinforce fair-minded behavior. Assertive behavior and sexual gratifications are rarely interfered with by guilt and remorse and are undertaken with a sense of responsibility toward self and others.	Reasonably realistic approval of ego's actions in terms of current and future consequences. Aspirations are harmonious with achievement capacity. Self-esteem regulation is internalized and not merely dependent on current feedback from others.
7	Guilt feelings, if any, are realistically based and do not impede adaptation. A realistic orientation toward rectifying errors where possible and tolerance of past mistakes is noted to the exclusion of blame, worrying, recriminations. No transformations	Ego-ideal corresponds closely to ego functioning potential. Self-evaluation and sense of worth are based on optimally reality-oriented self-observations.

Scale of Superego Adaptation (Continued)

Stop	a	b
7	or displacements are observed. S is flexibly accepting or rejecting of others, depending on considerations.	

Inconsistency-Consistency Ratings

The rater is also to rate the S on a four-point scale for integration and consistency of superego functioning:

1. Most maladaptive: extreme inconsistencies between behavior and standards, between standards, or between segments of behavior. "Swiss cheese" or corrupt, gap-ridden superego.
2. Tending toward maladaptive.
3. Tending toward adaptive.
4. Most adaptive: optimally unified superego. Relatively few contradictions between standards and behavior, between standards, or between different segments of behavior.

ID SCALES (DRIVE STRENGTH)

Instructions to Raters: Below are two scales: (A) rating strength of libidinal drive, and (B) rating strength of aggressive drive manifestations. We are attempting to rate instinctual drive derivatives and have used both behavioral and ideational reactions as criteria from which we can observe directly or make inferences about drive strength. A major difficulty with the scale is distinguishing behavior that is the result of high drive strength per se from apparent manifestations of drive strength that are a function of such various ego factors as lack of judgment about where drives are expressed or object-relations difficulties that determine maladaptive forms of drive expression. We shall attempt to take account of this source of unclarity by the specific scale-stop descriptions and by the way the id scales are constructed in relation to the regulation-and-control scale.

These two id scales differ specifically from the ego function scales in one important structural respect. Stop 3 in the scales for both libidinal and aggressive manifestations represents the highest drive strength, and stop 6 represents the lowest. Stop 0 would be considered as approaching "average." This ordering stands in obvious contrast to the ego scales in which stop 1 is low, 6 is average, and 7 is optimal. These are scales of drive strength, not ego adaptation.

On the rating sheet, an opportunity will also be provided to judge, on a 4-point scale, the extent to which libidinal and aggressive drives are sublimated and neutralized, 4 being optimal. For purposes of scaling, we will not differentiate between neutralization and sublimation. For a discussion of the concepts, see chapter on autonomous functioning.

A. Rating of Sublimation-Neutralization

One reflects minimal libidinal or aggressive sublimation-neutralization. There is behavioral evidence of any or many of the components, especially of pregenital, libidinal behavior, privately and (sometimes inappropriately) publicly. Perversions are the classical pathology of lack of sublimation. Psychotic behavior may involve smearing of feces, ingestion of any material, and so on. Classical lack of neutralization of aggression appears as major acting out in violent ways.

Two might represent unsuccessful ways of sublimation and neutralization as in primitive gratifications of oral drives, for instance, in gross obesity and anhedonia resulting from poor object relations, and poor neutralization of aggression in socially unacceptable voyeurism, such as spending much time in looking into apartment windows with a telescope.

Three would be consistent with isolated areas of failure of sublimation, such as inappropriate libidinization of flying and other customary activities resulting in anxieties that are troublesome but present in many people. Episodic failure of neutralization of aggression manifesting itself sometimes under stress in minor tics or frequent breakage of glassware or other accident-prone behavior might be suitable examples. Characterological manifestations might be, on the one hand, in the area of private indulgences in more pregenital behavior than is customary or, on the other, in such aggressive outlets as are not entirely socially accepted in some subcultures, as hunting or serving as a guard in a penal institution with chances for occasional breakthroughs of sadism.

Four represents a high degree of neutralization of aggression, as found in a surgeon, for instance, who treats his patients with utmost care, including their psychological sensitivities, without any breakthroughs of the original sadistic desires in any form of his behavior. A similar level of sublimation of voyeurism is attained professionally in well-functioning psychoanalysts or experimenters-for instance, microbiologists who might also have an interest in art.

B. Indications of Aggressive Drive Strength

This is a unipolar scale in which only presence-absence of aggressive drive manifestations is dimensionalized. Love, passivity, or any of the traditionally considered opposites do not here constitute the extremes indicating relative absence of aggressive drive.

Libidinal Drive Strength
(a,b,c,d,e = components)

Stop	a	b	c	d	e
	Overt sexual behavior: includes frequency and intensity of heterosexual contacts, intercourse, masturbation, pregenital behavior, homosexuality, perversions, etc. Only overt sexual *acts* are included in this category.	Associated and substitute sexual behavior: includes behavior short of overt sexual acts. Relevant behavior here would be voyeurism, exhibitionism, flirting, choice of occupation, hobbies and interests, and associated aspects of oral and anal and other pregenitally based behavior, as well as associated aspects of genital behavior.	Fantasies and other ideation: includes verbalization about sex; daydreams with overt or associated sexual content; sexualized ideational activities, such as reading pornography. Also includes inferences about unconscious fantasies other than dreams.	Dreams: includes frequency and intensity of any kind of sexual content in both the manifest dream and the latent dream thoughts.	Symptoms, defenses, and controls: this category is included only insofar as actual libidinal drive strength may be *inferred* from strength of counter-cathectic measures employed against it (e.g., impotence, frigidity or avoidance of sex would be strong indicators only if they reflect S's way of dealing with excessive sexual pushes). Repression would be a defense especially relevant to libidinal drive strength
+3	Overt sexual activity at its most excessive extreme. Sexual mode (e.g., intercourse, masturbation, fellatio, homosexuality) and selection of partner may be indiscriminate owing to *pressure of urges* (as opposed to a primary disturbance	Associated sexual activity at its most excessive extreme. May be public disrobing, exhibitionistic advances on subway, gluttony and obesity, drug addiction, and rituals like smearing feces, inappropriate rubbing of self and	Almost total preoccupation and/or fantasy about sexual matters; frequent reading of pornography, which nearly obliterates concern with other life issues.	Sexual themes in dreams extremely prominent — if not in manifest content, then in latent dream thoughts. Dreams contain almost no other content	Impotence, frigidity or blocking with respect to libidinal issues in the extreme so that *sexual behavior is markedly incapacitated*. When controls, defenses and symptoms are extreme, it is because of drive. With poor controls, may be symptoms of excessive sexual acting out.

537

Libidinal Drive Strength
(a,b,c,d,e, = components)

Stop	a	b	c	d	e
	in object relations or judgment). This pressure may, for example, be due to an excessive constitutional strength of the instincts. Activity is so frequent as to interfere markedly with other areas of functioning. Rape, etc., may lead to arrest.	others. Occupation may be stripteaser or other sexually oriented work, independent of the degree of primitivity or sublimation.			
+2	Excessive overt sexual activity. Frequent intercourse and masturbation, etc., where pressure of urges still makes it difficult to channel behavior appropriately.	Pronounced associated sexual behavior, such as concern with body preening, seductiveness, erotization of relatively nonsexual situations.	Very pronounced sexual preoccupation in *thoughts and fantasy*, except where very strong competing "pulls" prevent this.	Many dreams have sexual themes in manifest content and latent thoughts.	Symptoms, defenses and controls related to libidinal issues pronounced but not totally incapacitating.
+1	Intercourse, masturbation and other direct sexual activity more pronounced than	Associate or substitute behavior shows more than average concern with bodily functions,	Above average amount of sexual thought and fantasy.	More than average, but not excessive, number of "sex" dreams.	While not incapacitating or excessive specific symptoms, defenses or anxiety are elicited by

	average. Pressure of urges greater than usual.	contact needs, enjoyment of food and excretory activity. Above average seductiveness, interest in appearance for sexual reasons. More than average sexual motivation can be ascribed to choice of occupation and hobbies.			libidinal issues. Symptom-formation only sometimes replaces overt sexual behavior.
0	Intercourse and masturbation, etc., are moderately frequent. Promiscuity more likely to come from object-relations problems than from extreme pressure of urges.	Some seductiveness and flirting, but could not be considered out of bounds.	Moderate amount of preoccupation and fantasy about sexual matters.	Some dreams with sexual content.	Anxiety, symptoms, defenses, etc., occur in circumscribed situations indicating moderate strength of drive in need of defending against;
-1	Intercourse and masturbation and other overt sexual activity occur with less than average intensity and less than average overall urge toward sexuality.	Associated behavior, such as interest in appearance, bodily contact, and seductiveness are less than would be expected as compared with others of his age and his	Sexual fantasies only occasionally intrude upon thought. When they do, they relate more to associated than direct sexual activities.	Very few dreams have sexual content.	No specific symptomatic reactions can be readily associated with sexual urges, but there may be some occasional defensive operations or diffuse anxiety about sexual matters.

Libidinal Drive Strength
(a,b,c,d,e = components)

Stop	a	b	c	d	e
		situations. There may be some remote libidinal motivation in choice of hobbies or occupation.			
-2	Overt sexual activity of any kind is rare, even under conditions extremely stimulating to the average person. S experiences very little spontaneous or induced stimulation.	Associated sexual behavior is also rare. Coolness verging on frigidity in social contacts is typical, as opposed to warmth and seductiveness, which characterize strong drive. Hobbies and occupation have little sexual relevance, even taking neutralization and sublimation into account.	Sexual fantasies almost never intrude upon thought and they are rarely volitionally entertained.	Sexual content in dreams almost never occurs.	No symptoms and almost no defensive operations, controls, or anxiety relevant to sexual matters from which we could infer pressure of sexual drive.
-3	Overt sexual activity of any sort is almost never observed, and would thus appear *burnt out or dead*. Actual and psychological celibacy.	Practically no associated sexual behavior is observed. Occupation interests and hobbies imply a bland or "dead" basis to libidinal motivations.	No clear evidence of sexual fantasies.	No evident sexual content in dreams.	No symptoms, defenses, or controls are present to suggest significant underlying libidinal urges.

Aggressive Drive Strength
(a,b,c,d,e = components)

Stop	a	b	c	d	e
	Overt aggressive behavior: includes prominence and intensity of direct physical acts of aggression toward self, others, and inanimate objects, resulting from *pressure of destructive urges*.	Associated and substitute aggressive behavior: includes verbal expressions; various forms of primitive or more developed behavior associated with aggressive drives; degree of aggression associated with interests, hobbies, and occupation; behavioral manifestations other than direct physical acts of violence.	Fantasies and other ideation: includes conscious and unconscious thoughts and fantasies with aggressive content of any sort.	Dreams: frequency and intensity of aggressive content of any sort in both manifest dream and latent dream thoughts.	Symptoms, defenses, and controls: this category is included only insofar as actual aggressive drive strength may be inferred from strength of counter-cathectic measures employed against it. Especially relevant would be defenses of projection and reaction-formation, and severe or rigid superego formation to deal with guilt where they reflect underlying aggression.
+3	Overt aggressive activity most prominent and intense. Attempts to assault, murder, and destroy. The most extreme degree and kind of self-mutilation. May incite riots and throw bombs.	At this stop we would also generally expect sexual drive-derivative behavior to be fused with aggression. Intense sadomasochism as a drive component of object-relations; verbal abuse accompanied by the most extreme rage:	Fantasies about aggressive acts at their most frequent and intense level. "Morbid" preoccupation with death, murder, cruelty and wish to violently inflict harm.	Aggressive themes in dreams extremely prominent in manifest content and latent dream thoughts.	Symptoms, controls, defenses imply the highest level of aggression; all-persuasive delusions of persecution; withdrawal in the extreme to avoid killing.

Aggressive Drive Strength
(a,b,c,d,e = components)

Stop	a	b	c	d	e
+2	Excessive overt aggressive activity. Physical injury short of death inflicted on self and others results from pressure of destructive urges. Chronic suicide attempts. Arson and extreme assaultiveness may be common.	interests in violence, torture, and genocide. Occupation may be professional hangman, career military man with expressed preference for hand-to-hand combat. May talk about needs to destroy and devour. Interests may include hunting for the purpose of maiming; intense interest in offensive military strategy and tactics; all of these independent of the degree of adaptation but related only to strength of drive (not overlooking the fact that when drive strength is extreme, there may be little adaptation possible). Intense need to	Very pronounced aggressive thoughts and fantasies, often with others instead of the self, inflicting the harm.	Aggressive elements in dreams very prominent in manifest content and latent thoughts.	Symptoms, controls, defenses imply a very high level of aggression. Encapsulated delusions of persecution; extreme work or activity blocks; convulsive disorders with psychomotor rage equivalents.

	engage in competitive sports such as boxing, wrestling, Judo or karate to exclusion of other interests. May enjoy threatening strangers over the telephone.	More than average but not excessive number of aggressive dreams.	While not incapacitating or excessive, specific symptoms, defenses, or anxiety are elicited by aggressive issues. Somewhat exaggerated forms of protest against war, such as compulsive participation in protest marches; fiery missionary zeal for helping oppressed people; hand-washing and cleaning compulsions. Some oversensitivity to hostility or rejection by others.
+1	Overt acts of aggression more frequently intense than average. Presence of physical assaultiveness with intent to harm but not kill. Suicide gestures. Pressures of urges strong.	Associated or substitute behavior shows more than average concern with destruction. Hostile punning, witty repartee, self-righteous preaching are favored modes of verbal communication. Occupational choice may be lawyer, policeman. Interests may include hunting, competitive sports such as sportscar racing, football.	Above average amount of hostile and aggressive thought and fantasy, but these not totally intrusive or persuasive. Enjoys reading pulp stories and seeing monster movies.	

543

Aggressive Drive Strength
(a,b,c,d,e = components)

Stop	a	b	c	d	e
0	May be angered or enraged when sufficiently provoked and express this anger within average limits. Occasional self-chastisement or other self-directed aggression, such as moral masochism.	Humor contains average amount of aggression. Occasional biting sarcasm. Interest and/or participation in competitive sports; enjoyment of skiing, tennis, racing. Competes actively for jobs. Would be good soldier if drafted to defend country. Other interests coexist with aggression-ridden ones.	Moderate amount of fantasy about aggressive matters.	Some dreams with aggressive content.	Anxiety, symptoms, and defenses, etc. are sporadic and limited to circumscribed areas of conflict over aggressive drives indicating lower strength of drive in need of defending against.
-1	Overt expressions of aggression toward self and others are less frequent and intense than average. S's general vitality might seem less than average.	S ignores (although does not "make a point" of staying away from) many activities with aggressive connotations. If a pacifist, would have no particular interest in speaking out against aggression or in proselytizing.	Less than average fantasy about aggressive matters. When they do occur, they are easily relinquished and never significantly intrude upon other thinking.	Very few dreams have aggressive content.	No specific symptomatic reactions can be readily associated with aggressive urges, but there may be some occasional defensive operations or diffuse anxiety about circumscribed aggressive matters.

544

-2	Overt aggressive activity is very rare. There is a paucity of response even to severe provocations. Lethargy is characteristic.	Associated aggressive behavior is also very rare. Verbalizations are quite bland, choice of occupation indicates low aggressive drive level (e.g., sorting mail for post office). Competitive behavior is absent.	Aggressive fantasies almost never intrude upon thought, nor are they often volitionally entertained.	Aggressive content in dreams almost never occurs.	There are no symptoms and almost no defensive operations or diffuse anxiety relevant to aggression.
-3	No overt aggressive activity toward self, others, or inanimate objects is observed. S appears to have "no starch" in him at all.	No significant associated aggressive behavior is observed. Interests and hobbies convey blandness in the extreme, and occupations would be the least taxing possible, such as chronic loafing.	No important evidence of aggression in thought and fantasies.	No relevant aggressive content in dreams.	No significant symptoms, defenses or controls are present from which we could infer underlying aggressive urges.

APPENDIX C

Clinical Interview Rating Form

S Code_____
Rater _____

Date_____

CLINICAL INTERVIEW RATING FORM[a]

Please rate each Ego Function (and/or component factor), indicating the specific content used as the basis for the rating. Use mostly primary data. Inferences should be in parentheses.

I. REALITY TESTING

a. Distinction between inner and outer stimuli   Char ☐☐☐☐
    Cur ☐☐☐☐

b. Accuracy of perception   Char ☐☐☐☐
    Cur ☐☐☐☐

c. Reflective awareness and inner reality testing   Char ☐☐☐☐
    Cur ☐☐☐☐

LEVEL OF FUNCTIONING	
LOWEST	
HIGHEST	
CHARACTERISTIC	
CURRENT	

---

[a]For rating interviews from the *Manual for Rating Ego Functions From a Clinical Interview*

II. JUDGMENT

    a. Anticipation of consequences

         Char ▢
         Cur ▢

    b. Manifest in behavior

         Char ▢
         Cur ▢

    c. Emotional appropriateness

         Char ▢
         Cur ▢

LEVEL OF FUNCTIONING	
LOWEST	
HIGHEST	
CHARACTERISTIC	
CURRENT	

S Code _____
Rater _____
Date _____

III. SENSE OF REALITY

    a. Extent of derealization

         Char ▢
         Cur ▢

    b. Extent of depersonalization

         Char ▢
         Cur ▢

    c. Self identity and self esteem

         Char ▢
         Cur ▢

    d. Clarity of boundaries between self and world

         Char ▢
         Cur ▢

LEVEL OF FUNCTIONING	
LOWEST	
HIGHEST	
CHARACTERISTIC	
CURRENT	

IV. REGULATION AND CONTROL OF DRIVES, IMPULSES AND AFFECTS

a. Directness of impulse expression   Char ☐
     Cur ☐

b. Effectiveness of delay mechanisms   Char ☐
     Cur ☐

LEVEL OF FUNCTIONING	
LOWEST	
HIGHEST	
CHARACTERISTIC	
CURRENT	

S Code _____

Rater _____

Date _____

V. OBJECT RELATIONS

a. Degree and kind of relatedness   Char ☐
     Cur ☐

b. Primitivity — Maturity   Char ☐
     Cur ☐

c. Others perceived independently   Char ☐
     Cur ☐

d. Object constancy   Char ☐
     Cur ☐

LEVEL OF FUNCTIONING	
LOWEST	
HIGHEST	
CHARACTERISTIC	
CURRENT	

VI. THOUGHT PROCESSES

a. Memory, concentration, attention

Char [_____]
Cur [_____]

b. Ability to conceptualize

Char [_____]
Cur [_____]

c. Primary-secondary process

Char [_____]
Cur [_____]

LEVEL OF FUNCTIONING	
LOWEST	
HIGHEST	
CHARACTERISTIC	
CURRENT	

S Code _____
Rater _____

Date _____

VII. ADAPTIVE REGRESSION IN THE SERVICE OF THE EGO

a. Regressive relaxation of acuity

Char [_____]
Cur [_____]

b. New configurations

Char [_____]
Cur [_____]

LEVEL OF FUNCTIONING	
LOWEST	
HIGHEST	
CHARACTERISTIC	
CURRENT	

VIII. DEFENSIVE FUNCTIONING

    a. Presence of defensive indicators   Char [   ]
                                                  Cur [   ]

    b. Success and failure of defenses   Char [   ]
                                                  Cur [   ]

LEVEL OF FUNCTIONING	
LOWEST	
HIGHEST	
CHARACTERISTIC	
CURRENT	

S Code _____
Rater _____

Date _____

IX. STIMULUS BARRIER

    a. Threshold for stimuli   Char [   ]
                                                Cur [   ]

    b. Coping success   Char [   ]
                                                Cur [   ]

LEVEL OF FUNCTIONING	
LOWEST	
HIGHEST	
CHARACTERISTIC	
CURRENT	

X. AUTONOMOUS FUNCTIONING

    a. Degree of freedom from impairment   Char [   ]
        of primary autonomy apparatuses   Cur [   ]

    b. Degree of freedom from impairment   Char [   ]
        of secondary autonomy   Cur [   ]

LEVEL OF FUNCTIONING
LOWEST
HIGHEST
CHARACTERISTIC
CURRENT

S Code _____

Rater _____

Date _____

XI. SYNTHETIC INTEGRATIVE FUNCTIONING

a. Degree of reconciliation of incongruities
Char
Cur

b. Degree of active relating together of events
Char
Cur

LEVEL OF FUNCTIONING
LOWEST
HIGHEST
CHARACTERISTIC
CURRENT

XII. MASTERY COMPETENCE

a. Actual competence
Char
Cur

b. Sense of competence
Char
Cur

c. Discrepancy between performance and self-feeling
Char
Cur

Discrepancy Score (−, +, or =.) Competence _____

Sense of Competence _____

(Discrepancy) _____

LEVEL OF FUNCTIONING	
LOWEST	
HIGHEST	
CHARACTERISTIC	
CURRENT	

S Code _____

Rater _____

Date _____

SUPEREGO SCALE

a. Guilt (self-directed punishment, unconscious sense of guilt, blame-avoidance, talion principle)

Char [ ]

Cur [ ]

c. Ego ideal (self evaluation, sense of worth self-esteem regulation)

Char [ ]

Cur [ ]

LEVEL OF FUNCTIONING	
LOWEST	
HIGHEST	
CHARACTERISTIC	
CURRENT	

SUPEREGO FACTORS

INTERFERENCE OF SUPEREGO FACTORS WITH EGO FUNCTIONS

Severe	Moderate	Mild	Negligible
1	2	3	4

CONSISTENCY OF SUPEREGO
Basis for Ratings:

Most Maladaptive	Tending Toward Maladaptive	Tending Toward Adaptive	Most Adaptive
1	2	3	4

ID SCALE (Drive Strength)

Strength of:	+3	+2	+1	0	−1	−2	−3
Libidinal Drive							
Aggressive Drive							

Basis for ratings:
Libidinal Drive: Char _____

Cur _____

Aggressive Drive: 1   Char _____

Cur _____

Extent to which you judge Libidinal and Aggressive Drives to be sublimated and/or neutralized.

	Negligible	Somewhat Low	Moderate	Well Neutralized
Libidinal	1	2	3	4

Basis for ratings:

Aggressive	1	2	3	4

Basis for ratings:

Leopold Bellak, M. D., Principal Investigator
MULTIDISCIPLINARY STUDY OF SCHIZOPHRENIA
RESEARCH PROJECT
N.I.M.H. Grant #18395

Subject # _____
Group # _____
Rater(s) _____ _____
Date _____ __ _____

	I	II	III	IV	V	VI	VII	VIII	IX	X	XI	XII	Superego			Id scales			
	Reality Testing	Judgment	Sense of Reality	Regulat. & Cont. of Drives	Object Relat.	Thought Process	ARISE	Defensive Functs.	Stimulus Barrier	Auton. Functs.	Synthet. Functs.	Mastery—Cmptnc.	Interference (w/ ego functions)	Consistency of Superego	Overall Superego Adaptiveness	Libidinal Drive	Aggressive Drive	Sublimination (libidinal drive)	Sublimination (aggressive drive)
13																			
12																			
11																			
10																			
9																			
8																			
7																			
6																			
5																			
4																			4
3															3				3
2															2				2
1															1				1
															0				
					Ego functions										−1				
															−2				
															−3				

Author Index

Numbers in *italics* indicate pages on which full references appear.

Subject Index